Mechanisms and Concepts in Toxicology

Mechanisms and Concepts in Toxicology

W. NORMAN ALDRIDGE

Robens Institute of Health and Safety,
University of Surrey

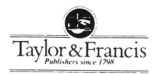

Taylor & Francis
Publishers since 1798

UK   Taylor & Francis Ltd, 1 Gunpowder Square, London EC4A 3DE

USA   Taylor & Francis Inc., 1900 Frost Road, Suite 101, Bristol, PA 19007

British Library Cataloguing in Publication Data

A catalogue record for this book is available from the British Library.

ISBN 0-7484-0413-9 (cased)
ISBN 0-7484-0414-7 (paperback)

Library of Congress Cataloguing Publication Data are available

Cover design by Youngs Design in Production

Typeset in Times 10/12 pt by Mathematical Composition Setters Ltd, Salisbury, Wiltshire, SP3 4UF

Printed in Great Britain by T.J. Press Ltd, Padstow

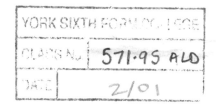

Contents

Preface   *page* ix

Acknowledgements   xi

1   Scope of Toxicology   1
   1.1   Toxicology and mechanisms of toxicity   1
   1.2   Definition of toxicology and toxicity   3
   1.3   Origin and types of exposure   7
   1.4   Discussion   8
   1.5   Summary   9

2   Stages in the Induction of Toxicity   10
   2.1   Introduction   10
   2.2   Five stages in toxicity   11
   2.3   Exposure and entry of chemicals   11
   2.4   Delivery of intoxicant   12
   2.5   Interactions with targets   13
   2.6   Early changes and clinical consequences   13
   2.7   Discussion   14
   2.8   Summary   15

3   Kinetics and End-points   17
   3.1   Introduction   17
   3.2   Reversible interactions   18
   3.3   Covalent interactions   20
   3.4   Michaelis constants   23
   3.5   Criteria to distinguish reversible from covalent interactions   25
   3.6   *In vivo* kinetics   26
   3.7   Discussion   27
   3.8   Summary   28

Contents

4   Acute and Chronic Intoxication   29
    4.1   Introduction   29
    4.2   Single exposure, rapid biological effect, rapid recovery   29
    4.3   Continuous exposure, rapid biological effect, slow but complete
           recovery   31
    4.4   Single exposure, rapid biological effect, slow but complete
           recovery   31
    4.5   Single exposure, latent intoxication, little or no recovery   32
    4.6   Single or repeated exposure, rapid intoxication, irreversible
           secondary changes   33
    4.7   Single exposure, latent intoxication, no recovery   34
    4.8   Discussion   34
    4.9   Summary   35

5   Delivery of Intoxicant: Decrease in delivery to the target   36
    5.1   Introduction   36
    5.2   Delivery (entry and distribution)   39
    5.3   Movement across membranes   41
    5.4   Distribution   46
    5.5   Factors which reduce the concentration of free intoxicant   47
    5.6   Discussion   55
    5.7   Summary   56

**6   Delivery of Intoxicant: Bioactivation and increase in delivery to the
    target**   58
    6.1   Introduction   58
    6.2   Bioactivation   60
    6.3   Delivery of bioactivated intoxicants   60
    6.4   Cytochrome P_{450}s   65
    6.5   Active transport of intoxicants   68
    6.6   Biliary excretion and enterohepatic circulation   71
    6.7   Methods to establish if *in vivo* bioactivation occurs   72
    6.8   Discussion   73
    6.9   Summary   75

7   Initiating Reactions with Targets   77
    7.1   Introduction   77
    7.2   Intoxicants which affect oxidative energy conservation (many
           tissues)   79
    7.3   Pyrethroids (nervous system)   81
    7.4   Paraquat (lung)   83
    7.5   Organophosphorus compounds and carbamates (nervous system)   86
    7.6   Organophosphorus compounds (delayed neuropathy;
           axonopathy)   90
    7.7   Acrylamide (nervous system; axonopathy)   93
    7.8   2,5-Hexanedione (nervous system peripheral and central
           axonopathy)   95
    7.9   Trichlorethylene (liver peroxisome proliferation)   97
    7.10   Glycol ethers (testis, embryonic and foetal development)   99

7.11	Beryllium and rare earths (liver, reticulo-endothelial system)	102
7.12	Triorganotins (nervous system; intramyelinic vacuoles and neuronal necrosis)	103
7.13	Cell death (necrosis and apoptosis)	105
7.14	Mutation and carcinogenesis	106
7.15	Immunotoxicity	109
7.16	Discussion	112
7.17	Summary	114

8 Biological Consequences of Initiating Reactions with Targets   **115**

8.1	Introduction	115
8.2	Functional without morphological change: perturbation of the cellular utilisation of oxygen	116
8.3	Functional without morphological change: perturbation of the cholinergic transmitter system	118
8.4	Functional without morphological change: perturbation of voltage-dependent sodium channels	119
8.5	Cell death: liver and lung damage and fibrosis	121
8.6	Cell death: neuronal necrosis in specific areas of the brain	122
8.7	Cell death: external stimuli and neuronal cell necrosis	124
8.8	Axonopathy: primary effects on the nerve axon	125
8.9	Chemical carcinogenesis: DNA adduct to tumour	127
8.10	Inflammatory response: toxic oil syndrome	130
8.11	Discussion	133
8.12	Summary	135

9 Exposure, Dose and Chemical Structure, Response and Activity, and Thresholds   **136**

9.1	Introduction	136
9.2	Essential and toxic compounds	137
9.3	Exposure–response for bioassay: the malathion episode in Pakistan	138
9.4	Exposure–response: chemical carcinogens	140
9.5	Structure– and dose–response: γ-diketones and acrylamide	141
9.6	Structure–response: triorganotins, phenols and phenylimino compounds	146
9.7	Thresholds	147
9.8	Discussion	150
9.9	Summary	151

10 Selective Toxicity, Animal Experimentation and *In Vitro* Methods   **153**

10.1	Introduction	153
10.2	Differences in metabolism: methanol	156
10.3	Differences in detoxification and reaction with target: chlorfenvinphos	157
10.4	Species difference in induction of peroxisomes in liver	159
10.5	Human chemical-induced disease with no animal model	160
10.6	The Ames test	160
10.7	*In vitro* techniques and the use of animals	162
10.8	Discussion	163
10.9	Summary	165

11 Biomonitoring 166
   11.1 Introduction 166
   11.2 Genetically determined susceptibility 168
   11.3 Succinyldicholine 169
   11.4 Exposure, dose and effect monitoring in humans 169
   11.5 Dose monitoring in humans: methylmercury (epidemic in Iraq) 170
   11.6 Dose monitoring in humans: ethylene oxide 172
   11.7 Dose and effect monitoring in humans: anticholinesterases 174
   11.8 Dose and effect monitoring in humans: dichlorvos 176
   11.9 Dose monitoring in experimental animals 177
   11.10 Effect monitoring 177
   11.11 Discussion 178
   11.12 Summary 179

12 Epidemiology 180
   12.1 Introduction 180
   12.2 General methodological approaches 182
   12.3 Epidemiological methods used in occupational exposures 184
   12.4 Smoking and lung cancer 185
   12.5 Toxic oil syndrome in Spain 188
   12.6 Health effects of environmental exposure to cadmium 191
   12.7 Discussion 193
   12.8 Summary 195

13 Environmental and Ecotoxicology 196
   13.1 Introduction 196
   13.2 Polychlorinated biphenyls 197
   13.3 Toxic chemicals produced by cyanobacteria (algae) 201
   13.4 Methylmercury: Minamata and Niigata episodes 202
   13.5 Chlorinated mutagenic agents in drinking water 204
   13.6 Discussion 206
   13.7 Summary 207

14 Reflections, Research and Risk 209
   14.1 Reflections 209
   14.2 Research 210
   14.3 Risk 213
   14.4 Summary 216

   References 218
   Index 249

Preface

Toxicology is the science of poisoning by chemicals, natural or man-made, small or large molecular weight. Historical studies have often been in essence descriptive but now we can define the early reactions and adverse consequences of the interaction of chemicals with biological systems in chemical terms. This chemical approach also requires a redefinition of some of the basic toxicological terms.

Biology is rapidly absorbing information from molecular biology and the control of biological processes is being defined in molecular terms. Research in toxicology aims to define the specific interactions of an intoxicant with molecular control points in living organisms. In biochemistry and physiology the control of biological systems by hormone and transmitters, and in pharmacology their modification by drugs etc. is now being described in terms of specific interactions with macromolecules (receptors). Although toxicity may be initiated by interactions with these same receptors there are other macromolecular components of cells (targets) whose physiological, biochemical and/or structural function is as yet unknown in detail but whose modification by a chemical causes toxicity.

Many advances in biology have resulted from the experimental and controlled manipulation of biological systems. Claude Bernard's famous quotation made in 1875 is explicit about the value to basic science of the understanding of the consequences of the perturbation of biological systems by intoxicants:

> Poisons can be employed as means for the destruction of life or as agents for the treatment of the sick but in addition there is a third of particular interest to the physiologist. For him the poison becomes an instrument which dissociates and analyses the most delicate phenomena of living structures and by attending carefully to their mechanism in causing death he can learn indirectly much about the physiological processes of life . . . .

Research in toxicology thus serves a dual purpose – it defines the factors determining the degree of interaction with the primary target and also illuminates the molecular aspects of the biological processes involved.

The focus of this book is research and not test procedures. Test procedures are to provide data on specific questions. In research, described by Medawar (1986) as 'that restless endeavour to make sense of things', experimental procedures are continually modified so that the results may prove or disprove a hypothesis. Mechanisms and concepts are illustrated as well as the research route by which they were established. Occasionally unproven mechanisms are presented which, because of our state of knowledge, stimulate working hypotheses leading to new research. The concepts of the 'biochemical lesion' and 'lethal synthesis' developed by Peters (1963) are milestones in toxicological research. Research on mechanisms in toxicology leads not only to greater understanding of the biology involved but also to the means to design substances with selectivity among species, for example pesticides with large differences between their toxicity to the pest and to humans.

Society now demands that reassurance be given prior to the introduction of a chemical that that chemical will not cause illness in those unavoidably exposed. Exposure can occur during medical treatment, at work or in the general environment. Governments have responded by increasing the extent of toxicity testing both *in vitro* and *in vivo*. However, the interpretation of the results of these tests in terms of the risk to humans may be difficult and often depends on other background information. Rational decisions on how a toxic chemical may be used safely, development of objective biological monitoring procedures, design of safer drugs and chemicals, development of quicker and more precise predictive tests (*in vitro* and using animals) for particular types of toxicity require more understanding of mechanisms in toxicity. A better definition of the factors which influence chemico-biological interactions and a greater knowledge of dose–response and structure–activity relationships enhance the intellectual climate necessary for the rational prediction of the hazards and risks of exposure.

Toxicologists, in the future, will have to utilise an increasing amount of information arising from expanding knowledge of the molecular complexity of biological phenomena. Experience gained in teaching postgraduate students with primary degrees in medicine, pathology, physiology, biochemistry, chemistry or physics (and more mature students wishing to gain a general view of principles and approaches) has shown that a conceptual framework helps in the assimilation of information from diverse disciplines. This book provides such a framework for interactions of any chemical with any biological system.

Although this book presents a chemist's view of mechanistic toxicology, other disciplines play an important role. Contributions from many disciplines are brought together and focused on the importance of understanding the molecular science of chemical-induced perturbations in complex biological systems for both practical and basic toxicology.

Norman Aldridge

Acknowledgements

The subject of toxicology is so wide and needs the expertise of so many disciplines that it is obvious that the author, before writing this book, has received help during his career from many colleagues including the staff of the Medical Research Council Toxicology Unit, UK, and many others from home and abroad who have taken part in discussions whenever we met.

For more immediate help I wish to acknowledge the following friends and colleagues who have given their time to read all or parts of the manuscript – many improvements have resulted.

Professor Ernst Cohen, formerly at the Department of Pharmacology, Leiden University and head of the Medico-Biological Laboratory, Rijswick, Professor Lewis Smith, Director of the Medical Research Council Toxicology Unit, University of Leicester and Dr Shirley Price, Pathologist at the Robens Institute of Health and Safety, University of Surrey who have acted as general readers.

The following have read specific chapters: Professor Gordon Gibson, School of Biological Sciences, University of Surrey (Chapters 5 and 6; delivery of intoxicant), Dr Peter Farmer, Medical Research Council Toxicology Unit, University of Leicester (Chapter 11; biomonitoring); Professor Sir Richard Doll, ICRF Cancer Studies Unit, Radcliffe Infirmary, University of Oxford, and Professor Benedetto Terracini, Department of Biological Sciences and Human Oncology, University of Turin (Chapter 12; epidemiology).

To all I am extremely grateful.

1

Scope of Toxicology

1.1 Toxicology and Mechanisms of Toxicity

Toxic substances have always been used by many species of animal including humans for defensive and offensive purposes. Textbooks of pharmacology are full of examples of such agents used by man, e.g. arrowhead poisons such as digitalis from *Strophanthus* and curare from *Strychnos* and *Chondrodendron*. Although there are many examples of man using natural toxins for his own purposes there are probably many more of one animal species using toxins to control another, to deter an attack by another, to immobilise a food source either for immediate or later consumption. Pharmacology has a rather positive image being concerned with the treatment of disease by natural products, structural modifications of natural products and by synthetic drugs designed for treatment of a particular disease. In contrast, toxicology is sometimes regarded in a negative way. This is a misconception, for in its wider context natural toxins have a respectable position in evolutionary development which has allowed the equilibrium between species to be attained and maintained. Man-made chemicals also have provided and will continue to provide protection by the control of disease vectors (in many species) and also enhanced comfort, convenience and security in modern society. Toxicology and pharmacology are complementary and the thought processes involved in mechanisms of toxicity are similar to those in pharmacology.

Novel therapeutic agents follow from new basic knowledge of disease processes and are now positively designed to interfere with a particular receptor. Even though it may be possible to design a chemical with a high affinity for a particular receptor it will not always result in an acceptable therapeutic agent. During the development of new chemical structures (drugs), undesirable and novel side-effects may appear in tests on experimental animals. Sometimes, even when a potential drug passes all safety checks, side-effects may appear during clinical trials or even after the drug's release for general use. Such side-effects highlight areas of biological activity about which little is known and new biological research is required.

The meaning of mechanistic and mechanisms when applied to toxicology is not always clear. It is often limited as if it were only research which established the primary interaction of a chemical with a macromolecule as the initiating event for the disease. This is an unhelpful and unnecessarily narrow view. Studies in the area of mechanisms are those whose purpose and intention is to provide a holistic view of the process of toxicity; there are many levels of biological complexity which, when combined, allow a reasonable hypothesis of each mechanism of toxicity to be stated.

In a historical context, mechanistic toxicology could not begin before a certain knowledge in basic biology. Research in the seventeenth and eighteenth centuries, largely on plants by Hooke and vøn Leeuwenhoek, led to the view that tissues consisted of many small entities, i.e. cells. The importance of the nucleus as a feature of all cells was promoted by Schwann, Purkinje, Brown and Schleiden followed by Virchow's clear statements:

1   All living organisms are composed of nucleated cells.
2   Cells are the functional units of life.
3   Cells arise only from pre-existing cells by dividing.

The foundation on which scientific toxicology developed probably derives from the work of Orfila who lived in times of great advancement in chemistry, physiology and pathology. In the early nineteenth century, Orfila was the first to treat toxicology as a separate scientific subject and introduced chemical analysis as an essential component. His first textbook on general toxicology laid the foundation of experimental and particularly forensic toxicology. During the same period Magendie was making many discoveries which became the basis for the experimental analysis of the site of action of poisons (for an extensive discussion of the contributions of Orfila and Magendie see Holmstedt & Liljestrand, 1963). Later in the nineteenth century it became clear that toxic substances could be useful as tools for the dissection of living tissues and thus to learn about the way they are organised in a functional sense (see Preface; Bernard, 1875).

Following such work and the ability to identify by histopathological techniques the tissue and cells attacked by a toxic substance, advances in many relevant sciences took place, e.g. methods for the separation of the active principles of plants, morphological detail of the structural arrangement of cells, the relationship between organ and cell function and the biochemical reactions occurring in them. The development of the electron microscope has led to understanding of intracellular organisation, e.g. subcellular organelles and the existence of other compartments. Methods for the separation by fractionation of tissues and of cells in a functioning state are now being devised so that reactions can be studied *in vitro* under controlled conditions separate from the controlling influences the whole organism. Analytical methods of great finesse are now available for the separation and identification of small and large molecules.

These advances in the biological sciences signalled that there was a reasonable expectation that mechanisms of toxicity should be able to be identified at the cell level and often down to changes in reactions occurring within cells and sometimes to a specific interaction with a macromolecule. The latter is an early event in contrast to changes in morphology which indeed may be a rather late consequence of the primary chemical event. The concept of a 'biochemical lesion' was first proposed by Rudolf Peters as a result of research on the effects of vitamin B (thiamine) deficiency (Gavrilescu & Peters, 1931) and was later used following research on the toxicity of vesicants such as the arsenical, lewisite (Peters *et al.*, 1945) and on the intoxicant fluoroacetate (Peters, 1963); in the latter the concept of 'lethal synthesis' was also introduced. Lethal synthesis is when the toxicity of a chemical is changed and increased by biological conversion of one chemical to another.

Thus understanding in toxicology depends on information derived from many other

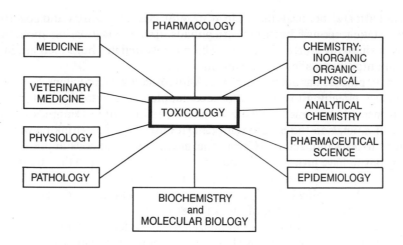

Figure 1.1 Areas of scientific study relevant to toxicology. These relationships imply that crucial steps catalytic for progress in mechanisms of toxicity may arise from research, not only in departments or institutes of toxicology but also in many other areas

disciplines, i.e. toxicology is an interdisciplinary subject (Figure 1.1). This is not exceptional for biological disciplines e.g. pharmacology, physiology, microbiology and so on. As in other areas of biology, in addition to the importance of the acquisition of new information, mechanisms of toxicity provide the intellectual climate for the solution of practical problems in toxicology and the subject moves from a descriptive to a predictive science.

1.2   Definition of Toxicology and Toxicity

1   Toxicity by chemicals is changes from the normal in either the structure or function of living organisms or both.
2   Chemicals causing toxicity are intoxicants or poisons.
3   Toxicology is the science of poisons.

These definitions are wide and open-ended with respect to organisms, responses and toxic chemicals.

1.2.1   *Organisms*

The aim of most studies is to provide safety for human beings. In the past half century there has been a radical change in public attitudes about exposure to chemicals. Prior to 1940 few chemicals were synthesised in large amounts and exposure often occurred during the mining of metals and their subsequent purification and fabrication. If illness resulted, then following medical advice conditions were improved. For a variety of reasons attitudes have changed; these include the advance of chemistry, the increased longevity due to treatment of infectious diseases and better nutrition, and an awareness through education of the possibilities of toxicity. It is now generally accepted that before (not after) a chemical (pesticide, drug, etc). is used, industry and governmental authorities take responsibility for ensuring that sufficient information about potential hazard is available to protect the public. This has resulted in a huge increase in the use of experimental animals for toxicity testing and for research.

Veterinary practice has always been faced with toxicological problems. Some are accidental as in the feeding to livestock of feed supplement containing polybrominated biphenyls instead of magnesium oxide (Dunckel, 1975). Other examples are the fatal exposure of animals in the Seveso episode (Holmstedt, 1980), drinking water contaminated by toxic cyanobacteria (Carmichael *et al.*, 1985) and consumption of feed on which organisms have grown and produced toxic metabolites as in the initial poisoning of turkeys with aflatoxin (Stoloff, 1977). Toxic plants in fields and pastures have always been a cause of poisoning in animals, e.g. consumption of ragwort containing the toxic Senecio alkaloids (WHO, 1988; Mattocks, 1986).

While the egocentric attitudes of humans have provided the main driving force for the evaluation of the toxicity of new chemicals in recent years there has been a growing view that the ecological balance in nature should be preserved. This view may be challenged and debated *in extenso*; it has resulted in greater attention being given to effects of chemicals on species other than the usual experimental and farm animals. For example, fish toxicity is now considered necessary before the introduction of most pesticides and the toxicity of effluent resulting from their manufacture is more carefully evaluated. The range of organisms which can be studied from a toxicological point of view is potentially very large. In many cases where exposure to chemicals is postulated to be the cause of the change in the population of particular organisms, proof that this is so often necessitates much more information and research (see Chapter 13).

The increase in the use of animals for experimental purposes has resulted in demands from some members of the public for the introduction of *in vitro* techniques to replace them or at least to diminish their numbers; they might utilise a pure enzyme, isolated animal tissues and in some cases model bacterial systems (see Chapter 10).

As a consequence of all the above demands, the range of species of organism and biological systems to be considered in a toxicological context is now very large and is increasing. This expanding range is mainly being driven by questions of a practical nature but, in another context, researchers in biological science have always been prepared to widen their studies to other species in order to solve particular academic problems (e.g. when an animal model is not available within the usual range of experimental animals; see Chapter 10).

1.2.2 Responses

Current perception is that the range of responses is almost infinite; any attempt to produce a useful list for the huge range of potentially affected organisms would fail. Sometimes the site of toxicity is decided by the route of exposure, e.g. through the skin, by inhalation or by absorption from the gastro-intestinal tract, when the toxicity evinced may be to the skin, to the lung, etc. However, all responses are not of equal practical importance. In most cases tissue damage (e.g. loss of cells) can be repaired by mitosis from remaining cells. Thus ingestion of the commonly consumed chemical ethyl alcohol no doubt from time to time causes the death of some hepatocytes but provokes few long-term consequences due to efficient repair processes. However, neuronal loss is permanent and although this may not be clinically significant owing to a large reserve capacity, a permanent change has taken place. Damage to long axons in the central (spinal cord) and peripheral (sciatic nerves) has different long-term consequences; peripheral nerves can be repaired and reach the end organ while axons of central nerves do not reconnect. Secondary consequences in the whole organism, such as scar tissue formation or long lasting inflammatory processes, clinical signs or symptoms which after a short exposure take a long time to appear or which require a long exposure, continue to present challenges to our current understanding in biology and toxicology (see Chapter 8).

Some chemicals cause toxicity following a reversible interaction with a tissue component, whereas others interact to yield a covalently bonded and modified tissue component. Biological consequences of such interactions can be very different but much remains to be explored, particularly in relation to chronic and long lasting toxicity (see Chapter 7).

Clinical responses are obviously emphasised but one of the most important tasks in toxicology is to identify early interactions which result in changes which are part of a chain of events leading to toxicity (a biological cascade). The identification of early changes may provide the basis for rational biomonitoring of human populations. The definition of such early changes, their dose–response relationships and the identification of longer-term consequences require a rather profound understanding of the biology involved. Sometimes current basic biology is inadequate for the task; thus the nature of a large human poisoning, known as toxic oil syndrome which in 1981 involved thousands of victims (Sections 8.10 and 12.5), is not yet fully understood at a biological level and the aetiological agent has not been identified.

1.2.3 Toxic Chemicals

Traditionally, material which causes toxicity has been divided into toxic chemicals and toxins. This division is arbitrary and is often based on molecular weight; sometimes it is based on whether toxicity is caused by a synthetic chemical or a natural product. Such a division is almost impossible to sustain when, for instance, an effluent is released into a river and then reacts with a natural constituent to produce a toxic entity. *Botulinum* toxin is not usually considered to be within the province of toxicology but plant lectins sometimes are. With few exceptions the toxic chemicals used in this book as examples of particular mechanisms have a molecular weight of less than 1,000; no distinction is made between those chemicals synthesised in chemical industry, mined, produced naturally by organisms in the environment or resulting from the release of synthesised chemicals or by-products into the environment.

There is a popular misconception that chemicals synthesised by chemical industry are dangerous and natural chemicals are not. This is untrue, for some of the most toxic agents occur in the natural world. Table 1.1 lists examples of both natural and synthesised chemicals. All have a molecular weight of less than 1,000. A wide range of toxicity is shown for both natural and synthetic chemicals, and extremely toxic chemicals occur in each group, e.g. with a toxicity of less than 0.1 μmol/kg. This selection of chemicals causes many types of toxicity by different mechanisms and illustrate a central fact in toxicology: chemicals are selective and specific in the toxicity they cause. In one example a natural product has been structurally modified to give a synthetic chemical with enhanced toxicity and properties. Natural pyrethrins derived from the Pyrethrum plant is an effective knock-down pesticide but is very unstable to light. Many pyrethroid

Table 1.1 Examples of natural and synthetic toxic chemicals

Toxic chemical (source)	Molecular weight	Tissue affected	Ref.
NATURAL TOXICANTS			
Aflatoxin B$_1$ (*Aspergillus flavus*: growth on nuts)	312	Liver necrosis and carcinogenesis	1
α-Amanitin (Mushroom: *amanita phalloides*)	902	Gastro-intestinal tract/liver necrosis	2
Anatoxin-a(S) (organophosphorus produced by cyanobacteria)	252	Nervous system: (anticholinesterase)	28,29
Fluoroacetate: Na (Plant: *dichapetalum cymosum*)	100	Heart/skeletal muscle/ nervous system	3,4
Monocrotaline (*Crotalaria spectabilis*)	325	Liver/lung	5,6
Ochratoxin A (*Aspergillus ochraceus*: growth on nuts/seeds)	403	Kidney	7,8
Pyrethrin I (Plant: *pyrethrum cinariaefolium*)	328	Nervous system: (nerve conduction)	9
Tetrodotoxin (Puffer fish)	319	Nervous system (nerve conduction)	10,11
SYNTHETIC TOXICANTS			
Deltamethrin (pyrethroid insecticide)	505	Nervous system (nerve conduction)	12,13
Ethylene glycol monomethyl ether (solvent)	76	Testis	14
Hexachloro-1,3-butadiene (intermediate)	267	Kidney	15
2,5-Hexane dione (bioactivated product from hexane)	114	Nervous system (long axons)	16,17
Methyl isocyanate (intermediate in synthesis of carbamates)	57	Lung/eye	18,19
Methylmercuric dicyandiamide (fungicide)	298	Nervous system (cerebellum)	20,21
MTTP: 1-methyl-4-phenyl-1, 2,3,6-tetrahydropyridine (impurity in pethidene derivative)	173	Nervous system (substantia nigra)	22,23
Paraquat (bipyridinium herbicide)	186	Lung	24,25
Pentachlorophenol (fungicide)	266	General metabolic poison	26
Soman: pinacolyl methylphosphonofluoridate (nerve gas)	182	Nervous system (anticholinesterase)	27

References: (1) Stoloff, 1977; (2) Weiland & Faulstich, 1978; (3) Peters, 1963; (4) Hayes, 1982; (5) McLean, 1970; (6) Mattocks, 1986; (7) Purchase & Theron, 1968; (8) Chu, 1974; (9) Elliot, 1971; (10) Kao, 1966; (11) Narahashi, 1990; (12) Elliott, 1979; (13) Verschoyle & Aldridge, 1980; (14) Thomas & Thomas,1984; (15) Hook *et al.*, 1983; (16) Divincenzo *et al.*, 1980; (17) Cavanagh, 1982a; (18) Nemery *et al.*, 1985; (19) Ferguson & Alarie, 1991; (20) Tsubaki & Irukayama, 1977; (21) Aldridge, 1987; (22) Jenner & Marsden, 1987; (23) Langston *et al.*, 1984; (24) Conning *et al.*, 1969; (25) Smith & Nemery, 1986; (26) Gaines (1969); (27) Black & Upshall, 1988; (28) Cook *et al.*, 1989; (29) Hyde & Carmichael, 1991.

structures have now been synthesised with high biological activity and stability to light (Elliott,1979; Hassall, 1990).

1.3 Origin and Types of Exposure

Exposure and toxicity occurs in different circumstances:

1 Medical and veterinary practice.
2 At work (occupational).
3 In the general environment (environmental).
4 Accidental or intentional (including forensic).

Other subdivisions have been used: environmental toxicity for incidental or occupational hazards; economic toxicity for intentional administration to living organisms, e.g. therapeutic agents for human and veterinary use, chemicals used as food additives or cosmetics and chemicals used by humans selectively to eliminate another species; and forensic toxicology including both intentional and accidental exposure.

1.3.1 Medical and Veterinary Practice

Modern-day therapeutics are often designed from knowledge of the way particular physiological functions are controlled and are thus intended to be specific in their action. Many are intended to rectify defects in normal control or to modify normal physiology and thus are also often prescribed for use for many years, e.g. treatment of hypertension or the contraceptive pill. Extensive animal studies are carried out so as to discard undesirable side-effects but, in practice, others sometimes emerge after the pre-marketing clinical trials or when the drug has been released for general use and the side-effect is recognised during post-marketing monitoring. Thus, experience indicates that drug side-effects continue to be a problem, as stated by Fingl and Woodbury (1966):

> Drug toxicity is as old as drug therapy and clinicians have long warned of drug-induced diseases. However with the introduction into therapeutic practice of drugs of greater and broader efficacy, the problem of drug toxicity has increased, and it is now considered the most critical aspect of modern therapeutics. Not only is a greater variety of drug toxicity being uncovered, but the average incidence of adverse effects of medication is increasing, and unexpected toxic effects occur relatively frequently. There is an urgent need for the development of methods in animals that accurately predict the potential harmful effects of drugs in man.

Although improvements have been made since 1966, problems remain. Side-effects which are novel forms of toxicity quite different from their therapeutic action may appear. Also, control of the dose necessary for the drug's therapeutic action is vital; this is the province of the pharmacologist and the clinician.

1.3.2 Exposure at Work

Exposure at work takes place during the development period, production on a pilot plant scale, full-scale production, formulation and use. In recent years there has been an irresistible centralising tendency in industry so that fewer places synthesise a

7

particular product or an intermediate for a future manufacture. This is beneficial for working conditions but the product then has to be transported in large quantities over great distances with a potentiality for accidents. In practice, the environments of formulation plants are often less controlled and exposure may be greater. It is difficult to generalise about the extent of the danger of exposure at work; however, during the dissemination of pesticides for agricultural pest control or vector control for public health purposes in developing countries, long hours of work under poor conditions, problems of diluting the concentrates and of disposal of empty containers often lead to high exposure.

1.3.3   Environmental Exposure

A major problem in environmental exposure is to reassure the public that long and perhaps life-time exposure to low residues of compounds in food and water, e.g. pesticides, food additives, fluoride in drinking water, will not cause undesirable effects. Neglecting the obvious problem of proving a negative, the potential for such a consequence can more confidently be predicted if a sound basis for mechanism of action is known and the scientific basis of threshold is established. From the results of basic research, dose- and biomonitoring techniques may be devised to follow up those people who are, during their work, exposed to a relatively higher concentration for a long time – such studies can be very useful for risk assessment.

1.3.4   Accidental and Intentional Exposure

As mentioned above there is always a potential hazard in the transport of the final product or the chemically active intermediates used in its synthesis. The use of a chemical for purposes for which it was not intended, failing to follow the recommended procedure for its use, the re-use of containers and the storage of a chemical in unsuitable and often unlabelled bottles has led to many fatalities by accidental poisoning. Experience shows that when a toxic chemical becomes available it will be used in suicide attempts, and even in the best regulated circumstances accidents will happen. Although such accidents are regretted when they happen they provide a source of information about the susceptibility of humans to poisoning by particular chemicals. Systems need to be available to collect and utilise this potential information (Aldridge & Connors, 1985). Expertise is required, as an immediate need, to care for those exposed and to contain the accident. However, others trained in epidemiology, analytical chemistry and experimental toxicology are needed at an early stage to ensure the conditions for the collection of relevant information and samples for analysis.

1.4   Discussion

The purpose of this chapter has been to outline the potential scope of toxicology both in the natural and industrialised environments. It is not intended to suggest demarcation disputes about what is and what is not toxicology. Perhaps more than other scientists, those who are engaged in studies on toxicity rely on information from many other scientific areas. Those engaged in research on mechanisms of toxicity are engaged in basic research in the biological sciences. While it is possible to limit research to projects with a predictable practical benefit, it is equally valid to choose an unsolved problem in mechanisms of toxicity which will throw light on some area of biology.

> We have to recognise the danger of being preoccupied with benefit rather than knowledge. Knowledge has a kind of inevitable priority, and our confidence in the expected benefit depends on the soundness of the knowledge. (Paton, 1984)

Over the past forty years due to inappropriate waste disposal and accidents involving chemicals ever more stringent regulations have been formulated to control the introduction of new chemicals to the market and to re-examine the safety of those materials already in use and a potential source for exposure of the public. While these regulations prescribe the quality and design of testing protocols, their execution is in essence a routine matter. However, the design of such tests and the interpretation of the results should be based on scientific principles. Regulation tends to be a national prerogative whereas the scientific aspects, and particularly mechanisms and concepts, are universal. The move forward in such basic science draws together research across the whole spectrum of physiological and biomedical sciences. The intention in this book is to provide for students a framework and mode of thought which will be useful to those who assess and apply the new hypotheses, for those who will be the future creators of new mechanisms and concepts and also for those who wish to learn more about the structure of toxicological science.

Because of advances in biological sciences, the unfolding specificity in molecular terms of all biological processes leads to endless possibilities of interference in individual steps by chemicals (both low and high molecular weight). Biological science and toxicology should advance in tandem; sometimes an unexpected toxic response begins the search for an unknown biological process and its control mechanisms, and sometimes the advance in biological science comes first. Although many disciplines contribute to the solution of mechanisms of toxicity an emphasis on the chemistry of the event is essential.

1.5 Summary

1 Toxicology is an interdisciplinary subject.
2 There is no fundamental distinction between natural and synthetic chemicals.
3 Studies in mechanisms of toxicity are research in basic biological science.
4 Exposure of humans and/or animals to chemicals occurs during medical and veterinary treatment, at work, in the environment and by accidental and intentional poisoning.
5 Organisms are targets for toxic chemicals in the environment.
6 Research on mechanisms of toxicity will produce new concepts and assist in the solution of practical problems.

2

Stages in the Induction of Toxicity

2.1 Introduction

In biological sciences, understanding of mechanisms of complex biological processes has resulted from dissection of the system into its component parts. It is now accepted that most controls of complex processes are mediated by the affinity and/or covalent reaction of specific substances with particular regions in macromolecules. These areas are now called receptors, which may be proteins with or without catalytic functions, lipoproteins, glycoproteins or nucleic acids. When intoxication occurs it is now accepted that it is initiated by interactions among particular macromolecular structures; in some cases these may be pharmacological receptors but not always. Therefore to make a distinction between beneficial (e.g. for hormones and drugs) and undesirable consequences (e.g. for toxic chemicals and side-effects of drugs), what the macromolecules interact with may be called receptors and targets respectively; sometimes reactions with receptors can cause toxicity, i.e. the receptor is the target.

In the development of new drugs, instead of requiring an animal model of the disease it is intended to treat, receptors in *in vitro* systems are increasingly being used for screening purposes to sift out potentially useful chemical structures. To be able to design out undesirable side-effects of chemicals to which humans and animals will be exposed, knowledge of targets is required (see Chapters 7 and 10).

In the control of physiological processes, e.g. by thyroxine, it is accepted that the route from essential element (iodide) to active hormone is extremely complex, as follows. Iodide is absorbed from the gut, transported via the blood stream and, by an energy-requiring process, is taken up by the thyroid gland and stored there. Iodide is bioactivated by oxidation by a peroxidase to iodine which then reacts with particular tyrosine residues in thyroglobulin to form tetra- (T4) and tri- (T3) iodothyronine by a complex reaction. T4 is preferentially released by proteolysis into the blood stream and before excreting its physiological and controlling action on metabolism it is de-iodinated to the more active T3 (i.e. by another bioactivation). Its action is terminated by metabolism and excretion. Each step of this complex pathway has its own structure–activity and dose–response requirements, and each step can be influenced by different inhibitors. Thus the relationship between exposure to iodide in the diet and the control

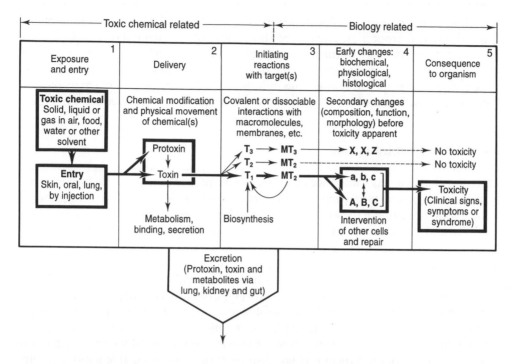

Figure 2.1 Five-stage scheme for developing toxicity due to chemicals. Heavy lines = developing toxicity; light lines = less or no toxicity; T_1, T_2, T_3 = targets; MT_1, MT_2, MT_3 = modified targets; A,B,C,X,Y,Z,a,b,c = independent or linked changes. Acute or chronic intoxication differ by the time in one or more phases. (*Sources*: Aldridge, 1981, 1986)

of metabolic rate in the whole animal tells us nothing about the details of this complicated pathway.

The same kind of complexity exists in the influence of toxic substances on whole organisms. As an aid to coherent thought what occurs between exposure and clinical signs of poisoning can be divided into five stages (Figure 2.1).

2.2   Five Stages in Toxicity

In this scheme the stages 2–5 which follow exposure to a toxic chemical are: (2) all the processes before the delivery of the chemical to the target (or the proximal toxic agent if it is bioactivated); (3) the reactions of the biologically active chemical with its target; (4) before clinical disease is seen the discreet biochemical, physiological and pathological consequences which follow, and (5) the signs, symptoms or the syndrome of the illness in the organism.

2.3   Exposure and Entry of Chemicals

In addition to stages 2–5, entry (stage 1) into the organism may be by many routes such as the mouth, stomach, duodenum, or by inhalation, through the skin or more directly by various routes of injection. The penetration of the chemical is influenced by its chemical and physical properties. The rate of absorption will be affected by its lipophilicity and ionic state as well as, by the oral route, by competition in binding to food. Unless the chemical gains access to the internal milieu, toxicity will not occur. Even for skin toxicity the final response is often due to influence of the chemical on particular cell types. For a discussion of the routes of access and the factors involved see Chapter 5.

2.4   Delivery of Intoxicant

Once the chemical has gained access to the organism many factors influence whether it reaches a potential target and the concentration which does so. Many processes are known which contribute to delivery, including physical and chemical properties of the chemical and its derivatives due to enzymic metabolism. Such metabolism may be beneficial to the organism if the chemical becomes less toxic. The substance may also be bioactivated so that a chemical which is inactive in an *in vitro* system becomes toxic *in vivo*. The bioactivated species will also be subject to enzymic metabolism thus reducing the concentration available to cause toxicity (Figure 2.2). The major route of excretion of exogenous substances and their metabolites is usually by the kidney but a number of other routes are possible. Recirculation of chemicals occurs when they are secreted into the bile or by the salivary glands into the saliva, bound to proteins in such a way that their physiological function is not disturbed or when lipophilic substances are concentrated in the body fat. Many factors and processes contribute and interact with

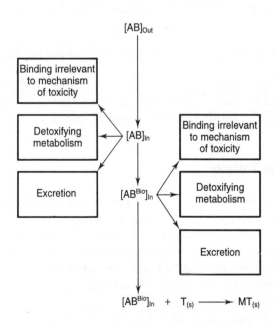

Figure 2.2   Illustration of pathways which influence the *in vivo* concentration of a chemical which is bioactivated. [AB] = concentration of the chemical; $[AB^{Bio}]$ = concentration of the bioactivated chemical; Out = outside the organism (exposure); In = within the organism; $T_{(s)}$ or $MT_{(s)}$ are subcellular macromolecular target(s) or modified target(s) at or within the target cell

each other to influence the concentration of the toxic substance reaching its primary target. For acute intoxication these have often been defined; however, rates of metabolic reactions may become very different when the exposure to the substance is to a low concentration over a long time. These determinants of the progress of the toxic chemical to its target are described in Chapters 5 and 6.

2.5   Interactions with Targets

After the delivery of the toxic chemical to its site of action an interaction between it and a target (T_1) initiates processes which develop and may culminate in the signs, symptoms or syndrome of toxicity. These interactions can be by reversible reactions defined by dissociation or affinity constants or by covalent interactions which may or may not be irreversible (in a biological rather than a chemical sense). The rates of covalent reactions are defined by rate constants. Sometimes the product of this interaction may be unstable and the parent target may be reformed. The crucial point is that when covalent interaction takes place between target and toxic chemical the route by which it is reformed is not the reverse of the route by which the modified target (MT_1) was formed but by an entirely different reaction. Sometimes MT_1 may be sufficiently stable for the biosynthesis of the new macromolecule to be the major route for the formation *in vivo* of a new target.

In Figure 2.1 the reaction with target T_1 is designated as that which leads to toxicity. Reaction with other targets $(T_2$ and $T_3)$ is also shown in Figure 2.1; these are reactions which do not lead to toxicity although they may cause non-hazardous changes in the biochemistry, physiology or morphology of the cell or tissue. Many or perhaps most interactions with targets such as proteins or enzymes etc. have no biological consequences (either undesirable or beneficial). Some interactions, although non-toxic, have been utilised in dose monitoring techniques to determine the amount of the chemical circulating *in vivo* or occasionally that presented to the target (see Chapter 11).

A discussion of the kinetics of interaction of chemicals with targets and examples of specific initiating interactions leading to toxicity are discussed in Chapters 3 and 7 respectively.

2.6   Early Changes and Clinical Consequences

There may be many consequences to a complex organism of the interaction of a chemical with, for example, an enzyme. There are many common systems in the metabolic pathways of different cells and the main energy-yielding reactions through the energy conservation systems are, in mammals, brought about in all cells by mitochondria. An interaction of a chemical with a component of mitochondria may therefore lead to changes in many organs. Depending on whether interference in energy-yielding reactions in particular organs is more vital for the immediate function of the organ will influence the nature of the toxicity and its time of onset. Sometimes a particular neurotransmitter is used to control a wide variety of functions. Interference with the production of the transmitter or with its metabolism (which controls the transmitter's duration of effect) will clearly have many consequences, some of which can be immediately life-threatening or may be of little long-term consequence. Thus there may be many subtle consequences following the interaction of a chemical with a target but only a few may contribute to the final expression of toxicity.

Although some of the aforementioned changes may be irrelevant to the final toxicity, knowledge of them is not useless. If these effects can be measured in accessible tissues then they may be very useful as indicators of the consequence of exposure of target to a particular concentration of the toxic chemical.

Biological changes before frank disease are of two general types: they may be functional without or with morphological change sometimes leading to cell death. The extent of and/or rate in which either or both occur determines the speed of onset of toxicity. If no morphological change occurs then, if death does not occur, recovery is usually complete. If morphological changes occur then recovery may or may not be complete.

This phase of developing toxicity is the biological cascade (i.e. it is not toxic chemical related) initiated by the primary chemical interaction with a target. Sometimes the cascade is straight and uncomplicated, sometimes one cascade has to be supplemented by another by chemical interaction(s) with other target(s), and sometimes repair processes initiated by the first response may lead to loss of function, for example as in the formation of scar tissue after severe tissue damage and cell loss. These biological consequences are discussed in detail in Chapter 8.

2.7 Discussion

Besides its application to toxicology the five-stage scheme may be used for other disciplines when bioactive substances are involved. Figure 2.3 shows other areas of science which also involve delivery, interaction with target or receptor and the biological consequences. The mode of thought is identical for the development of pesticides or bacteriocides with organisms other than mammals (insects, plants, micro-organisms, etc.). The scheme is also directly applicable for the mechanism of action of therapeutic drugs.

The control of cell function and metabolism is often brought about by chemical substances such as hormones, neurotransmitters, etc. The same phases are involved although penetration of the organism does not occur since such endogenous bioactive chemicals are synthesised *in vivo*; i.e. equivalent to intravenous injection of chemicals. With essential exogenous elements or substances (e.g. metals or vitamins in nutrition) the scheme is also applicable.

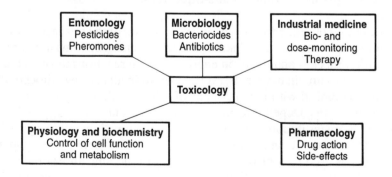

Figure 2.3   Scientific disciplines other than toxicology for which the five-stage scheme (Figure 2.1) is applicable

New methods are becoming possible, e.g. ascertaining the extent of reaction with targets for measurement of internal dose (dose monitoring) and detection of biological effects (effect monitoring) utilising both reaction with targets and its biological consequences. Monitoring of individuals is now sometimes possible; this is preferable to the statistical approach involving measurement of average exposure and numbers showing clinical effect (studies of populations). The relationship between these two kinds of monitoring is discussed in Chapter 11. An important area requiring more research is the discovery of rational measures for the treatment of chemical poisoning. No matter how well risk assessment has been carried out to protect people exposed in their occupation and in the environment generally, accidental or intentional poisoning will always occur and means for the treatment of such poisoning cases should be available. The scheme serves to illustrate in which phase prophylaxis, therapy or the amelioration of symptoms may take place by measures influencing reactions occurring in the different phases (Chapter 8).

One implicit assumption in toxicity testing of drugs and chemicals in experimental animals is that the essential physiological make-up of the animal species resembles that in humans. Thus it is assumed that in the various species used (in practice these are few – rat, mouse, rabbit, guinea pig, dog and, for special purposes, chicken and monkey) the mechanisms involved in intoxication are the same. While this is often so there are many exceptions. An ideal situation is when intoxication is brought about by the same initiating interaction of the chemical and target in the animal species as in humans (stage 3, Figure 2.1). Even though this may be the case, the toxicity of the chemical in different species can differ by several orders of magnitude. Quantitative differences in the rates of systems which affect the delivery of the chemical to its target are often, but not always, the most important factor (stage 2, Figure 2.1). Species differences and difficulties in using data from animal experimentation for the prediction of human susceptibility are discussed in Chapter 10.

All the reactions (events) occurring between exposure and clinical signs of poisoning are not compound (toxic chemical) related. The rates and extents of reactions in stages 1 and 2 are determined by the chemical and physical properties of the toxic chemical and modification of the structure (homologous series) will often result in huge changes in the dose required to cause toxicity. Such structure–activity and dose–response relationships are discussed in Chapter 9. In stage 3, the rate and degree of interaction of the intoxicant with the initiating target is influenced both by the properties of the chemical and the target; stage 3 is the meeting place of the chemistry and biology directly relevant to the subsequent biological and clinical responses. However, stages 4 and 5 are not compound-related and are solely mediated by endogenous biology. Thus the toxic chemical by its reaction with its target initiates biological changes which may be rapid or prolonged (biological cascade). It is from these biological events that new knowledge in basic biology can arise, i.e. by experimental studies of the consequences of controlled modification of specific points in a physiological process (see Preface and Chapters 5, 8 and 10).

2.8   Summary

1   Intoxication by chemicals is a five stage process:

   • Exposure and entry of chemical (stage 1)
   • Delivery of intoxicant to the target cell (stage 2)

- Interaction of intoxicant with the target(s) (stage 3)
- Early consequences of stage 3 (stage 4)
- Clinical consequences (stage 5)

Stages 1 and 2 are intoxicant-related and stages 4 and 5 are biology-related. In stage 3 the rate and degree of interaction are dependent on the properties of the chemical and the target.

2 The same scheme is applicable to endogenous control mechanisms, the mode of action of therapeutic agents (on pathogenic organisms, modification of physiology) and chemicals used to control exogenous agents (insects, weeds, organisms pathogenic to agricultural plants), etc.

3

Kinetics and End-points

3.1 Introduction

The control of homeostasis and the signals accelerating or reducing various functions are mediated by chemical interactions at the molecular level, often between small molecules and macromolecules. There are two rather different types of interaction involved. Combination of various substances, e.g. transmitters with receptors, is usually by a reversible interaction, whereas the control of the rate of some enzymic processes takes place by the attachment of a chemical grouping by a covalent bond, e.g. as in phosphorylation of many proteins (TIBS, 1994). These two forms of interaction (Figure 3.1) are also involved in the action of therapeutic and toxic agents. The degree and rate of interaction are important determinants of their activity.

In biological control the action of transmitters, hormones, etc. must be selective; affinity for a small molecule resides in specific areas in the macromolecule brought together by its tertiary structure. Such areas may be hydrophilic and close to the aqueous environment or, in some cases, lipophilic so that reactions can take place somewhat isolated from the aqueous medium. Much has been learnt about such areas, e.g. receptors, catalytic centres, etc. from the structure of protein crystals. However, in an aqueous environment there will undoubtedly be small but highly significant changes in the macromolecules' structure with a degree of flexibility not possible in the crystal. Micro changes in the juxtaposition of interacting groups can make huge differences in affinity and in rates of reaction. New techniques of study of macromolecules in water such as nuclear magnetic resonance are helping to throw new light on these problems. However, although it may now be possible to predict that a particular chemical will have an affinity for or react with a particular protein at a particular place in its structure, it is still difficult to predict the rate at which reactions will take place.

In reversible and covalent interactions a complex, [M–AB], is formed from the chemical and the macromolecule (Figure 3.1). In wholly reversible reactions the parent macromolecule is reformed by the reverse of the forward reaction; this usually happens in biological systems by the removal of the chemical by dilution, excretion or metabolism to products which have no affinity. In covalent interactions after the formation of a similar complex an intramolecular reaction follows leading to the breakdown of the

17

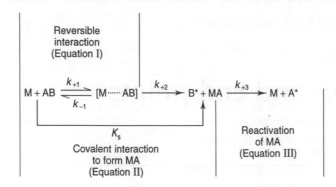

Figure 3.1 Reversible and covalent interaction of chemical AB with a macromolecular target M. B* and A* indicate that during the reaction the products are different chemical entities

chemical AB and the formation of a macromolecule derivative MA in a form unable to carry out its biological function. The formation of the parent macromolecule M from its inactive derivative MA depends on a forward reaction different from those involved in its formation. The difference between these two types of interaction is of great importance in biology, pharmacology and toxicology. In reality most of the reactions involved are much more complicated than this and they have been studied extensively. Additional steps involving molecular rearrangements have been and are being postulated, but details of these are beyond the scope of this volume (for discussions of enzymic reactions see Gutfreund (1965) and Jencks (1969)).

3.2 Reversible Interactions

Reversible interactions are defined by their affinity (K_{Aff}) or dissociation (K_{Diss}) constants. When the chemical AB (often called a ligand) has a moderate affinity for the macromolecule M, i.e. $[AB] \gg [M]$ so that its concentration is not substantially decreased by binding to M, then K_{Aff} and K_{Diss} are respectively:

$$K_{Aff} = \frac{k_{+1}}{k_{-1}} = \frac{[M\cdots AB]}{[M][AB]} \tag{1}$$

$$K_{Diss} = \frac{k_{-1}}{k_{+1}} = \frac{[M][AB]}{[M\cdots AB]} \tag{2}$$

Thus when $[M]/[M\cdots AB] = 1$ (i.e. 50% of molecules of M are associated with AB) then $K_{Aff} = [AB]^{-1}$ and $K_{Diss} = [AB]$.

Techniques of equilibrium dialysis or centrifugation are used for the determination of the affinity or dissociation constants for such reversible combinations and the data are analysed by various methods including that of Scatchard (1949).

By a simple rearrangement of equation 1 the following is obtained:

$$\frac{[M\cdots AB]}{[AB]} = K_{Aff} \ ([M]_T - [M\cdots AB]) \tag{3}$$

in which $[M]_T$ is the total concentration of binding sites.

In operational terms this becomes,

$$\frac{B}{F} = nk - \text{Bound } K \tag{4}$$

in which K is the affinity constant, B is the total bound ligand, F is the concentration of free ligand and n is the number of binding sites per mol if the molecular weight of the macromolecule is known; otherwise n is the mol of ligand bound per unit of macromolecule (often mol/unit of protein).

As shown in Figure 3.2a, a plot of B/F against B yields a linear plot indicating one class of binding sites with the same affinity constant (K) and n the concentration of binding sites. A straight line parallel to the horizontal axis indicates a very large number of binding sites of very low affinity for the ligand (i.e. at its limit this becomes a distri-

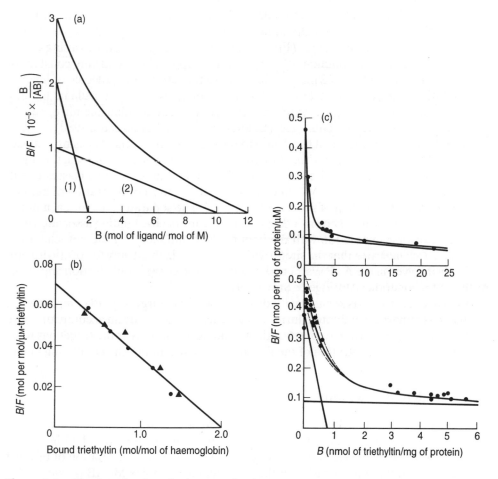

Figure 3.2 The Scatchard method (1949) for the evaluation of the dissociation constant and concentration of ligand binding sites. (a) Theoretical: The two straight lines (1) and (2) have been calculated for B_1, $n_1 = 2$ and $K_1 = 10^5\ M^{-1}$ and for B_2, $n_2 = 10$ and $K_2 = 10^4\ M^{-1}$. The curved line represents binding sites of different affinity on the same molecule. See text for explanation terms. (b) Binding of triethyltin to cat haemoglobin. (c) Binding of triethyltin to rat liver mitochondria. See text for details. (*Sources*: data from Aldridge and Street, 1970; Elliot and Aldridge, 1977)

bution coefficient between two phases). Between these two extremes are curves indicating that there is more than one class of binding site, i.e. the binding sites have different affinities for the ligand.

From equation 4 the relationship becomes:

$$\frac{B}{F} = n_1 (K_1 - B_1) + n_2 (K_2 - B_2) + \ldots + n_x (K_x + B_x) \tag{5}$$

in which $n_1, \ldots, n_x$ are the amounts of binding per unit of macromolecule; $k_1, \ldots k_x$, and $B_1, \ldots, B_x$ are the affinity of constants and the binding to respectively the sites 1, $\ldots, x$. In practice it is experimentally difficult to obtain accurate measures for binding to more than two sites owing to errors inherent in the analytical methods even though the iterative calculation methods are much easier with the use of computers. For a more extensive discussion of this and other methods of analysing data from binding experiments see Tipton (1980), and Edsall & Wyman (1958).

Figures 3.2(b) and (c) illustrate examples of the use of the Scatchard method. Binding of triethyltin to pure cat haemoglobin has been determined using radioactive ^{113}[Sn]-triethyltin and equilibrium dialysis (Figure 3.2b). The linear plot indicates a single class of sites (i.e. they have a common affinity) and the slope yields an affinity constant of 3.5×10^4 M^{-1} for binding of 2 mol of triethyltin to the tetrameric molecule of haemoglobin. Other research has established that the binding involves 5-coordinate binding to a site containing the sulphydryl of a cysteine residue and a imidazole nitrogen of a histidine residue in the α-subunit only (Elliott *et al.*, 1979; Taketa *et al.*, 1980).

In contrast for the binding of triethyltin to rat liver mitochondria also using radioactive ^{113}[Sn]-triethyltin and centrifugation to separate bound and free ligand, the line is not linear (Figure 3.2c). Analysis by an iterative method indicates two classes of site of affinities, namely 4.7×10^5 M^{-1} and 1.4×10^3 M^{-1}, and a concentration of binding sites of 0.8 and 66 nmol/mg of protein respectively. The separate lines for each of the two classes of site are also shown. The latter may be unspecific binding associated with weak electrostatic interaction with the lipoprotein components of the mitochondria; other research indicates that the site(s) with a relatively high affinity for triethyltin are probably involved in the ATP synthetase reaction in the energy conservation apparatus of the mitochondrion (Aldridge & Street, 1970).

Analytical problems associated with dissociation of the target-ligand complex when the tissue is removed and diluted during homogenisation preclude an accurate measure of the bound ligand *in vivo*. In practice the bound ligand at or near the target has to be derived from the concentration of the ligand in the tissue and/or the circulating blood.

3.3 Covalent Interactions

The reacting chemical (AB) is usually in excess compared with the macromolecule (M) and the rate equation is that for a bimolecular reaction (see equation II, Figure 3.1) with one component in excess (i.e. first order); often the rate of formation of product MA is such that the concentration of the intermediate complex M–AB is low:

$$M + A \xrightarrow{k_a} B^* + MA \quad \text{(see Figure 3.1)} \tag{6}$$

$$k_a = \frac{1}{[AB]t} \ln \frac{[M]_t}{[M]} \tag{7}$$

in which $[M]_t$ is the total concentration of macromolecule (100%), [M] is the concentration of macromolecule at any time t.

A plot of ln or log [M] against time t yields a straight line passing through the origin (Figure 3.3a). Similarly a plot against concentration of reacting chemical [AB] also gives a straight line and the concentration × time([AB]t) dependence of the reaction is linear (Figure 3.3b).

When the concentration of the intermediate complex M····AB is not negligible as shown (see equation II, Figure 3.1) the rate of reaction (formation of MA) is exponential and first order for each concentration of [AB] but the concentration dependence does not conform to that described above. As the concentration of [AB] is raised the

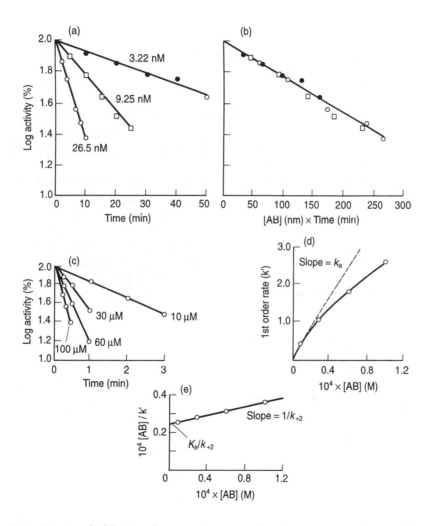

Figure 3.3 Kinetics of inhibition of esterases by organophosphorus compounds. a and b Esterase in rat intestinal mucosa homogenate and diethyl 4-nitrophenyl phosphate. The derived rate constant is 5.3×10^6 M^{-1} min^{-1} at pH 7.2 and 37°C (Aldridge and Reiner,1972). c, d and e Acetylcholinesterase and phosphostigmine. See text for details. The derived constants are k_{+2} 8.3 min^{-1}, K_a 2×10^{-4} M and the initial second order constant 4×10^4 M^{-1} min^{-1}. (*Source*: data from Aldridge & Reiner, 1972)

rate of reaction increases to a maximum when all the available macromolecule is in the form of the intermediate complex M····AB. The following equation then applies:

$$\frac{[AB]}{k} = \frac{K_a}{k_{+2}} + \frac{[AB]}{k_{+2}} \tag{8}$$

in which k is the first order rate concentration at a given $[AB]$ and K_a is a constant which has some similarity to the Michaelis constant K_m in enzymic reactions. Like K_m it is an operational constant and cannot be assumed to approximate to the dissociation constant for the formation of the intermediate complex. It is defined:

$$K_a = \frac{k_{-1} + k_{+2}}{k_{+1}} \tag{9}$$

From equation 8 it follows that a plot of $[AB]/k$ against $[AB]$ yields a straight line with a slope of $1/k_{+2}$ and an intercept on the vertical axis of K_a/k_{+2}. In Figures 3.3(c)(d) and (e) the inhibitor is phosphostigmine which like the natural substrate for acetylcholinesterase (acetylcholine) has a positive nitrogen in the molecule and has a high affinity for the enzyme. In Figure 3.3(c) the first-order plots are individually linear but when the first-order rate constants are plotted against each concentration of inhibitor $[AB]$ then it is clear that a linear relationship (Figure 3.3d) is not obtained. When the results are plotted as shown in equation 8, K_a and k_{+2} can be evaluated (Figure 3.3e).

In equation III (Figure 3.1) an additional step, k_{+3}, the rate of breakdown of the product MA is included, i.e. the reactivation step to regenerate M analogous to an enzyme substrate reaction. There is, however, no fundamental reason why this should not occur after reactions with non-enzymic macromolecules. When the macromolecule derivative MA is unstable then the linear kinetics shown in Figure 3.3 are not obtained. In Figure 3.4a comparison of the rate of reaction of dimethyl and diethyl 4-nitrophenyl phosphate with acetylcholinesterase in rabbit erythrocytes indicates that the diethyl compound shows the expected first-order kinetics but for the dimethyl

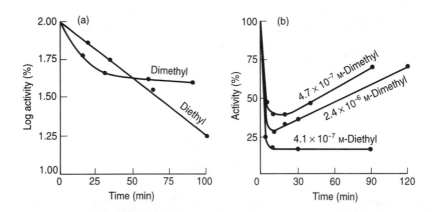

Figure 3.4 Inhibition of acetylcholinesterase by dimethyl or diethyl 4-nitrophenyl phosphates. (a) During incubation of washed rabbit red cells the inhibitors are stable. (b) During incubation of whole rabbit blood the inhibitors are hydrolysed to inactive compounds by a plasma esterase. (*Source*: Aldridge, 1953)

compound a curved relationship is obtained. In this experiment both inhibitors are stable in the incubation medium. When whole blood is used, both compounds produce curves (Figure 3.4b); plasma contains an esterase which hydrolyses both compounds thus destroying their inhibitory power and under this condition another difference emerges when the incubation is prolonged. The percentage inhibition by the diethyl compound remains the same for the two-hour incubation but for the dimethyl compound activity slowly returns. Thus when all active inhibitor has been hydrolysed the diethyl phosphorylated enzyme is stable. In contrast, the dimethyl phosphoryl derivative is unstable with a half-life of approximately 90 minutes.

Thus there are many factors which will influence the rate of reaction of chemicals with macromolecules (Figures 3.3 and 3.4 and section 3.5). For the experimentalist one of the most important features of covalent interaction is that the reaction product is usually stable both *in vitro* and also *in vivo*. This simplifies deductions about cause and effect in mechanisms of toxicity.

3.4 Michaelis Constants

The Michaelis constant for an enzyme reaction is the concentration of substrate when the reaction proceeds at half its maximum rate. Such a constant may be used for any reaction in which there is an intermediate step. Thus when all the macromolecule, i.e. the enzyme in catalysed reactions, becomes occupied with the substrate and all the enzyme is in the intermediate Michaelis complex form, the maximum rate of the reaction is attained (V_{max}). The Michaelis constant is an operational constant and may have different meanings depending on the complexity of the reaction. Thus if we consider the reactions given in Figure 3.1, the Michaelis constants for the whole and parts of the reaction are given by:

From equation I:

$$K_m = \frac{k_{-1}}{k_{+1}} \tag{10}$$

From equation II:

$$K_m = \frac{k_{-1} + k_{+2}}{k_{+1}} \tag{11}$$

From equation II and III

$$K_m = \frac{k_{-1} + k_{+2}}{k_{+1}} \cdot \frac{k_{+3}}{k_{+2} + k_{+3}} \tag{12}$$

Thus the more complex the catalysed reaction the more rate constants must be included in the definition of the Michaelis constant. In equation 10 it is an affinity constant; whether the others in equations 11 and 12 approximate to the dissociation constant of the first step in the reaction depends on the relative rates of the other steps.

The standard Michaelis equation postulates that enzyme and substrate form a complex which can either dissociate into free enzyme and substrate or decompose into free enzyme and products (see Figure 3.1). The velocity equation is:

$$v = \frac{V[S]}{K_m + [S]} \tag{13}$$

Rearrangements of this equation into forms for graphical presentation of experimental results due to Lineweaver and Burke (equation 14) and Hanes (equation 15) are:

$$\frac{1}{v} = \frac{K_m}{V[S]} + \frac{1}{V} \tag{14}$$

$$\frac{[S]}{v} = \frac{K_m}{V} + \frac{[S]}{V} \tag{15}$$

in which $[S]$ is the substrate concentration, v is the rate of production of products or loss of substrate, K_m is the Michaelis constant which defines the concentration of substrate when the reaction proceeds at $V_{max}/2$.

The form of the graphs are shown in Figure 3.5. That derived from equation 15 is the most satisfactory since it avoids the spreading out of the data inevitable when using reciprocals (equation 14); a procedure for the statistical evaluation of constants has been described (Wilkinson, 1961). For other graphical and statistical methods see Dixon & Webb (1966).

Such a constant can be applied to any system in which there is a limiting concentration of an intermediate component of the reaction, e.g. not only all reactions catalysed by enzymes, but also other systems such as carrier-mediated transport of a chemical from one side of a membrane to the other. Indeed, if there is experimental evidence to show that as the concentration of chemical is increased the rate of transport approaches a maximum then this is usually taken as evidence of such an intermediate carrier-mediated step. Thus the 'Michaelis' constant is that concentration of the chemical which allows transport at one-half its maximum rate; it is, as for enzyme reactions, an operational constant the meaning of which in mechanistic terms requires more information.

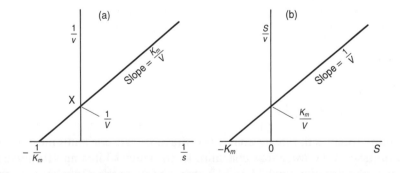

Figure 3.5 Graphical procedures for the estimation of the Michaelis constant (K_m) and the maximum rate (V_{max}) for reactions involving an intermediate complex. For the definition of symbols see section 3.4; graph a is the Lineweaver–Burk plot and b is due to Hanes

3.5 Criteria to Distinguish Reversible from Covalent Interactions

The general kinetic properties of reversible and covalent interactions have been discussed. There are, however, many factors which may make it difficult to decide which type of product has been produced. For example, breakdown of the chemical because of its chemical instability or by biological agents, or breakdown of the covalent product and other factors prevents the demonstration of the clear kinetic picture expected (equation 6 and Figure 3.3a). Instability of the product can make it very difficult to distinguish whether a reversible reaction has taken place or whether a covalent reaction has produced an unstable product. For example, carbamoyl choline produces a transient effect *in vivo* and it would be natural to deduce that this results from a reversible interaction with acetylcholinesterase. This is not the case since an unstable but covalently linked carbamoyl cholinesterase is produced (approximate half-life of 2 minutes at 25°C). Carbamoyl choline therefore fits in the the reaction mechanism as other carbamates, organophosphorus compounds and organosulphur compounds and kinetic behaviour, structure–activity and dose–response relationships can be correctly interpreted.

Both reversible and covalent interactions are affected by the composition of the medium (e.g. pH, composition and concentration of salts) but they may be distinguished from one another if sensitive analytical methods are available (e.g. using radiolabelled material) by precipitation of protein by acids and washing of the precipitates, by extensive dialysis or by removal of radioactivity by treatment with unlabelled reactant or by destruction of the ligand by enzymic means. If the radiolabelled material is not removed by such treatment it is probable that a covalent reaction has taken place. However, there are many instances when covalently attached groups are removed because of the instability of the product; also some ligands attached by high affinity bonds are difficult to remove by dilution or other methods.

Two properties are crucial: the effect of time and the temperature of incubation. Reversible interactions (equation I, Figure 3.1) usually reach an equilibrium rapidly and it is generally accepted that such interactions are diffusion-controlled. For small molecules the second-order rate constant for diffusion is of the order of 10^{12}–10^{13} M^{-1} min^{-1} and, with the assumption for macromolecules that only a small area of the molecule will be involved in binding, the rate constant should be at least 10^{10}–10^{11} M^{-1} min^{-1} (Gutfreund, 1965; Jencks, 1969). Changes of temperature exert a small influence on the equilibrium position.

For covalent interactions when the product is unstable, an apparent steady state is produced at a rate which depends on the rates of the formation and loss of product (equations II and III, Figure 3.1). Covalent interactions are progressive and temperature-dependent. If the modified macromolecule is unstable and reactivates to give the parent macromolecule then the rate of reactivation is also progressive and temperature-dependent. The interpretation in detail of the influence of temperature is complex and beyond the scope of this book. The reader is referred to Gutfreund, 1965; Dixon & Webb, 1966; Laidler, 1958; Simeon *et al.*, 1972; Aldridge & Reiner, 1972. Reversible interactions (equation I) are rapid and diffusion limited and little affected by temperature. Covalent interactions, in contrast, show a marked time and temperature dependence not only for the formation of the macromolecule derivative (equation II) but also for the modified macromolecule's reactivation if it is unstable (equation III, Figure 3.1).

Table 3.1 lists of some of the types of chemical which have been shown to interact with specific groups in macromolecules.

Table 3.1 Examples of chemicals which will react covalently with macromolecules

Chemical	Groups or residues involved
Diethyl pyrocarbonate	Histidine
2,5-alkanediones (6 or more carbons in the alkane)	Lysine
Organophosphorus compounds (phosphates, phosphonates or phosphinates)	Serine
Organosulphur compounds	Serine
Esters of carbamic acid (unsubstituted or substituted on the nitrogen of the carbamic acid)	Serine
Pyrroles	Many residues in protein and nucleic acids
Epoxides	Many residues in protein and nucleic acid
Unsaturated compounds (double or triple bonds)	Cysteine and valine
Alkylating agents	Cysteine, histidine and valine

3.6   In vivo *Kinetics*

Interpretation of dose–response and structure–activity relationships require information on the concentration of chemical reaching the tissue and/or cell and/or target (see Chapter 9). In practice the values for the cell and/or target are rarely available and predictions must often be made from overall tissue or circulating blood concentrations.

The relationship between therapeutic effect and blood or plasma concentrations is an essential component of clinical trials of drugs. To ascertain the toxic effects of drugs or other chemicals, similar relationships must be worked out. The rates of detoxification and bioactivation pathways often show larger species variation than the species variation of affinity for receptors or targets. The relationship between circulating concentration of the actual intoxicant at various times versus the appearance of toxicity must be established.

Two factors are particularly important: the apparent volume of distribution and rate of disposal of the toxic chemical from the blood. The apparent volume of distribution of a substance (V_d) is the fluid volume in which it seems to be distributed. Ideally its determination is simple; a known amount is injected intravenously and, after allowing sufficient time for it to distribute, a sample of blood is taken and the concentration determined. Thus if AB is the amount of substance administered and the resulting concentration in the blood is [AB] then [AB] = AB/V_d or V_d = AB/[AB]. In practice, estimating V_d is not so simple because ideal behaviour is rare – the substance is metabolised, excreted and bound to various macromolecules, no real distribution plateau is reached and the concentration [AB] continues to fall. Most detoxification reactions occurring *in vivo* follow first-order kinetics and disposal curves are usually analysed by fitting successive first-order kinetics to experimental data. Both the volume of distribution and the rate of detoxification of the chemical/intoxicant are influenced by many factors, e.g. concentration into certain cells often by energy-requiring processes, binding, metabolic modification to enhance excretion and/or reduce biological activity and bioactivation to produce compounds with higher biological activity (see Chapters 5 and 6). To obtain an estimate of the volume of distribution, extrapolation to zero time of a logarithmic plot of [AB] in blood at different times is used. Sometimes linear plots are obtained, but sometimes curves result because of differences in the rate of mixing with different tissue compartments.

Standard substances are used to estimate the volume of different compartments, e.g. Evans blue for the vascular compartment, radioactive sodium, chloride or bromide for the extracellular fluid and D_2O or ^3H_2O or antipyrine for the total body water. Although the concepts seem attractively simple, interpretation of the analyses can be misleading. The reasons for this are many and include the complexity of the equilibration between different tissue compartments, plasma concentrations in which some of the substance may be bound to proteins instead of the desired concentration in plasma water, and so on. Nevertheless, analyses for AB in relation to time after administration, together with tissue concentrations, provide useful background information with which to consider estimates of [AB] dose at the target. An approximate value for the total body water is 60% of the body weight, for the extracellular water 16–18%, for the whole blood volume 8–9% and for the plasma volume 4–5%.

Knowledge is sometimes adequate to derive the *in vivo* distribution and persistence of the intoxicants from the individual constants of the processes involved (see discussion of physiologically based pharmacokinetic modelling in Chapter 6).

3.7 Discussion

A potential research topic emerges with the discovery that exposure to a chemical leads to a new phenomenon, e.g. a unique clinical picture, functional deficits, etc., which may be extended in a suitable experimental model to morphological correlates for the signs of poisoning. This is the vital qualitative information for the definition of a new problem. To follow this by research on mechanisms in all five stages of toxicity (see Figure 2.1) requires quantitative results derived from the use of many analytical techniques and experimental approaches. Most of the steps in each stage may be characterised by affinity (K) or rate constants (k), Michaelis constants (K_m) and maximum rates (V_{max}) derived from studies of the effects of concentration of intoxicant, time and sometimes temperature. The first three stages (1–3 in Figure 2.1) are chemical intoxicant related and involve direct measures of the chemical and its metabolites, e.g. rates of penetration, detoxification pathways, bioactivation, reaction with target, etc. The last three stages (3–5 in Figure 2.1) – the biological cascade – are biology-related and may involve many factors such as rates of loss and recovery of activity of an enzyme or receptor, rates of macromolecular resynthesis, cell turnover, recruitment of other cells, etc. Many of the rates will be determined from *in vitro* studies; confirmation of a potential mechanistic hypothesis requires adequate proof that the concentration and time relationships are similar *in vivo* and *in vitro*. Examples given in this chapter have been chosen because they provide relatively simple systems, illustrate the principles involved and can easily be worked through from the original papers.

Health may be regarded as a kind of 'steady state' (homeostasis) in which all the competing and collaborating reactions operate at controlled and adaptable rates.

Clinical signs and symptoms of disease appear when, through the action of an intoxicant, this 'equilibrium' is sufficiently perturbed to disrupt homeostasis. Perturbation of the rates of many individual steps contribute to the dose(exposure)–response relationships. Knowledge of what happens to the intoxicant and what it does to the biology often leads to biomonitoring techniques for dose (internal) and early biological effects. In the following chapters the contribution of these kinetic parameters to understanding of mechanisms in all five stages in developing toxicity (intoxication) will be elaborated.

As emphasised above, time dependence of reactions of the chemical with biological systems and the relationship between such reaction and the development of disease is a vital part of mechanistic studies. Pathological (morphological) examination of tissue is often concerned only with end-points, i.e. with the cause of death, but, from the mechanistic point of view, morphological changes at early stages of the poisoning are particularly important. With current and developing finesse in defining early changes, e.g. using the electron microscope, much more attention must be given to early times after exposure; such studies have been termed 'pathokinetics' (Aldridge, 1976; Cavanagh, 1982b).

Using whatever discipline is relevant, time dependence is one of the most important variables to manipulate in experimental studies of the five stages and the different steps involved in developing toxicity.

3.8 Summary

1 Reversible interaction of intoxicant (ligand) and macromolecule usually takes place rapidly and the final extent of reaction is defined by a dissociation or affinity constant (K). The forward and reverse reactions are identical.

2 Covalent reactions between intoxicant and macromolecule are defined by rate constants (k). During the reaction, which often involves several steps, one molecule of chemical is destroyed and usually a stable derivative of the macromolecule is formed. If this is unstable then reactivation occurs by a different reaction, not by the reverse of the forward reaction.

3 Reversible and covalent interactions are distinguished by experiments involving dilution, dialysis or the addition of substrates (for enzymes) or competitive ligands or destruction of the reacting chemical say by enzymic means. For a reversible interaction, active macromolecule reappears. In contrast, a progressive covalent reaction is usually stopped but reactivation does not occur.

4 Reversible interactions are rapid and usually neither progressive nor temperature-dependent.

5 The rate and extent of covalent reactions are time- and temperature-dependent. If the product is unstable then reactivation is also time- and temperature-dependent; the latter is usually accepted as proof that covalent bonding has taken place.

6 Knowledge of the rates and extent of reactions *in vivo* (pharmaco- and toxicokinetics) and concentrations of intoxicant in blood and tissues is essential for the understanding dose–response and structure–activity relationships (see Chapters 6 and 9).

7 In addition to the reaction of the chemical with components of the affected cell(s), the time relationships of the appearance of clinical signs and symptoms, morphological changes and changes in physiological and biochemical functions are essential components of hypotheses of mechanisms of toxicity.

4

Acute and Chronic Intoxication

4.1 Introduction

Probably the most used terms in toxicology are 'acute' and 'chronic'. Although they are often combined with the word 'toxicity' this is incorrect because toxicity indicates a quality of a substance. Since toxicology is concerned with the nature of the biological effect the correct term is 'intoxication'.

Activity of toxic substances is influenced by the route of exposure or administration of chemicals and the description of the effect includes the time taken for signs and symptoms and their persistence. Many of these factors are listed in Table 4.1. Chronic intoxication and chronic or continuous administration must be distinguished from one another because there are many examples of chronic intoxication in which a long-lasting or irreversible biological change results from a single exposure to an unstable substance. The following examples are discussed under headings stating the three main parameters involved (mode of exposure, latency and nature of the biological effect) and serve to illustrate some of the complexities involved.

Throughout this book dose is defined as the amount of intoxicant which reaches the internal milieu, i.e. dose may be used for various routes of injection (subcutaneous, intraperitoneal, intravenous, etc.; stages 2 and 3 of the five-stage scheme) but exposure is limited to the oral, dermal and via the lung routes (stage 1). Medical convention is to use the term 'dose' for any route of drug administration; in toxicology a conscious effort should be made to distinguish between exposure and dose; for mechanisms of toxicity probably the most important parameter is the concentration of intoxicant reaching the target (i.e. dose; stage 3).

4.2 Single Exposure, Rapid Biological Effect, Rapid Recovery

Hydrocyanic acid is a weak acid with a pK of 9.31 (K_a 4.93 × 10^{-10}). Thus at physiological pH of plasma (7.4) it will be less than 1% in the ionised CN^- form and almost all will be the unionised and volatile (BP 26°C) hydrocyanic acid. Thus to humans and animals hydrocyanic acid will be presented to absorbing surfaces by inhalation or by

Table 4.1 Descriptive parameters in intoxication by chemicals

Administration	Time taken to signs and symptoms of poisoning	Consequences of poisoning
Exposure	Immediate	PRIMARY
Single	Latent (short	Morphological
Repeated	or prolonged	Physiological
Continuous	silent period)	Biochemical
Route		
Oral (food or intubation)		TIME
Intravenous		Transient with
Intraperitoneal		complete recovery
Subcutaneous		Long-lasting or
Percutaneous		permanent effect
Outer surface (skin or eye)		
Carrier		SECONDARY
Food		Biological effects
Solution (hydrophobic or lipophilic		following single
solvents)		or repeated chemical
Dispersion (hydrophobic or		insult
lipophilic solvents)		
Vapour		
Particulate material		

mouth as an alkaline salt soon neutralised by stomach acids. Being unionised and soluble in solvents and lipid it penetrates membranes and equilibrates with the body water very rapidly.

The affinity of cyanide for cytochrome oxidase is high (K_{Aff} 3×10^5 M^{-1}; Wainio & Greenlees, 1960). Since cyanide gains rapid access to the intracellular components of the cell cytochrome oxidase, the final step of the electron transport chain is inhibited and oxidative metabolism and the supply of ATP produced by energy conservation in the mitochondria are rapidly reduced. The circulating concentration of cyanide required to cause death is approximately 5 μg ml^{-1} (1.8×10^{-4} M) (Aldridge & Lovatt Evans, 1946). Assuming a uniform distribution between plasma, brain and the mitochondria in brain, such a concentration would produce approximately 98% inhibition of cytochrome oxidase. Thus the rapid absorption of cyanide by several routes of exposure, the rapid equilibration throughout the body water and its rapid inhibition can lead to rapid death.

The inhibition of cytochrome oxidase by cyanide is a reversible reaction. For doses which are not lethal, there are several ways whereby the concentration of cyanide can be reduced and reversible dissociation of cyanide from cytochrome oxidase can be brought about as soon as exposure ends. Cyanide, or more accurately hydrocyanic acid, is removed by the normal physiological methods of excretion (via the kidneys and lungs) and also by metabolism to the essentially non-toxic thiocyanate; the enzyme responsible is rhodanese which utilises thiosulphate as the sulphur source. Thus, after a single acute dose of cyanide, recovery is rapid and, provided the patient or animal was not unconscious for a protracted period, there is complete recovery with no pathological sequelae.

Cyanide thus satisfies criteria for an acute intoxicant; it is rapidly absorbed and rapidly distributed, it rapidly reacts with an enzyme vital for immediate survival, and after a non-lethal dose there is complete recovery. In circumstances when animals are exposed to almost lethal amounts for longer times, permanent neuronal necrosis may result (section 4.6).

4.3 Continuous Exposure, Rapid Biological Effect, Slow but Complete Recovery

Inhalation of carbon monoxide can lead to rapid death if the concentration is high, but exposure to a low concentration results in an insidious appearance of symptoms. The affinity of carbon monoxide for haemoglobin is approximately two hundred times that of oxygen; with 30–40% of haemoglobin in the carboxymonoxy form little effect is seen, but at around 50%, headache, weakness, vomiting and often collapse occur. At higher concentrations coma, convulsions, respiratory failure and death may result.

Recovery from carbon monoxide poisoning is slow owing to its high affinity for haemoglobin (Roughton & Darling, 1944) and the absence of metabolic processes for its removal. It is mainly removed by exhalation after its slow displacement by the high oxygen tension in the lung. The rate of exchange of oxygen for carbon monoxide can be increased by an increase of the oxygen tension in the inhaled gases.

Thus poisoning by cyanide and by carbon monoxide are superficially similar and both cause a decrease in cellular oxidative processes. However, this is brought about by reactions with two different macromolecules: cytochrome oxidase and haemoglobin. The reaction between these two macromolecules and their respective ligands is by reversible and dissociable interactions. See Chapter 7 for a more detailed discussion of the nature of the combination of carbon monoxide with haemoglobin.

4.4 Single Exposure, Rapid Biological Effect, Slow but Complete Recovery

Most organophosphorus compounds are lipophilic and readily absorbed after oral administration. If they are volatile or dispersed as a fine spray, they can be inhaled, but they are also absorbed through the membranes of the mouth, lung or eye. Organophosphorus compounds are acutely toxic because they inhibit acetylcholinesterase, the enzyme present to remove the neurotransmitter acetylcholine released at nerve endings and elsewhere. As organophosphorus compounds enter the tissues from the circulation, reaction with acetylcholinesterase is usually rapid. Consequently, the activity of the enzyme is reduced, the concentration of acetylcholine raised and symptoms of acetylcholine poisoning begin to appear. Initially the symptoms are headache, blurred vision, weakness, excessive perspiration, nausea, abdominal cramps, tightness of the chest and constricted pupils. These are followed by incapacitating nausea, cramps, discomfort in the chest, muscular twitching (fasciculation) and may lead to respiratory collapse and death. Inhibition of the acetylcholinesterase by 50% can be tolerated for a long time with only slight expression of the symptoms outlined above; death occurs with 90–95% inhibition. The reaction of organophosphorus compounds leads to a phosphylated esterase with the phosphorus moiety attached by a stable covalent bond (Aldridge & Reiner, 1972). In most cases the inhibited enzyme is stable and return of activity is due to the biosynthesis of fresh enzyme by the normal pathways involved in enzyme turnover. Thus recovery from poisoning is slow and, unlike after poisoning by cyanide or carbon monoxide, is due to the biosynthesis of new enzyme. In most cases the original organophosphorus compound is inactivated by a variety of detoxification pathways. Recovery from acute organophosphorus poisoning is usually complete with no residual disability or morphological change (Koelle, 1963; Ballantyne & Marrs, 1992).

Some types of intoxication may be produced by a single exposure, dose or by repeated administration over a long period. Kidney dysfunction results from a single or small number of doses of a cadmium salt. It can also be produced by a slow accumulation of cadmium in the kidney by the ingestion of low concentrations in food. The excretion of cadmium once it is absorbed is slow – it has a half-life of 16–20 years. Eventually the concentration of cadmium in the kidney is high enough to cause damage and kidney dysfunction. The nature of the lesions after acute and chronic administration is in essence the same. Recovery and repair of the morphological changes in the kidney are slow and depend on a reduction of the concentration of cadmium (Webb, 1979).

It is extremely difficult to bring about toxic effects by a single or a few exposures of a suspension of DDT in water. DDT is very insoluble in water but very soluble in oils and solvents. If an oral exposure to DDT in oil is given to a rat, some is absorbed but symptoms are rare even though when administered in a detergent by intravenous injection the lethal dose is less than 10 mg/kg body weight. From the gastro-intestinal tract DDT is rapidly taken up by the adipose tissue where it is biologically inert. If the animal is starved then the adipose tissue is reduced in size by metabolism and DDT is released and causes symptoms originating from the central nervous system which are identical to those following an intravenous dose. Thus, provided DDT reaches the nervous system, toxicity appears. If the animal does not die, recovery is complete with no histopathological changes.

In all the examples cited in sections 4.2–4.4 an acute intoxication has been caused, i.e. an intoxication which can be produced rapidly and from which, dependent on the exposure, complete recovery is possible. The administration can be by many routes and can be by a single exposure, a few exposures or even by a slow uptake over a long time. Provided the toxic chemical reaches and accumulates at its site of action or reacts to cause a persistent chemical change, signs or symptoms of poisoning will appear. Recovery occurs by removal of the toxic chemical and/or by repair of the damage to the biological system.

4.5 Single Exposure, Latent Intoxication, Little or No Recovery

Some organophosphorus compounds also cause a delayed neurotoxicity sometimes accompanied by immediate symptoms as described in section 4.4 and sometimes not. The lesions caused are a dying back of the axons in the long nerves in both the central and peripheral nervous systems; the nerves therefore become disconnected from their end-organs. After the administration of the compound there is a silent period when no sign or symptom appears for up to three weeks. The first sign of poisoning in humans is unsteadiness in walking which then progresses to effects in the arms and sometimes to complete paralysis. If the morphological lesions which are in the axons (axonopathy) are present in the peripheral nerves then a slow return of function can be expected. This is due to reformation and growth of the axon and reconnection to its end-organ.

If the damage is in the long axons in the central nervous system (e.g. in the spinal cord) then little recovery will take place. Apparently the repair facility which occurs in the peripheral nerves does not exist in the central nerves. Thus a long-lasting or permanent effect has been produced and this is clearly chronic intoxication. However, such an intoxication can be caused by a single exposure of an organophosphorus compound which is rapidly detoxified to inactive compounds. It has been established that, for the disease to appear, reaction of the organophosphorus compound must take place with an esterase (not acetylcholinesterase as in acute toxicity) which has been called neuropathy target esterase (NTE). Thus the initiating chemical reaction with this esterase takes place very rapidly and initiates some biological change(s) which take three weeks to be expressed as clinical signs of poisoning (Johnson, 1975a, b).

4.6 Single or Repeated Exposures, Rapid Intoxication, Irreversible Secondary Changes

Permanent and adverse effects are sometimes brought about by the activation of processes which, in normal circumstances, would be repair processes. The most common example is the formation of scar tissue following injury, i.e. space-filling by collagen instead of by cells. Persistent consumption of ethanol, carbon tetrachloride, aflatoxin or dimethylnitrosamine leads to the necrosis of hepatocytes. During the replacement of these cells by cell division, other activated cells, the fibrocytes, are producing collagen. Following the first and later insults to the liver, there is each time an irreversible increase in collagen. Eventually this so reduces the proportion of metabolically active and functioning liver that clinical cirrhosis results.

Paraquat when ingested or injected causes damage to the lung. This condition, which sometimes leads to death from respiratory insufficiency, is initiated by necrosis of type 2 followed by loss of type 1 pneumocytes (alveolar cells). If the early damage is not severe enough to cause death, then fibrocytes are activated and a fibrotic lung results which, in human poisoning, is often so extensive that gas exchange is reduced to such an extent that the patient dies (Smith & Heath, 1976).

Sometimes the dying-back lesions (axonopathy) caused by several structurally different chemicals such as organophosphorus compounds, acrylamide and 2,5-hexanedione are of such severity that the lesion includes the cell body in the spinal roots. If the cell body is intact then the axon grows from it and connects to its end-organ, e.g. muscle endplate. If the cell body is lost then there will be no recovery and secondarily, the denervated muscle wastes away with a permanent loss of function.

In all of the above examples the initial lesion includes cell death (necrosis) and the permanent dysfunction is caused by secondary processes which lead to non-functioning tissue. These changes are not due to the presence of the initial toxic chemical. Whether cell death is a necessary feature for the induction of inflammatory conditions which with other cell recruitment cause diverse and sometimes permanent tissue dysfunction is not always clear.

If hydrocyanic acid or carbon monoxide, discussed earlier as causing acute intoxication, are administered in doses that will reduce to a low level for some time the oxygen utilised by the brain tissue, irreversible neuronal necrosis will occur with a pattern similar to that produced by anoxia (low oxygen tension). Thus substances causing an acute intoxication can, with certain dosing regimes, cause permanent chronic intoxication.

4.7 Single Exposure, Latent Intoxication, No Recovery

Carcinogenesis is the classic case of chronic intoxication with a permanent biological change. Although there are many examples of tumours appearing after repeated administration of a chemical, repeated administration is not always necessary for the induction of carcinogenesis. The dose– or exposure–response relationships for carcinogenesis are fully discussed later and probably indicate that there is little or no threshold, i.e. the relationship between delivered dose and induction of cancer by low doses is linear towards the origin.

There are well documented instances of carcinogenesis being brought about by a single dose of a carcinogen. Dimethylnitrosamine, a water- and lipid-soluble compound which mixes with the body water, is metabolised to a reactive intermediate which alkylates the genetic material, DNA. The dimethylnitrosamine is removed or metabolised entirely within 24 hours and yet tumours appear months later. If the diet of rat is modified so that the metabolic bioactivation systems are reduced in the liver but maintained in the kidney, experimental conditions are possible that ensure that after a single exposure to dimethylnitrosamine all rats develop kidney tumours at approximately 10 months (Swann & Maclean, 1968; Hard & Butler, 1970a, b). The initiation step is brought about by a reaction of an alkylating moiety with DNA which is completed within one day, thus beginning the biological cascade leading to tumour formation and clinical cancer.

It is now accepted that carcinogenesis is a multi-stage biological process (Berenblum, 1974) and the initiation step outlined above is but one of these steps. Presumably, compounds which produce tumours in most of the animals after a single dose are 'complete carcinogens' capable of initiating all of the essential steps. A permanent biological change (chronic intoxication) results from chemical events which cause an irreversible change in the DNA template, e.g. mutation, carcinogenesis and sometimes teratogenesis.

4.8 Discussion

The commonly used terms 'acute toxicity' or 'chronic toxicity' are ill-defined and, as normally used, contain elements of the type of exposure to the substance and also the type of toxicity which ensues. If these are separated into acute or chronic administration and acute or chronic intoxication then definitions can be made. Such operational definitions require arbitrary decisions. For instance, when acute administration ceases to be acute and becomes chronic, is acute reserved to single doses given by injection or by mouth or is it the administration achieved in 1, 2 or more days? A similar problem arises when we try to define when administration becomes chronic. These problems indicate that there is no system which is rational enough to be used routinely which would cover all the different modes of administration (Table 4.1).

The only solution is to state exactly what has been done in the experiments or, when man has been exposed, what has happened. Examples of different modes of exposure are: substance A was administered by a single intravenous injection in glycerol formal (methylidinoglycerol, a useful solvent for the administration of lipid-soluble chemicals) or by the oral route as a single exposure of a solution in oil, was volatilised in a closed chamber and the animals exposed for 3 minutes, was applied as a solution in ethanol to the skin, covered for 2 hours and then removed by washing, was added to the diet and fed to the animals with continuous or limited access to the food, and so on. It is possible that all these routes of administration will produce the same type of toxicity but the exposure required will be different. The different routes can only be linked when information is available about the absorbed dose, the rate of penetration and the rate of excretion. Calling one or other of them acute or chronic is not helpful.

There is less ambiguity about acute and chronic intoxication when the definitions are based on clinical descriptions. Chronic is reserved for long-lasting intoxication, and therefore acute is for those forms for which complete recovery or death is reasonably fast and complete. Chronic intoxication lasts for a reasonably long time or is permanent; a decision of what is reasonable in both cases is quite arbitrary. What is the correct term if, after the administration of a single exposure, illness is detected which then appears to diminish and even disappear for a time followed by a secondary stage which then leads to a permanent disability? There is no rational way of defining acute and chronic intoxication except at the extreme ends of the range of possibilities; for example a single dose of a compound which causes illness in ten minutes and recovery within one day contrasting with a single dose of a compound which caused illness in three weeks which lasted for one year. Everything between is a problem.

The use of such terms can inhibit rational thought and lead nowhere in the development of understanding of mechanisms and concepts. As understanding develops, the meaning of the terms becomes more disseminated and even illusory. For example, if after a chemically induced neurological illness there is an apparent clinical recovery, detailed histopathology may demonstrate that a substantial number of neurones have been lost and cannot be replaced. The experimentalist should be asking questions which will illuminate the problem. The toxicologist faced with practical decisions must take into account all the experimental data and strive to bridge the gap between animal data and the probability of similar effects occurring in humans and the risk of their occurrence after a defined exposure. There may be a reason to use 'acute' or 'chronic' toxicity or similar terms in the context of defined protocols for toxicity testing but they have no place in mechanisms and concepts.

4.9 Summary

1 The terms 'acute' and 'chronic' toxicity are confusing since they do not distinguish between the type of administration and biological effect. Their use is not recommended.

2 Acute and chronic intoxication refer unambiguously to the type of biological effect.

3 Exposure is the amount or concentration applied to the external milieu as in the oral, dermal or inhalation routes.

4 Dose is the amount or concentration reaching and being distributed within the internal milieu.

5 Exposure or administration should always be defined by route, number and concentration of applications, nature of exposure (in solvent, as a suspension or particulate) and type of repeated application (continuous or divided).

6 Intoxication should always be characterised by the nature of the signs and symptoms, the time the signs/symptoms appear, how long they persist or at what time they become permanent.

5

Delivery of Intoxicant

Decrease in delivery to the target

5.1 Introduction

This chapter concerns many factors which, after exposure, can influence entry and delivery of the intoxicant to the cells (stages 1 and 2 in Figure 5.1). For many substances the route is circuitous, and the type of exposure and the properties of the chemical influence entry to the internal milieu. The processes discussed decrease the concentration of intoxicant gaining access to the target.

The essence of organised biological systems is the integrated structure within which various functions are exercised by specific organs and within which many reactions occur in specific cells and specific compartments within the cells. While the membranes surrounding these compartments are essential for the orderly function of the organism, they can provide barriers for the penetration of exogenous chemicals. Cellular membranes have a complex structure and are constructed so that some substances are excluded and for some entry is facilitated. In higher organisms the constitution and properties of membranes cover a huge range, for example those from the gastric mucosa, the hepatocyte, alveolar cells of the lung. The skin allows organisms to establish an internal environment separate from their surroundings. Animals need skin for structure, preservation of water and essential nutrients and for protection against the environment, i.e. strong against physical attack, to resist penetration by chemicals (predominately hydrophilic). To serve these functions the skin possesses a non-vascularised keratinous layer. The underlying dermis is more permeable and vascularised but, to reach the circulation through the skin toxic substances have to travel through and between layers of cells – contrast the relatively short distance that a toxic substance has to go in absorption from the gastro-intestinal tract. Even with this diversity of structure and function, the essential common feature of biological membranes is layers of proteinacious and lipophilic material.

Where exposure of humans to chemicals is concerned, the usual routes of entry are via the skin, the mouth (mouth, oesophagus, gastro-intestinal tract) and the lungs (trachea, bronchus, bronchioles, alveolar tissue). In experimental toxicology, administration can be by other routes in procedures designed to answer particular questions.

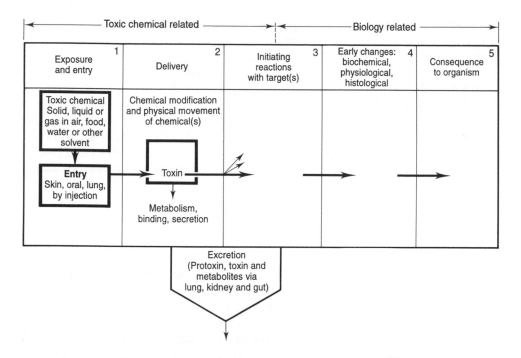

Figure 5.1 Exposure, entry and delivery of intoxicant to its site of action. (Stages 1 and 2 from Figure 2.1; see legend.)

Rapid penetration of chemicals is best achieved when the substance has both lipophilic and hydrophilic properties.

Oils penetrate the skin and, provided they or their solutes have sufficient solubility in water, reach the blood and are generally distributed throughout the body. Oils as solvents of other substances are used as a reliable way of administering substances. Drug administration via absorption through the skin is now often used (for example, the use of patches applied to the skin in order to supply a small dose of nicotine to those who are trying to break the habit of smoking). Fully ionised substances are poorly absorbed. Most of the body is covered by a dry skin but there are breaks in it, such as the hair follicles, which can provide a point of entry for extraneous applied chemicals. Skin damaged by physical and sometimes chemical attack also may lead to rapid absorption of substances largely excluded by intact skin.

The intermediate tissues involved in entry are those of the mouth and alimentary tract and of the nose and lung; these are kept functioning by secretions and are always wet. Penetration of hydrophilic and lipophilic substances is rapid. All gases are somewhat lipophilic and upon inhalation are rapidly taken into the blood stream, e.g. the inert gases, diethylether, anaesthetics. Droplets of liquid (aerosols or particulates) can only reach the alveolar regions of the lung provided they have the correct aerodynamic diameter; the rate of absorption will depend on the volatility and solubility in water of the liquid. If an aerosol contains a solute then its absorption will depend on its physical and/or chemical properties and the rate of uptake into the circulation will be directly proportional to the concentration gradients between each side of the relevant membranes.

Following absorption from the intestine, lipids may form large droplets (chylomicrons) which enter the intercellular spaces and ultimately pass via the lymphatic capillaries, larger lymph vessels and the thoracic duct to enter the general circulation. Some chemicals may be transported dissolved in the chylomicrons.

If the chemical is highly reactive, e.g. strong acids or bases, powerful alkylating agents or lipophilic chemicals such as tri n-butyltin chloride which possess biological properties affecting all cells, then local toxic effects will be produced on all the external surfaces described above. The term 'general toxicity' should be reserved for this type of indiscriminate cell destruction brought about by chemicals. All other toxicity is specific and is a consequence of selective interactions at the cellular and macromolecular levels.

Two examples – DDT and methyl isocyanate – illustrate the many 'delivery' factors which influence whether toxicity occurs.

5.1.1 DDT

DDT (1,1,1-trichloro-2,2-di(4-chlorophenyl)ethane) is a highly effective insecticide and exerts its toxic action by a modification of Na^+ channel activity in the nervous system (Narahashi, 1992). Under certain circumstances it is toxic to rats and, like some pyrethroids, the toxicity is characterised by the appearance of a fine tremor which gradually becomes more severe until the animals become prostrate with whole body tremor (T- or Type 2 syndrome as described by Vershoyle & Aldridge, 1980; Narahashi, 1992). By careful intravenous injection of DDT dissolved in the detergent Tween 60, DDT's intrinsic toxicity is quite high (approximately 10 mg/kg body weight). DDT has unusual physical and chemical properties and is chemically unreactive, stable to chemical attack, solid (melting point 108°C), lipophilic and soluble in most organic solvents including food oils, and has an extremely low solubility in water. It is often described as insoluble but careful measurements have shown that its solubility in water is approximately 1.7 parts per billion (4.8×10^{-9} M; 4.8 nM; Biggar *et al.*, 1967). As a suspension of fine particles in water, DDT is almost non-toxic to humans (as is well known to sprayers in malaria control programmes to eradicate mosquitoes). It is almost impossible to produce signs of poisoning in rats by the administration by mouth of suspensions of DDT in water. The application of DDT in organic solvents, rather than the usual suspensions in water, would lead to its absorption through contaminated skin. If the DDT is dissolved in food oils such as olive or ground nut oil, some DDT is absorbed from the gastro-intestinal tract via the usual routes of absorption of lipids (small intestine and the lymphatic system). If DDT is administered to rats by mouth in small amounts in food, the rate of partition into the fat depots (adipose tissue) is high and takes precedence over partition in toxic amounts into the nervous system. DDT stored in the fat may be mobilised when rats are deprived of food and the lipids in adipose tissue are required as a source of metabolic energy; under these circumstances symptoms of intoxication may well appear.

Thus intoxication may be entirely prevented by the form in which the chemical is presented to humans or animals. When presented as a suspension of fine particles the insolubility of DDT in water prevents its entry into the body.

5.1.2 Methyl Isocyanate

Methyl isocyanate ($CH_3-N = C = O$) is a volatile liquid (MP -45°C; BP 40°C; VP 300 torr at 20°C). It is soluble in water and in organic solvents. It is highly reactive, reacts rapidly with water and amines and is used as a chemical intermediate in the synthesis of methyl carbamate insecticides.

In December 1984 an industrial accident occurred in Bhopal, India, when a large quantity of methyl isocyanate was released. At the prevailing temperatures a cloud of the gas flowed along the ground into the town. Over two thousand people died and it is estimated that over twenty thousand were exposed (Kamat *et al.*, 1985a,b). The effects seen after human exposure were severe irritation of the eyes, nose and throat followed by irritating cough, chest pain, sensation of choking and death in the more severely affected people. Many have recovered completely but many survivors show symptoms of chronic obstructive lung disease. These signs of poisoning have also been demonstrated in animals (Nemery *et al.*, 1985; Ferguson & Alarie, 1991). Systemic disease other than that which can be ascribed as secondary to severe fibrotic changes in the upper bronchial tree seems not to occur.

Toxic amounts of methyl isocyanate, therefore, do not reach the blood stream in sufficient concentration to cause damage to internal organs. The toxicity seen in humans and animals is due to reaction of methyl isocyanate with tissues with wet surfaces, e.g. eyes, mouth, nose, throat and the lung bronchus, bronchioles, and extending to the alveolar regions if the exposure was severe. The chemical's speed of reaction with local tissue components and water is so high that little is available for movement into the systemic circulation. Such poisoning is one of the few examples which may be considered to be general toxicity; however, when methyl isocyanate reaches the lung its reaction in the airways is selective for the respiratory region and cell type (Kennedy *et al.*, 1993).

5.2   Delivery (Entry and Distribution)

The many factors which influence and decrease the rate of delivery of the intoxicant to its site of action in an active form are discussed in more detail here. Some of the systems may, depending on the chemical, increase instead of decrease intoxication by bioactivation or by concentration within particular cells (see Chapter 6 and Discussion for a general assessment of Chapters 5 and 6).

The concentration which reaches the affected cell is a result of many competing reactions, including the rate of penetration, binding to other toxicologically irrelevant sites, transport mechanisms and metabolism to inactive, less active or more active chemicals (see Chapter 6), excretion and secretion. The influence of such systems or factors is different for reversible and covalent interactions. The difference is illustrated by considering the two situations when there is a constant infusion of intoxicants (Figure 5.2).

With a constant rate of entry of the intoxicant AB a steady state concentration, $[AB]_{free}$, is reached both in the circulation and in the cell affected. This is a steady state with many other processes competing for AB. The concentration of the complexed target $[T\cdots AB]$ is also in steady state with respect to $[AB]_{free}$ as shown in the reversible reaction a in the diagram. When entry of AB ceases or increases $[T\cdots AB]$ dissociates or increases respectively. If entry of AB is stopped long enough for all AB to be cleared from the organism by excretion, metabolism, etc. then when exposure to AB is restarted the organism should have the same sensitivity as for the first infusion. These principles are exactly the same as for the treatment of disease

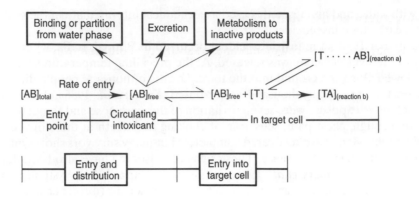

Figure 5.2 Systems or factors influencing the delivery of active (free) intoxicant to its target cell. $[AB]_{total}$ is the total concentration presented at the entry point to the internal environment. $[AB]_{free}$ is the free and unbound intoxicant in circulation, in unaffected cells as well as in the target cells. The items in the boxes operate in stages 1 and 2 from Figure 5.1

when a constant concentration of circulating drug is maintained to produce optimal therapeutic effect.

When a covalent reaction takes place (reaction b in Figure 5.2) a steady state is not attained. Although a steady state concentration of $[AB]_{free}$ may be attained, the concentration of TA (the product of the covalent reaction) continuously increases with time. Depending of the proportion of T converted to TA, signs of intoxication will be seen, and with more reaction the signs will become more severe. When entry of AB ceases and its concentration falls by excretion, metabolism, etc., the concentration of TA is unaffected and the organism remains sensitive to further entry of AB. If the rate of entry of AB is increased and $[AB]_{free}$ increases, the rate of reaction with AB will increase and signs of poisoning will appear earlier.

The above statements are for an idealised and simple situation and illustrate that even though two substances may gain entry at the same rate the response to changes in the rate of disposal is different depending on the chemical properties of the intoxicant. In practice there are many other complicating factors which are considered later. It is rare for a toxic chemical to be perfused into animals or man but the principles outlined above apply to other situations. Different rates and mechanisms of penetration of the toxic chemical for different routes of exposure (see Table 4.1) will greatly influence the rate of appearance of signs and symptoms of and recovery from intoxication.

Although many enzymic reactions may take place at catalytic centres within hydrophobic pockets within proteins, the rate at which these reactions take place is determined by the concentration of the substrate within the water phase. In the same way, whether intoxication occurs (involving initiating reaction with targets) depends on the concentration of free toxic reactant. Thus, $[AB]_{free}$ is the concentration of free reactant (Figure 5.2) which will be in equilibrium with all other reactions sequestering it in non-reactive forms. The measurement of this important parameter of internal dose, i.e. $[AB]_{free}$ of the proximal intoxicant in the circulating blood or in the tissue or cells affected is often difficult and in many cases an estimate of its magnitude has to be derived from other measurements.

5.3 Movement across Membranes

Chemicals may pass across cell membranes in a variety of different ways:

1 Passive diffusion
2 Filtration
3 Facilitated diffusion
4 Active transport
5 Pinocytosis
6 Phagocytosis

Sometimes the substance may not be in the same chemical form when it moves through the membrane as when it was administered. This may be due not to metabolism which changes the administered chemical to another but to the association of anions/cations with the ionised intoxicant. Such changes brought about by ionisation or combination with other ions can change significantly the substance's properties and render them more or less lipophilic/hydrophilic and sometimes increase their molecular weight. Such changes are frequent in the organometal series of compounds (see section 5.4.)

5.3.1 Passive Diffusion

Passive diffusion is probably the most common mechanism of penetration of membranes and depends on the diffusion of the substance through the lipid–protein bilayer down a concentration gradient with the partition of it from the water phase on one side to the water phase on the other. The physical properties which allow this to be rapid are solubility in water, organic solvents and/or lipids. If the substance is miscible both with water and organic solvents then conditions are optimal. Substances which are charged do not easily pass membranes by passive diffusion and indeed the previous condition of miscibility excludes charged molecules. The following is a short list of chemicals which possess the former properties:

Dimethylnitrosamine	$(CH_3)_2N–N = O$
Dimethyl sulphoxide	$(CH_3)_2S = O$
Dimethyl formamide	$HC(=O)N(CH_3)_2$
sym-Dimethyl hydrazine	$(CH_3)NH–NH(CH_3)$
OSS-Trimethylphosphorodithioate	$(CH_3O)(CH_3S)_2P = O$
Ethanol	CH_3CH_2OH
2-Ethoxyethanol	$C_2H_5OCH_2CH_2OH$
Acrylamide	$CH_2 = CHC(=O)NH_2$
Hydrocyanic acid	$HC = N$
Antipyrine (1,5-dimethyl-2-phenyl-3-pyrazolone)	

All the above are soluble in water and organic solvents and, except for hydrocyanic acid, are uncharged at all pHs. However, this is not really an exception because HCN is a weak acid (pK 9.3) and under all physiological conditions it is unionised.

The properties which facilitate the absorption or entry into the organism of the above compounds will also ensure their rapid penetration into all cells because the general make-up of all cell membranes is the same. One example is dimethylnitrosamine, a potent carcinogen for the liver and kidney of rats, which rapidly enters and is distributed throughout the body water of rats. The relationship between the blood concentration of dimethylnitrosamine and time after intravenous administration is shown in Figure 5.3. The first-order rate of the chemical's removal from the blood is 0.13 h^{-1} with a half-life of 5.3 h; the intercept on the vertical axis is the extrapolated concentration at zero time (64.5 μg/ml plasma); this is the expected concentration if dimethylnitrosamine is uniformly distributed in the whole body water.

Passive diffusion can also take place when the state of ionisation of the chemical differs on either side of the membrane. Using the Henderson–Hasselbach equations:

For an acid, $pH = pK_a + \log \dfrac{A^-}{HA}$ where $HA = H^+ + A^-$

For a base, $pH = pK_a + \log \dfrac{B}{HB^+}$ where $B + H^+ = HB^+$

it is a simple computation to determine the degree of ionisation of acids and bases at the pH of 1–3, mean 2, for rat stomach and at the pH of 7.4 for the internal milieu (see Table 5.1). In the middle of the list devoted to acids most of them would be unionised at pH 2 and ionised at pH 7.4 thus providing a very large concentration drop for the unionised form between the external and internal milieu. The strong acids at the top of Table 5.1 will not pass through the mucosa by passive diffusion, whereas those towards the end of the acid section will be unionised at both pH and will be absorbed rapidly due to their lipophilicity and water solubility. Weak bases (top of the list) will be absorbed readily in the unionised form in the stomach and intestinal tract. With

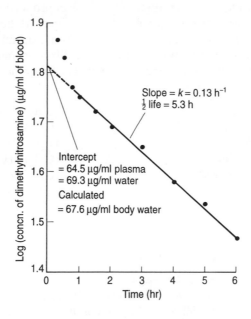

Figure 5.3 Clearance of dimethylnitrosamine from rabbit blood. A rabbit (1.6 kg) was injected intravenously with dimethylnitrosamine (50 mg/kg body weight). The water content of rabbit plasma is 93% and of a whole rabbit 74% of the body weight. (*Source*: figure and results from Magee, 1956)

Table 5.1   Degree of ionisation of a selection of acids and bases at the pH of rat stomach contents and the internal physiological pH

Acids	pK_a	A⁻	HA	A⁻	HA
		(pH 2.0; %)		(pH 7.4; %)	
Hydrochloric	–	Completely ionised			
Trichloracetic	0.70	95.2	4.8	100	0
2,4.6-Trichlorophenol	0.80	94.0	5.0	100	0
Dichloroacetic	1.48	76.8	23.2	100	0
Chloroacetic	2.85	12.3	87.7	100	0
Acetylsalicylic (aspirin)	3.49	3.1	96.9	100	0
2,4-Dinitrophenol	3.96	1.1	98.9	100	0
Ascorbic (1)[a]	4.10	0.79	99.2	99.9	0.05
Acetic	4.75	0.18	99.2	99.8	0.2
4-Nitrophenol	7.15	0	100	64.0	36.0
Hydrocyanic	9.31	0	100	1.2	98.8
Phenol	9.89	0	100	0.3	99.7
Ascorbic (2)[a]	11.79	0	100	0	100

Bases		B	HB⁺	B	HB⁺
		(pH 2.0; %)		(pH 7.4; %)	
Acetanilide	0.61	96.1	3.9	100	0
Physostigmine (1)[a,b]	1.76	63.5	37.5	100	0
Nicotine	3.15	6.6	93.4	100	0
4-Chloroaniline	3.93	1.2	98.8	99.9	0.03
Aniline	4.80	0.16	99.8	99.7	0.26
Triethyltin	6.81	0	100	79.5	20.5
Physostigmine (2)[a,b]	7.88	0	100	11.7	88.3
Ammonia	9.25	0	100	1.4	98.6
Paraquat[c]	–	Completely ionised			

[a] The two entries for ascorbic acid and physostigmine are for the two ionising groups in the molecule.

[b] Physostigmine is an anticholinesterase and is the monomethylcarbamyl ester isolated from the calabar bean (see Chapter 7).

[c] Paraquat is the herbicide 1,1'-dimethyl-4,4'-bipyridinium (see Chapter 7).

stronger bases (end of the list) penetration of membranes throughout the gastro-intestinal tract will be difficult. If such positively charged molecules are readily absorbed the mechanism is likely to involve facilitated diffusion or active transport.

Diffusion through a membrane is influenced by the concentration gradient; sometimes the rate is limited by the rate of presentation of the penetrant to the membrane, i.e. penetration is perfusion-limited.

5.3.2   Filtration

In contrast to passive diffusion, filtration relies on movement through the pores of the aqueous channels in biological membranes and is restricted to hydrophilic substances soluble in water and of a low molecular weight. Foreign compounds move through these channels at a rate which is dependent upon the flow of water which is itself dependent on the size of the pores. Pore sizes vary from tissue to tissue and may be quite large, as in the glomerulus of the kidney, but in general they are around 7 Å in diameter: transport by this route is therefore usually restricted to hydrophilic molecules with molecular weights of around 100.

Recent advances are indicating the kind of tertiary/quaternary structures in enzymes facilitating the movement of small molecules (substrates and products) in and out of the catalytic centre area (Sussman *et al.*, 1991). Acetylcholinesterase has a rather rapid catalytic centre activity ($>10^6$ molecules of acetylcholine hydrolysed per catalytic centre per minute). Much kinetic information is available about the potential rates of the chemical steps in the hydrolysis and it has always been assumed that the positive nitrogen of acetylcholine was held in the correct orientation by a negative charge embedded inside the protein but near the reacting groups involved in the hydrolysis. Such rapid catalysis poses logistical problems of how the substrate reaches the catalytic site and after hydrolysis how the products move out. Recent studies have thrown some light on these problems. The 'anionic' site does not exist and is a cage of aromatic groups in which Van der Waal's forces predominate and the channel to and from the active site is made up of hydrophobic residues. This recent research (Sussman *et al.*, 1991) on pure enzymes may have a wider significance for the biology of the 'catalysed' and directed movement of small molecules. These emerging principles may well be applicable to the movement of exogenous chemicals across membranes, to attachment to receptors and into the catalytic centres of enzymes.

5.3.3 *Facilitated Diffusion and Active Transport*

Both facilitated diffusion and active transport are carrier-mediated. The chemical enters the membrane and becomes attached to a 'carrier' for which it has a reasonably high affinity. The chemical/carrier complex then moves across the membrane and releases the chemical which has thereby moved from one side of the membrane to the other. Facilitated diffusion is carrier-mediated transport down a concentration gradient whereas active transport is against a concentration gradient and therefore requires a source of energy. Both facilitated diffusion and active transport are much more specific than passive diffusion and filtration which depend mainly on the physical form of the moving chemical. Since both require combination with a carrier, the rate of transport will be influenced by the affinity of the chemical for the carrier and its concentration in the membrane. Transport of chemicals across membranes with and without carriers may be readily distinguished by the kinetics of the processes. Without a carrier the rate will not reach a maximum and will be solely dependent on the concentration on either side of the membranes. In contrast, where carrier-mediated processes are concerned, increasing proportions of carrier become converted to carrier/chemical complex and the process reaches a maximum rate. The kinetics have been described in Chapter 3 and are identical to those seen for many enzymic reactions. The molecular structure of a carrier defines the specificity of the process. Active transport requires a source of energy, usually ATP, and may be distinguished from facilitated diffusion by the effects of removing or depleting the energy source. This is usually achieved by the addition of inhibitors of the energy reactions of the cell such as uncouplers or inhibitors of mitochondrial energy conservation reactions (see section 7.2). Competition between different chemicals will occur when they compete for the same carrier. Transport of a competing chemical can occur through its high affinity for the carrier but the carrier can also be immobilised if the affinity of a competing chemical is too high, i.e. the carrier is not released. A competing chemical may even take part in facilitated diffusion down a concentration gradient instead of via an energy-requiring system.

5.3.4   Endocytosis: Pinocytosis and Phagocytosis

Endocytosis is an important process for the movement of small volumes of liquid. If the membrane is endocytosed in the form of vesicles containing a small amount of plasma, the uptake of plasma and solutes is called pinocytosis. Pinocytosis involves small invaginations of the membrane which pinch off and close up to form free fluid-filled vesicles within the cell cytoplasm. This is thought to be a mechanism for active transport of fluid and solutes across cell membranes.

Endocytosis which leads to the selective uptake of particles of size up to several microns is phagocytosis. Steps in this process are specific recognition of particles, adherence to the cell membrane, invagination around the particle followed by pinching off of the cell membrane at the neck of the vesicle to form a phagosome. The phagosome may fuse with lysosomes which can lead to digestion or solubilisation. Particles can be of many types and when inorganic are probably recognised by their protein covering. This may be a means of transport of absorbed solutes or of particulates which slowly go into solution within the cell either after digestion within the lysosomes or directly, e.g. beryllium and rare earth phosphates.

5.3.5   Absorption from the Gastro-intestinal Tract

Although the principles have been outlined in the preceding sections the rate and extent of absorption from the gastro-intestinal tract are often difficult to predict.

Conditions of experimental studies are designed for particular purposes; the administration may be by a single dose, to animals from whom food has been withheld during the preceding 24 hours, with the intoxicant in special solvents, etc. Most of the processes take place with the effective concentration being that of the free molecule in solution in the aqueous phase. Food contents of indeterminate composition will often reduce the concentration of free intoxicant and thus the rate of absorption. For example, inorganic ions such as beryllium can produce insoluble phosphates which are extremely insoluble in water. It is therefore difficult to demonstrate the toxicity of beryllium when it is administered by the oral route even though it is a rather toxic metal when injected. Cadmium may complex with food constituents and there may also be a competition with complexes of iron, calcium, copper and zinc with carrier transport systems for these essential inorganic ions (Bremner, 1979). Methylmercury forms lipid-soluble chloride and hydroxide *in vivo* thus aiding absorption. It also complexes with high and low molecular weight thiols; reaction with the former may reduce absorption whereas the latter may increase it and the complex, say with cysteine, may circulate as such *in vivo*.

The quaternary compounds pralidoxime (2-PAM), used for the treatment of organophosphorus poisoning, and the herbicide paraquat would not be expected to be absorbed through the gastro-intestinal tract since they are fully ionised at physiological pHs. 2-PAM and other aldoximes which are taken by mouth as a prophylactic before exposure to organophosphorus compounds (Leadbetter, 1988) have been shown to pass through the intestinal wall (Levine & Steinberg, 1966). Paraquat is toxic to the

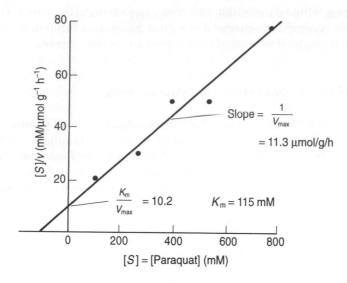

Figure 5.4 Evidence for carrier-mediated uptake of paraquat through rat intestinal mucosa. The results presented have been recalculated from Heylings (1991) for intestinal mucosa at 37°C. Paraquat uptake was much reduced in experiments at 4°C or under nitrogen

lung when administered by the oral route. This may be a special case since high doses are required and the lung possesses an active transport system which can raise the concentration of paraquat in specific cell types in the lung many times the concentration in the circulating plasma (Rose *et al.*, 1974, and see Chapters 6 and 7). In a recent study it has been shown that the mechanisms of movement of paraquat across the mucosa in the intestine are more complex than in the lung. Absorption was highest in the jejunum although the processes are saturable (Figure 5.4) and, although part seems to be energy-dependent it is not clear what the proportion is. Direct damage to epithelial cells by paraquat may cause an increase in mucosal permeability or effects of paraquat on energy yielding systems are complicating factors.

Many substances (chemicals and drugs), e.g. organotin and organolead compounds administered in oil, cause damage in the gastro-intestinal tract (Verschoyle & Little, 1981).

All these uncertainties emphasise the difficulties of the interpretation of intoxication resulting from tests when the administration is by the oral route in internal dose–response terms. Prediction from one species to another is also a problem. For these reasons there should be much more emphasis on measurement of absorbed and internal dose after different routes of administration and less reliance on definition of the exposure, oral dose, etc., i.e. there is need for good pharmacokinetic and toxicokinetic studies.

5.4 Distribution

The general principles which influence and govern the movement of chemicals from the gastro-intestinal tract also apply to their movement around the body and into cells. Substances with physical properties which allow them to pass through biological membranes, i.e. solubility in water and lipids, rapidly penetrate all cells and become equally distributed in the body water (see section 5.3.1). The differences in the extremes of pH seen between the contents of the stomach and the intracellular fluids such as blood are not seen in the internal milieu. Thus carboxylic acids are fully ionised and their movement into cells by passive diffusion is restricted. However, even a small amount of an acid in the unionised form will allow diffusion through a membrane at a rate determined by the concentration gradient across it. If the material moving across the membrane is further metabolised then this gradient will be dependent upon its rate of conversion to other substances. It is perhaps not an accident that many of the substances present in intermediary metabolism are fully ionised acids. Thus penetration of the cells and metabolism of the unionised glucose proceeds through many steps involving acidic intermediates which are retained intracellularly or inside subcellular organelles. The metabolism of exogenous chemicals to more water-soluble and ionised acids may also require specific transport mechanisms to extrude them from cells on their way to the kidney for excretion. For general texts consult Parke (1968), Timbrell (1982), Sipes & Gandolfi (1986) and Klaassen (1986).

5.5 Factors which Reduce the Concentration of Free Intoxicant

In vivo many factors influence and reduce the concentration of free chemical in the circulation and in the cell cytoplasm. The following are examples which result in significant reductions of the concentration of intoxicant:

1 Extracellular proteins; albumin.
2 Intracellular proteins; haemoglobin.
3 Intracellular proteins; ligandin (glutathione transferase).
4 Intracellular proteins; metallothioneine.
5 Adipose tissue.

Many of these factors involve reversible binding to macromolecules or partition between lipid and water; the concentration in the water phase will be in free equilibrium with the bound form or that partitioned into lipid.

All of the above factors, which are discussed individually in more detail, retain the intoxicant in its original form and although the intoxicant's concentration within cells and in the circulation may be reduced, the time that it stays in the organism may be prolonged. Other effective systems involve the metabolism (detoxification) of the intoxicant and its conversion to less or non-toxic agents. These systems include:

6 Metabolism (detoxification): phase 1.
7 Metabolism (detoxification): phase 2.
8 Reaction with small and large molecules which have no toxic consequences.
9 Excretion of the intoxicant or of phase 1 and 2 metabolites.

5.5.1 *Albumin*

Albumin is the most abundant protein in plasma and is present at a concentration of 4–5 g/100 ml (60% of the total protein). The other 40% is made up of the globulins and fibrinogen. The concentration of albumin (molecular weight 69,000) is 0.6–0.7 mM whereas the total globulins with their higher molecular weights (160,000–300,000) are only approximately 0.08–0.19 mM. In addition to its higher concentration, albumin appears to act as a depot or transport protein for many endogenous substances such as bilirubin and long chain fatty acids. However, it has a broad affinity for many chemicals including both therapeutic drugs and intoxicants. Although in common with many proteins albumin possesses many acidic and basic groups which no doubt take part in the binding of some compounds, the major binding takes place in association with hydrogen bonding and Van der Waal's forces as for chloro or nitro substituted phenols. It has particular affinity for lipophilic compounds and binds, for example, the non-ionic chlorinated pesticide dieldrin. For a review on the mechanism of binding of small molecules to albumin see Kragh-Hansen (1981).

Albumin is clearly important in sequestering intoxicants and by so doing reducing the effective (from a toxicological point of view) concentration of free agent in the circulation and in the cell water. Interaction with other plasma proteins may play a minor role. Binding to plasma proteins should not be confused with binding of exogenous substances to protein which has a specific physiological role in the transport of particular essential substances. Such binding may be significant in the initiation of toxicity and as such may be regarded as a target (see Chapter 7). A recent example is the interference of a hydroxy metabolite of 3,4,3',4'-tetrachlorobiphenyl with the retinol-binding proteins in rats (Brouwer *et al.*, 1988; see Chapter 13).

5.5.2 Haemoglobin

Haemoglobin is an abundant protein and is present in blood of mammalian species at approximately 15 g/100 ml, which is in molar terms 2.3 mM. Haemoglobin contains many groups or residues not directly involved in its physiological function as a carrier of oxygen to the tissues. These residues can and do react with toxicants; the determination of this bound intoxicant or the adduct formed by reaction of electrophilic chemicals with its nucleophilic residues are used for dose monitoring (see Chapter 11).

Two molecules of triethyltin or trimethyltin bind to one molecule of rat haemoglobin with an affinity constant of 3.5×10^4 M^{-1} (see Figure 3.2). The binding is to the α-subunits of the tetramer and involves a cysteine and histidine residue in a 5-coordinate combination (Table 5.2.; Rose & Aldridge, 1968; Elliott *et al.*, 1979; Taketa *et al.*, 1980). This combination has no effect on the spectral characteristics of haemoglobin and causes a minor increase in the affinity for oxygen which is not significant toxicologically. At doses which cause toxicity to the nervous system the binding sites of the α-subunits are only 12% and 5% saturated with trimethyltin and triethyltin respectively. However, 72% and 20% of trimethyltin and triethyltin respectively of the administered dose are bound to haemoglobin thus reducing the concentration available for toxicity to the nervous system. These observations also provide an example of unexpected species specificity since up to the present only rat and cat haemoglobin has been found to bind the trialkyltins in this way – human haemoglobin and that of other species do not. It seems that the capacity to bind these organotin compounds is a biological accident in that the relevant groups are in the correct positions in haemoglobin only of the rat and cat.

Mercurials have a strong affinity for sulphydryl groups. For both small and large molecules containing thiol groups the affinity for methylmercury can be as high as 10^{15}–10^{16} M^{-1}. Both haemoglobin and albumin possess free thiol groups and in the erythrocyte there are millimolar concentrations of glutathione. There will thus be competition between these different thiols based on their affinity constants. In Table 5.2 results are quoted showing that after ten daily doses of methylmercury 32% of the total dose can be recovered from the blood of the rat largely bound to haemoglobin – there is 22–159 times more methylmercury in red blood cells than in plasma. Thus binding of methylmercury to thiol containing macromolecules is significant in reducing methylmercury's concentration in the nervous system in both rats and humans. For a full discussion of the factors involved in the distribution of mercury and organomercurials see Gage (1964) and Magos (1981).

5.5.3 Ligandin (Glutathione S-transferase)

While it had long been known that various substances were bound to proteins present in the liver cell cytoplasm it was not until 1971 that it was shown that most of the binding was due to one protein which was then called ligandin (Litwack *et al.*, 1971; Tipping *et al.*, 1976). This protein, which is 4–5% of the total cell sap protein, binds a wide variety of lipophilic and anionic substances including bilirubin, oestradiol, bromosulphophthalein, methylcholanthrene and azodye carcinogens, and is present in fully developed amphibia, reptiles, birds and mammals including monkeys and humans. It is absent from gill-breathing invertebrates and is low in foetal liver of mammals but increases rapidly postpartum; it is also low in hepatoma. In kidney tubular cells and mucosal cells of the small intestine ligandin constitutes 2% of the soluble protein. Conjugates with glutathione are also bound to ligandin.

The protein has a molecular weight of 45,000–46,000, consists of two subunits of approximately 23,000 each and is a basic protein with an isoelectric point of about 9.1. Ligandin is now known to be the same protein as glutathione S-transferase, the enzyme

Table 5.2 The binding of trimethyltin, triethyltin and methylmercury to haemoglobin after administration to rats

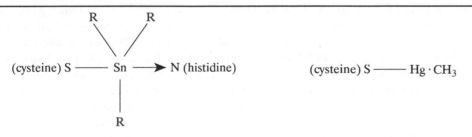

Compound	Triorganotin complex		Methylmercury complex	
	Dose (μmol/kg)	Blood (nmol/kg)	Saturation of binding sites (%)	Dose bound to haemoglobin (%)
Trimethyltin[a]	50	538	12	72
Triethyltin[a]	79	230	5	20
Methymercury[b]	50[c]	241	–	32

[a] Taken from Aldridge, 1992a.
[b] Taken from Friberg, 1959.
[c] Given as 10 daily doses of 5 μmol/kg body weight.

which catalyses the reaction of the thiol group of glutathione (GSH) with electrophilic substrates of a very wide range of structures (Habig *et al.*, 1974; Ketley *et al.*, 1975). The substrates which bind to ligandin also bind to glutathione S-transferase and in many cases inhibit the enzymic action of the enzyme (e.g. when the substrates are GSH and 1-chloro-2,4-dinitrobenzene) although kinetic studies have shown that the characteristics of the binding are not always as competitive as might be expected.

The GSH-S-transferases are a wide range of different isozymes consisting of dimers formed by reaction between six different subunits of around 23,000 molecular weight (see for discussion and nomenclature Jakoby, 1978; Jakoby *et al.*, 1984; Mannervik *et al.*, 1992). The ligands which bind to ligandin also bind to most of the transferases although usually with less affinity than with the most prevalent transferase (Fleischner *et al.*, 1972).

It has been suggested that ligandin/GSH-S-transferase(s) is a protein(s) with a dual function, one concerned with binding and cellular transport of many lipophilic substances and the other with the removal of electrophilic reagents by catalysing their reaction with the nucleophile GSH. Its intracellular binding function has been compared with that of extracellular albumin.

5.5.4 Metallothionein

The uptake of cadmium by animals and humans results in cadmium's accumulation in liver and kidney where it is bound to a soluble protein, metallothionein. This protein, first discovered in Vallee's laboratory (Margoshes & Vallee, 1957; Kagi & Vallee, 1960), has a molecular weight of 10,000–12,000, is probably a dimer, and has a structure well designed to bind metals; it contains 25–35% cysteine, 7–17% serine, 10–15% lysine and no tyrosine; in metallothionein from a few species an aromatic amino acid, phenylalanine, is present (Webb, 1979). Free thionein devoid of a metal does not seem to exist in liver, kidney and small intestine which are the major tissues containing this protein. After the administration of cadmium, thionein's synthesis is stimulated but the mechanism of the initiation of this biosynthesis is not clear. The stimulus may be the zinc displaced by cadmium from existing zinc metallothionein or some other zinc complex. There is a relatively high concentration of zinc and copper metallothionein in the neonate (Kagi *et al.*, 1974) which is consistent with the need for an effective buffer against the toxicity of zinc and copper while there is a need for these elements during active cell proliferation. Probably thionein has a physiological function concerned with the biologically essential elements zinc and copper; it is a fortunate accident that it combines with cadmium and mercuric mercury (Pulido *et al.*, 1966) and reduces their toxicity. Little or no toxicity is seen in cadmium contained in liver, but when the concentration of cadmium in kidney exceeds 200 μg/g tissue, damage to the kidney may be observed (see Chapter 12).

For a full review of the properties of the metallothioneins and the structure of the metal complexes consult Webb (1979) and Weser & Rupp (1979).

5.5.5 Adipose Tissue

Adipose tissue can provide a sink for a high concentration of lipophilic compounds (see section 5.1.1). The distribution of lipophilic toxicants is by simple partition and the maintenance of this concentration is dependent on a variety of factors. If the compound is highly lipophilic, rather insoluble in water and stable, i.e. slowly metabolised, then after a single dose the intoxicant distributes into adipose tissue and persists *in vivo*. Examples are DDT and the polyhalogenated biphenyls. Their persistence and ready partition into fat depots has been the means of passage via the food chain from one species to another.

Many intoxicants are lipophilic, e.g. pyrethroids, organophosphorus and carbamate pesticides, but high concentrations of these substances are not usually maintained in the fat depots. The main reason is probably a combination of the size of the partition coefficient (fat/water or fat/plasma) and the existence of systems capable of metabolising them to more water soluble and often less toxic compounds.

In recent years it has been generally accepted that the release of stable highly lipophilic compounds into the environment is undesirable even though there may be no known or no universally accepted untoward biological consequences of a wide distribution in the environment. These views are now incorporated into the development of new pesticides for agricultural use and the control of insect and other vectors of human and domestic animal diseases. An example of the need for care and vigilance is the widespread contamination of the environment by the polychlorinated biphenyls brought about by the careless disposal of the fluid in electrical transformers.

5.5.6 *Excretion*

It is often asserted that the major route of excretion of foreign toxic compounds of low volatility is the kidney. Other routes are via the bile, the lungs (for volatile compounds) and secretion into the gastro-intestinal tract or in fluids such as saliva, sweat, milk and semen. In fact the kidney often does not excrete the intoxicants but is the major route for the elimination of metabolites (see sections 5.5.7 and 5.5.8).

The kidney is a complex anatomical organ with additional functions unconnected with its excretory activity. Its primary physiological function is the excretion of waste while retaining important metabolic material. The functional unit is the nephron, a highly vascular structure including afferent and efferent arterioles associated with the glomerular and tubular elements. A substantial proportion of the cardiac output passes through the kidney and first reaches the cortex which contains the glomerulus and the proximal convoluted tubule of the nephron. The medulla contains the proximal straight tubule (pars recta), the descending and thin and thick ascending loop of Henle, the distal convoluted tubule and collecting ducts. The anatomical distribution of these various elements vary and some glomerular/tubular elements are almost entirely within the cortex while in others the loops of Henle run deep into the medulla. The filtration system of the nephron begins in the glomerulus, a relatively porous capillary, and is a selective filter of the plasma. Depending on the size and charge of the components of the plasma, certain material will move into the tubules which reabsorb the bulk of the filtrate and up to 99% of the salts and water moves back into the circulation. There is also virtually complete reabsorption of filtered sugars and amino acids. In contrast, waste materials such as urea arising from the degradation of purines and the ammonia released during protein catabolism is selectively eliminated. It also has other vital biological functions including production of hormones, e.g. erythropoietin (in erythrocyte formation), activation of vitamin D (in calcium metabolism), renin (in formation of aldosterone and angiotensin) and prostaglandins and kinins (in inflammatory processes). The kidney is thus physiologically an important organ in the maintenance of homeostasis and aspects of normal endogenous metabolism in animals and humans. For a discussion of the anatomy and function of the kidney see Brenner & Rector (1976), Gottschalk (1964) and Hook & Hewitt (1986).

The excretion of non-nutritious exogenous chemicals (mainly as metabolites) to which all mammals are continuously exposed in their diet takes place via the kidney. In normal circumstances such 'natural' exposure is far in excess of the minor exposures to synthetic chemicals, for example exposure via residues of pesticides in food and water. To give one example, brassica vegetables such as cabbage, brussel sprouts, swedes, turnips and cauliflower contain glucosinolates, derivatives of the reactive and potentially toxic isothiocyanates (Fenwick *et al.*, 1983; Sones *et al.*, 1984); The excretion of the primary exogenous chemicals will depend on their physicochemical characteristics and the dose. In most cases this is a minor component and the chemical is excreted as a non- or much less toxic and more water-soluble metabolite suitable for rapid elimination in the urine. Such metabolism is by enzymic systems usually divided into two classes, phases 1 and 2 discussed in the next section. While these processes are often efficient as detoxification systems, some metabolites are further metabolised (bioactivated; see Chapter 6) in the kidney to produce intoxicants for the kidney. Passage through the kidney of metals bound to circulating protein and in equilibrium with metal/small molecular weight thiols is a delivery system whereby the metal becomes attached to functional areas of the tubule (possibly via thiol groups).

The rate of clearance of exogenous chemicals is an important factor to be taken into account in risk assessment. This is done using suitably radiolabelled material with measurements at various times of the radioactivity in the urine, blood and other tissues. While this provides useful information for the purpose it is intended, for mechanistic purposes it is rarely enough. The chemical identity of the radioactively labelled material in the various biological materials is a prerequisite for understanding and for the derivation of meaningful dose–response relationships (see Chapter 9).

5.5.7 *The Enzymes and Chemistry of Detoxification*

Living organisms contain enzymic systems whose function is to convert food constituents into a source of carbon, nitrogen, sulphur, metals, etc. Other exogenous chemicals whose lipophilic properties allow absorption into the organism are also likely to be retained. There will be, without other interventions, a tendency to accumulate unwanted chemicals. Many higher organisms possess an array of enzymes with rather broad specificity capable of preventing such an accumulation; in evolutionary terms this is biologically very satisfactory.

Table 5.3 lists enzymes of detoxification which metabolise chemicals gaining entry into less toxic forms which ultimately results in the excretion of the less toxic and more water-soluble products. The pathway of metabolism prior to excretion may involve several enzymes in more than one tissue. For example, glutathione conjugates produced in the liver by glutathione S-transferase are degraded in the kidney sequentially by γ-glutamyltransferase, cysteinyl glycinase and N-acetyl transferase to yield mercapturic acids ready for excretion.

It is physiologically sound that liver and kidney are the most active tissues since the liver is often the first organ to receive the chemical, sometimes in high concentration, from the gastro-intestinal tract and the kidney is the exit route of water-soluble products

Table 5.3 Examples of enzymes of which detoxify some xenobiotics

Phase 1 enzymes	Phase 2 enzymes	Other enzymes
Flavin monooxygenases	Glutathione transferases	Alcohol dehydrogenase
P_{450} monoxygenases	UDP-glucuronyl transferases	Aldehyde dehydrogenase
Monoamine oxidase	Phenol sulphotransferase	Esterases and amidases
Aldehyde oxidase	Tyrosine-ester sulphotransferase	Rhodanese
Xanthine oxidase	Alcohol sulphotransferase	Glutathione peroxidase
Quinone reductase	Amine N-sulphotransferase	Catalase*
Carbonyl reductase	Cysteine conjugate N-acetyl	Superoxide dismutase*
Dihydrodiol dehydrogenase	transferase	
Epoxide hydrolase	Catechol O-methyltransferase	
	Amine N-methyltransferase	
	Thiol S-methyltransferase	
	Acetyltransacetylase	
	Organic acid CoA ligase*	
	/N-acyl transferase*	

Note: With the exception of those marked * the list of enzymes is taken from Jakoby and Ziegler, 1990.

produced from chemicals whatever was the route of entry. Other tissues – the small intestine, lung, skin, nose, oesophagus – contain some of these enzymes. These are all organs of first contact by the relevant route of exposure to exogenous chemicals. In contrast to the liver, which contains predominately one cell type, in the above tissues these enzymes are often located in particular cell types. Although, when compared with liver, the overall activity of the enzyme per unit weight of tissue may be low, the specific cellular activity can be as high and sometimes higher when calculated per unit weight of the cell containing it. However, hepatocytes are not uniform and contain different concentrations of various drug-processing enzymes dependent upon their position in the liver lobule.

Some chemicals, instead of being detoxified, are metabolised by the same enzymes to more toxic compounds (bioactivation; see Chapter 6). Such bioactivated metabolites may be further metabolised by 'detoxification' enzymes, their biological activity being reduced and their excretion enhanced. Whether toxicity is seen after a particular exposure or dose of compound depends on complex relationships between the rate of many competing and sequential enzyme-catalysed reactions. The rate at which most of these reactions take place is defined by constants K_m and V_{max} for each enzyme and each chemical. Since these enzymes act on a rather broad range of substrates there is much opportunity for competition between substrates and for inhibition by structural analogues (see Chapter 6 and Figure 2.2).

For convenience many of these enzymes are classified into two groups: phase 1 and phase 2. Phase 1 is enzymes which by an oxidative process add a hydroxyl group to lipophilic compounds thus making them more water-soluble. Other groups enhancing water solubility become available by the action of esterases and amidases and by the conversion of epoxides to diols by epoxide hydrase. The products of these reactions thus become available for conjugation by phase 2 enzymes when, via energy-requiring reactions, glucuronic acid, sulphate, methyl, acetyl and various amino acids are conjugated with functional groups in the intoxicant or the intoxicant modified by phase 1 reactions. Glutathione conjugates are also formed without a requirement for energy (see section

5.5.7). Table 5.3 lists enzymes which play a part in reducing toxicity. Some are easy to classify as phase 1 or phase 2 whereas others are not.

5.5.8 *The Detoxification of Electrophiles, Oxidants and Active Oxygen Metabolites*

The nucleophile glutathione is present in all mammalian cells often in concentrations approaching 1 mM and in many tissues glutathione S-transferases are present and catalyse reactions with electrophiles which are often a cause of intoxication following their reaction with, for example, the catalytic centres of enzymes and nucleic acids. Glutathione S-transferases exist as many isozymes (eight in rat liver; Jakoby *et al.*, 1984) and all have a broad specificity. The mechanism of catalysis requires a lipophilic substrate which binds to the enzyme thus bringing it into the correct orientation for reaction with an activated glutathione molecule attached to the catalytic centre. All substrates seem to react slowly non-enzymically but the rate is greatly enhanced by catalysis (Jakoby, 1978). Glutathione adducts are exported from liver and other cells, probably by specific energy-dependent transport systems, into the circulation on their way to the kidney where they are metabolised via the mercapturic acid pathway (see above) prior to excretion. Glutathione turnover is rapid, taking just over an hour in rat liver. Glutathione adduct formation is thus a powerful enzymic system for the detoxification of a continuous supply of potentially toxic electrophiles (Table 5.4; Meister & Anderson, 1983; Larsson *et al.*, 1983; Orrenius & Moldeus, 1984).

Glutathione is also a reducing agent and can be readily oxidised to the disulphide by many oxidants and by-products of oxidative metabolism such as organic hydroperoxides, hydrogen peroxide, superoxide, etc. Glutathione reductase with NADPH readily reduces the oxidised glutathione to the original thiol. Other enzymes such as catalase, superoxide dismutase and glutathione peroxidase also detoxify active oxygen species which may arise during the metabolism of xenobiotics, oxidation of lipids in peroxisomes and even in low concentration during normal oxidative metabolism. Figure 5.5 shows some of the relationships between these protective mechanisms and serves to illustrate the number and scope of catalytic mechanisms available.

Although glutathione plays an important role in detoxification, recent research has demonstrated that, following reaction with certain chemicals, new intoxicants are produced, i.e. reactions with glutathione can lead to bioactivation (see Chapter 6).

Table 5.4 Examples of catalysis of reactions of glutathione with xenobiotics by glutathione S-transferases

Reactant	Product
Alkyl halides	G–S -methyl
3,4-dichloro-1-nitrobenzene	G–S – in 4-position
Benzyl chloride	G–S – on side chain
Acrylamide	G–S – on C–3
Epoxides (–C–C–)	–C(OH)–C(SG)–
Methylisothiocyanate	CH₃NHC(S)–S–G
Trialkyl phosphorothioates	G–S -alkyl (from alkyl-*O*-)

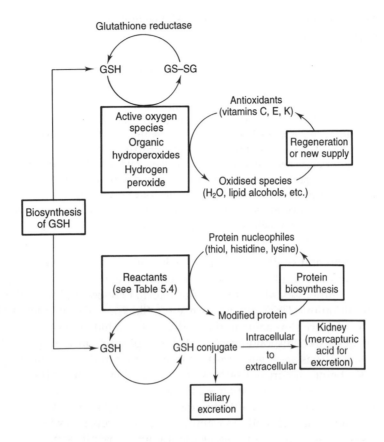

Figure 5.5   The role of glutathione and metabolic pathways involved in the protection of tissues against intoxication by electrophiles, oxidants and active oxygen species.

5.6   Discussion

The general principles of the processes which, following exposure to a chemical, influence their entry into the organism have been discussed. These are many and vary with the physicochemical properties of those chemicals soluble in lipid and water for rapid entry to those with a very low solubility in water and those soluble in water but completely ionised whose entry will be slow.

After entry there are many systems which can decrease the effective concentration of free intoxicant by binding to macromolecules and/or metabolism to less toxic and readily excreted metabolites. Mammals are well endowed with an array of enzymes capable of metabolising xenobiotics, whether they arise from natural constituents of foods, flavours and spices or from synthetic chemicals. These enzymes are usually specific in the reactions they catalyse (oxidation, reduction, group transfer, ester hydrolysis) but are effective on a wide range of substrates. As enzymes they are not particularly efficient, with rather low catalytic centre activity (CCA). Nevertheless the capacity of a cell to metabolise many xenobiotics is often considerable owing to the presence of a large amount of enzyme even though its CCA is low; its efficiency is further enhanced if it has a low Michaelis constant (K_m) so that at most exposures it is working at full capacity.

Mammals are therefore well organised to act as a remover of non-nutritious and potentially toxic material, as has recently been succinctly stated:

> Instead of the vast array of highly specific enzymes that are distributed among large numbers of bacteria, each capable of converting a small group of compounds to potentially useful metabolites, animals have evolved systems adapted for elimination, rather than utilisation, of toxic compounds. Each animal comes equipped with its own trash disposal system which includes a finely honed means of transport and excretion.
>
> ... the group [of enzymes of detoxification] has several related characteristics in common: the enzymes have a preference for lipophilic compounds although all polar compounds are not excluded; each has a phenomenally broad substrate range; and, as a group, they are relatively more concentrated at major points of entry to either the body (liver, lung, intestinal mucosa) or to a specific organ (the choroid plexus for the brain). Many also appear to be inducible ... (Jakoby & Ziegler, 1990)

Many experimental studies are with a single and/or at a relatively high exposure. Whether intoxication occurs depends on the relationship between the rate of entry and the sum of the processes which reduce the internal concentration of the intoxicant (binding, partition into lipids, metabolism, etc.). Skin provides an effective barrier so that rates of entry are slow compared with the oral or inhalation route and skin application toxicities are correspondingly low. As the exposure concentration is decreased, similar considerations apply with the the concentration of the relevant enzymes, their CCA and K_m being the crucial factors. With even lower concentration of reactive intoxicant the rate of reaction with macromolecules (even with the target responsible for initiating toxicity) can be an effective detoxification pathway. Whether it is detoxification or intoxication depends on whether the rate of reaction with macromolecule/target is less or more than its turnover (removal and biosynthesis).

These 'detoxification' pathways are similar in principle to the mechanisms utilised for the switching on and off of receptor–hormone interactions, e.g. cholinergic receptor–acetylcholine and the recently postulated mechanism of production and inactivation of the active epoxide leucotrienes and the unsaturated prostaglandins (West, 1990; Ishikawa, 1992).

The same systems with their broad substrate acceptance also metabolise chemicals, which because of their chemical structure, yield metabolites which are more not less toxic. This is the subject of Chapter 6.

5.7 Summary

1 Entry of intoxicants into the internal circulation after exposure is influenced by the physicochemical properties of the substance. Whatever is the route of exposure the rate of entry is facilitated for those chemicals which are soluble in both water and lipids.

2 The rate of entry of intoxicants varies with the different routes of exposure.

3 Nearly all forms of toxicity are selective (see Chapter 7): the term 'general toxicity' should be reserved for those substances which are so reactive and corrosive that they destroy all cells they contact.

4 Movement of small molecules across membranes can take place by passive

diffusion, filtration, facilitated diffusion, active transport, pinocytosis and phago-cytosis (particulates of low solubility). Passive diffusion and filtration are physical events governed by the concentration gradient across the membrane. Facilitated diffusion and active transport involve a carrier mechanism and have a maximum rate.

5   The concentration of the free (unbound and in solution in water) intoxicant may be limited by the extent of binding to macromolecules, distribution into lipids and enzymic detoxification.

6   Detoxification enzymes are usually classified as phase 1 (oxidative systems which add oxygen, esterases, epoxide hydrolase which render the intoxicant more water soluble) or phase 2 (conjugation to add groups which facilitate excretion). This clas-sification is becoming more difficult to sustain as knowledge increases.

7   Glutathione as a nucleophile is a biological reagent for reactive electrophiles and also, as a reductant, protects from the toxicity to oxidants or active oxygen species.

8   Detoxification enzymes have a broad substrate acceptance, are specific for the general reaction they catalyse, are mostly of low catalytic activity and may be present in large amount. They are thus well organised as a protective mechanism against the continual exposure and entry of non-nutritious substances in a normal diet. (Incidentally, they metabolise man-made synthetic chemicals if they 'fit' the broad substrate patterns of these enzyme systems.)

9   After high or low, single dose or continuous exposures, the circulating concen-tration of intoxicant (free) is determined by the relationship between the rate of entry, the extent of binding and the rate of detoxification determined by the K_m and V_{max} of the relevant enzymes.

10   For continuous exposure to low concentrations of most intoxicants, when the rate of reaction of the intoxicant with macromolecules (including initiating targets, see Chapter 7) is less than the macromolecules' turnover rate (removal and biosyn-thesis), then no intoxication will ensue.

11   Some natural and man-made chemicals are made more toxic rather than less by the 'detoxification' enzymes (see Chapter 6).

6

Delivery of Intoxicant

Bioactivation and increase in delivery to target

6.1   Introduction

In the previous chapter some of the factors contributing to the detoxification process were described and characterised by either converting the intoxicant to something less toxic or binding the chemical to macromolecules so as to reduce the concentration of free and effective agent. These events are beneficial to the organism and have led to

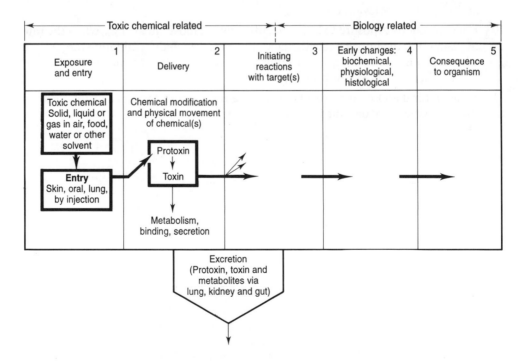

Figure 6.1   Bioactivation of absorbed chemicals and delivery of intoxicants to their site of action (Stages 1 and 2 from Figure 2.1; see legend.)

much philosophical discussion of the function of the enzymes involved. It is now clear that there are many examples where the action of enzymes leads to increase of toxicity (Figure 6.1). Among these are bioactivation when a substance is converted to a more toxic chemical and active transport increasing the concentration of an intoxicant in particular cells above the circulating concentration. For discussion of the 'rationality' of such events see 'Discussion', section 5.6.

Table 6.1   Examples of chemicals which have been shown to be bioactivated *in vivo*

Compound	Reactive pathway or intermediate	Toxicity	Ref.
2-Acetylaminofluorene	*N*-hydroxy-2-acetyl-aminofluorene: conjugates	Liver	1
Aflatoxin B$_1$	Aflatoxin-2,3-oxide	Liver	2
Allyl alcohol	Glycidol and acrolein	Liver	3
Benzene	Arene oxides	Bone marrow	4
Bromobenzene	Epoxides	Liver	4
Chlorinated aliphatic hydrocarbons	Various electrophilic species	Mutagens	5
Diethyl 4-nitrophenyl phosphorothionate	Diethyl 4-nitrophenyl phosphate	Nervous system	6
Dimethylnitrosamine	Carbonium ion $(CH_3)^+$	Liver	7
Fluoroacetate	Fluorocitrate	Heart, nervous system	8
Hexane: 6 carbon compounds	2,5-hexane diol	Nervous system	9
Hexachloro-1,3-butadiene	Reactive thiol from glutathione conjugate	Kidney	10
4-Ipomeanol	Furan ring oxidation	Lung	11
Methanol	Formaldehyde	Eye	12
Monocrotaline	Dihydromonocrotaline	Liver, lung	13
3,4,3',4'-Tetrachloro biphenyl	5-hydroxy derivative	Vitamin A metabolism	14
Tetraethyllead	Triethyllead	Nervous system	15
OSS-Trimethyl phosphorothioate	Unidentified	Lung	16
Tri 2-tolyl phosphate	Di 2-tolyl saligenin phosphate	Nervous system	17

References: (1) Hanna & Banks, 1985; (2) Swensen *et al.*, 1974; Martin & Garner, 1977; (3) Patel *et al.*, 1980; Reid, 1972; (4) Kaminsky, 1985; (5) Henschler, 1987; (6) Gage, 1953; Kamataki *et al.*, 1976; (7) Magee & Farber, 1962; Lijinsky *et al.*, 1968; (8) Peters, 1957; Peters & Wakelin, 1957; (9) DiVincenzo *et al.*, 1976; Spencer & Schaumberg, 1975; (10) Nash *et al.*, 1984; Jaffe *et al.*, 1983; (11) Minchin & Boyd, 1983; (12) Tephly, 1991; (13) Mattocks, 1986; Glowaz *et al.*, 1992; (14) Brouwer *et al.*, 1988; (15) Cremer, 1959; (16) Verschoyle & Aldridge, 1987; (17) Eto *et al.*, 1962.

6.2   Bioactivation

Bioactivation consists of those biological processes occurring *in vivo* which change the structure of a chemical in such a way as to increase its toxicity. In Table 6.1 are a few examples of chemical changes which are associated with enhanced toxicity. Most involve oxidation but there are other possibilities; we should keep an open mind that other systems can be utilised, e.g. the formation of glucuronides which are more biologically active than the original compounds (Mulder, 1992). Occasionally a substance may become activated by chemical changes taking place without the intervention of enzymes, e.g. the conversion of metrifonate into dichlorvos (see section 6.3.6). For full accounts of bioactivation systems see Gillette (1982) and Anders (1985).

6.3   Delivery of Bioactivated Intoxicants

All systems previously discussed which reduce the concentration of intoxicant are also active in detoxification of the bioactivated product. Depending on chemical reactivity, intoxication may take place at the cell site of bioactivation or at some distance in other cells or organs. The following examples illustrate the range of possibilities.

6.3.1   *Dimethylnitrosamine*

Dimethylnitrosamine is metabolised in the liver and causes liver necrosis. In the reaction mechanism one of the methyl groups is oxidised by the cytochrome P_{450} system to a monohydroxy derivative which rapidly loses formaldehyde to give an unstable monomethylnitrosamine which breaks down to a carbonium ion (Magee, 1956; Lijinsky *et al.*, 1968).

$$
\begin{array}{ccc}
CH_3 & HOCH_2 & \\
\diagdown & \diagdown & \\
N=N=O \xrightarrow{+0} & N=N=O \xrightarrow{-HCHO} [CH_3-NH=N=O] \longrightarrow [CH_3]^+ \\
\diagup & \diagup & \\
CH_3 & CH_3 &
\end{array}
$$

This is very chemically unstable and little escapes from the liver. Thus anything available in the cell becomes methylated – proteins, DNA, RNA (Magee & Farber, 1962). If the dose is high enough then the animal dies from chemical hepatectomy. An animal surviving a lower dose may eventually develop tumours in the liver (Magee & Barnes, 1956). Cytochrome P_{450} in the liver metabolises most of the dimethylnitrosamine but other tissues are active even though at a lower rate and capacity. If the activity of the cytochrome P_{450} system in rat liver is reduced by a low protein diet then a larger proportion of the dose is metabolised by the kidney than is the case in rats on a normal diet. Using this experimental protocol it is possible to organise experiments so that all the animals develop tumours in the kidney. This has provided a valuable experimental method for an extensive study by electron microscopy of the progression from initiation to the appearance of tumours (Hard & Butler, 1970a,b, 1971a,b,c; see also Chapter 8, section 8.9).

Since dimethylnitrosamine is bioactivated to a product that is so reactive that almost none escapes from the tissue where it was produced, if methylated residues in macromolecules are found in tissues then a bioactivation system must be present in that tissue.

6.3.2 Monocrotaline

Monocrotaline is a member of a large class of pyrolizidine alkaloids found in numerous plants (Figure 6.2). These alkaloids with an 1,2-unsaturated bond are hepatotoxic as a result of bioactivation in the liver. However, in addition to causing hepatotoxicity, monocrotaline is also toxic to the lung and causes pulmonary hyperplasia, pulmonary arterial hypertension and right ventricular atrophy in man. The pneumotoxicity of monocrotaline was recognised in early studies and the mechanism was suggested to originate with damage to the endothelium cells. The pyrolizidine alkaloids are unreactive with proteins and nucleic acids but, when administered to animals, adducts may be found and therefore they are bioactivated *in vivo*. Two particular problems remain for monocrotaline: (1) the identity of the reactive metabolite and (2) whether the metabolite is produced only in the liver or whether the lung makes a contribution (Mattocks, 1968, 1986; Smith & Culvenor, 1981; Huxstable, 1990; Plestina & Stoner, 1972).

Recent research has now established that when monocrotaline is added to a rat liver microsomal system dehydromonocrotaline (see Figure 6.2) is produced. Although this is rapidly hydrolysed in a few seconds to dehydroretronecine, it will react with a trapping agent such as thiosepharose and the expected products can be identified (Glowaz *et al.*, 1992; Mattocks *et al.*, 1990).

Since dehydromonocrotaline causes pneumotoxicity when added to the perfused rat lung it seems probable that this is the species responsible for the *in vivo* lung toxicity. Attempts to demonstrate bioactivation of monocrotaline by lung tissue have been unsuccessful. In this instance, therefore, bioactivation occurs in the liver, causing hepatotoxicity, but some of the bioactivated product is sufficiently stable to leave the liver and reach the lung causing damage to the endothelial cells in the first organ it reaches.

6.3.3 Tri 2-tolyl phosphate

During February 1930 an unusual disease began to appear in the mid- and southwestern USA. During the course of the epidemic around fifteen thousand cases were reported, the majority of which were adult males of average age 40. The signs and symp-

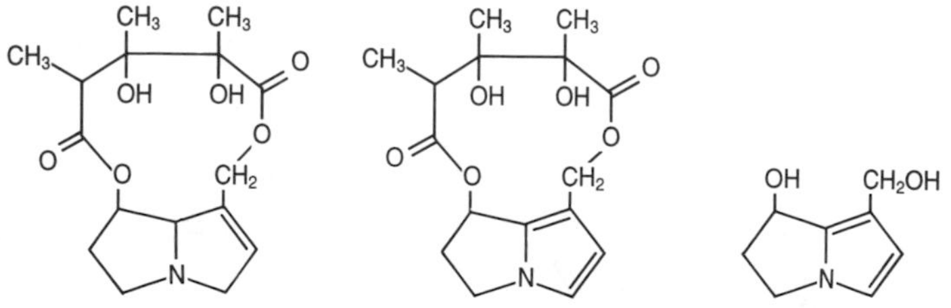

Figure 6.2 The chemical structures of (I) monocrotaline; (II) dehydromonocrotaline; (III) dehydroretronecine

toms of the disease were initial soreness in the muscles of the arms and legs and occasional numbness of the fingers and toes which progressed to a flaccid paralysis with no sensory disturbances. The neuropathy was first characterised as a primary demyelination but is now established as a primary axonopathy somewhat similar to Wallerian degeneration (after nerve section). The long nerves are most affected in both the central and peripheral nervous system; regeneration to the nerve's end-organ occurs in peripheral but not central nerves. In this epidemic there was much involvement of the central nervous system since recovery was slight and many were permanently disabled (Smith & Elvove, 1930; Smith *et al.*, 1930; Lillie & Smith, 1932; Bouldin & Cavanagh, 1979a,b).

It was quickly established that this was a disability caused by poisoning and not an infection; a strong correlation was found between those affected and their consumption of a USP fluid extract of ginger purchased from local dealers. Such potions were much in demand at this time of prohibition in the USA. In a series of outstanding and now classical papers it was described how, by the use of animal bioassay procedures (the chicken was found to be the best species) alongside chemical separation methods, it was established that the ginger extracts contained triaryl phosphates (see Figure 6.3) with a proportion of the aryl groups *o*-cresyl (sometimes called *o*- or 2-tolyl). A typical analysis was USP extract of ginger 3.3%, tricresyl phosphates 2.7% and alcohol 85.5% (Smith & Elvove, 1930; Smith *et al.*, 1932).

Although it was established beyond doubt that the disease was caused by the consumption of tri *o*-cresyl phosphate and it could be reproduced in the chicken, the mechanism of the disease remained unknown until much later. The main problem was that this compound is not very reactive and, when pure, is not an *in vitro* inhibitor of esterases. However, if pure material was administered to rats, rabbits or chickens, substantial inhibition of plasma cholinesterases occurred thus indicating a real possibility that a metabolite of tri *o*-cresyl phosphate was the active agent. Other research has now shown that tri *o*-cresyl phosphate is bioactivated to mono *o*-cresyl saligen phosphate which causes the disease in much smaller doses when administered to chickens.

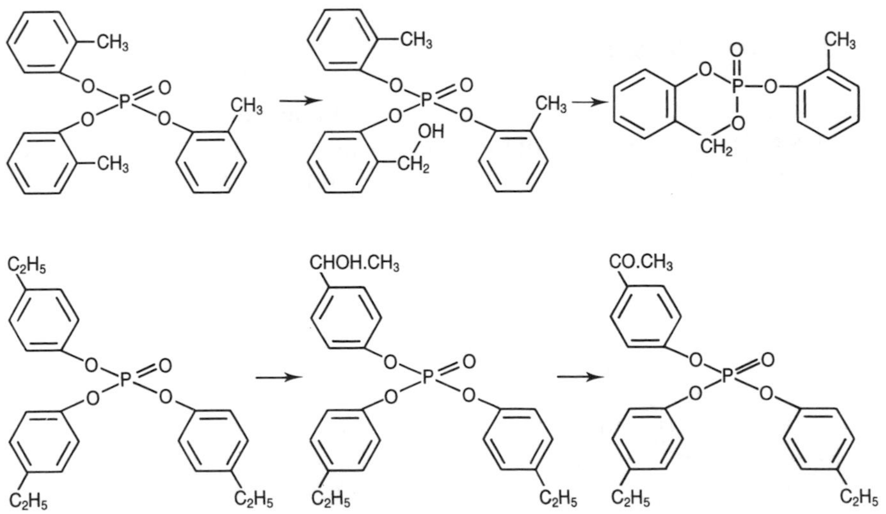

Figure 6.3 The route of oxidative metabolism of tri *o*-cresyl phosphate and tri 4-ethylphenyl phosphate

This metabolism by the liver cytochrome P_{450} system consists of oxidation of the methyl group of one *o*-cresyl group followed by an intramolecular rearrangement with loss of another *o*-cresyl group thus forming the saligenin phosphate (see Figure 6.3; Aldridge, 1954; Eto *et al.*, 1962).

Other aryl phosphates cause this disease which is now called delayed neuropathy because there is always a delay of 10–20 days before signs or symptoms appear. Compounds with ortho or 2- substituents on the ring are bioactivated by the above mechanism, e.g. tri *o*-ethylphenyl phosphate. However, although tri *p*-cresyl phosphate has no such biological activity tri *p*-ethylphenyl phosphate does. This is bioactivated to an active esterase inhibitor by oxidation of the *p*-ethyl group to a methyl keto group (see Figure 6.4). If an organophosphorus compound causes delayed neuropathy in chickens or other species and does not inhibit esterases *in vitro* then it may be concluded that it is bioactivated *in vivo* (Aldridge & Barnes, 1961; Eto *et al.*, 1971).

For discussion of the mechanism of initiation of delayed neuropathy see Chapter 7, section 7.6.

6.3.4 Tetraethyllead

Many fatal cases of tetraethyllead poisoning have been reported. The signs and symptoms indicate neurological involvement and include headache, irritability, hypoactivity, confusion, impairment of memory, ataxia, nystagmus and tremor. Although the physical properties of tetraethyllead are such as to promote absorption by any route and rapid penetration of the nervous system, tetraethyllead's chemical structure does not suggest that it would interact in a specific way with macromolecules. Tetraethyllead is converted *in vivo* into triethyllead and this stable metabolite causes the same clinical pattern of poisoning as tetraethyllead. Metabolism takes place in the liver by an oxidative reaction catalysed by a cytochrome P_{450} system and the product is transported via

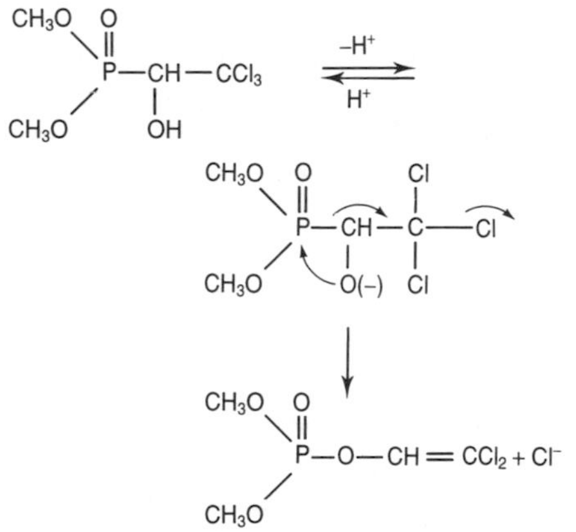

Figure 6.4 Pathway of the non-enzymic conversion of metrifonate to dichlorvos. The chemical structures of metrifonate and dichlorvos are O,O-dimethyl 2,2,2-trichloro-1-hydroxyethylphosphonate and O,O-dimethyl 2,2-dichlorovinyl phosphate respectively. (*Source*: reaction mechanism taken from Hofer, 1981)

the circulation to the brain as lipophilic hydroxide or chloride. Following oxidative attack on one ethyl group the proportion of the two products, ethanol and ethylene, depends on the extent of attack on the α and β carbons respectively (Fish *et al.*, 1976a).

$$(CH_3CH_2)_4Pb–(CH_3CH_2)_3Pb^+ + [CH_2 = CH_2/CH_3CH_2OH]$$

Triethyllead is also converted by successive dealkylation into di- and monoethyllead but the rates are slower than for the loss of the first ethyl group; neither of the lower metabolites are toxic to the nervous system (Cremer & Callaway, 1961; Casida *et al.*, 1971; Bridges *et al.*, 1967; Aldridge & Brown, 1988).

The same oxidative reactions remove the alkyl groups from tetraethyltin. Oxidation of longer chain alkyl groups may yield stable compounds with hydroxy or keto groups in the alkyl chain (Cremer, 1958; Kimmel *et al.*, 1976; Fish *et al.*, 1976a,b).

The mechanism of the toxicity of the trialkyltin and -lead compounds is discussed in Chapter 7, section 7.12.

6.3.5 *Hexachloro-1,3-butadiene*

Hexachloro-1,3-butadiene is a liquid at room temperature and is a by-product of the chlorination of hydrocarbons to produce useful solvents. It is nephrotoxic to rats; damage occurs in the straight portion of the proximal tubule which is involved with the organic anion transport system. Early evidence for damage can be detected by an examination of slices of renal cortex from rats 24 hours after dosing; they accumulate *p*-aminohippurate much slower than control slices, while accumulation of tetraethylammonium ion is unaffected. If hexachloro-1,3-butadiene was added *in vitro* to slices from control rats, no changes in either *p*-aminohippurate or tetraethylammonium ion uptake were seen even when concentrations as high as 0.1 mM were used (see Table 6.2; Lock & Ishmael, 1979).

These findings suggest that bioactivation of hexachloro-1,3-butadiene may be taking place but prior administration to rats of substances which induce or inhibit the activity

Table 6.2 The accumulation of *p*-aminohippuric acid (PAH) and tetraethylammonium (TEA) by rat renal cortical slices in the presence of hexachloro-1,3-butadiene (HCBD) added *in vitro* and by slices taken from rats dosed *in vivo*

Addition or treatment	Accumulation[a] (slice/medium ratio)	
	PAH	TEA
Control	7.37 ± 0.22	20.1 ± 0.7
HCBD *in vitro*: 0.1 mM	7.32 ± 0.31	21.8 ± 2.8
0.01 mM	6.31 ± 0.47	26.0 ± 2.8
HCBD *in vivo*: 200 mg/kg	$3.46^b \pm 0.35$	17.0 ± 1.2
100 mg/kg	$4.85^b \pm 0.38$	23.0 ± 3.2
50 mg/kg	$4.93^b \pm 0.35$	17.6 ± 1.1
25 mg/kg	6.27 ± 0.32	20.3 ± 1.2

[a] Mean $\pm$ standard error.
[b] Result is significantly different from control ($p < 0.05$).
Source: Data from Lock & Ishmael, 1979.

of cytochrome P_{450} monooxygenase systems failed to influence the susceptibility of the kidney to hexachloro-1,3-butadiene. Glutathione administered in excess of the hexachloro-1,3-butadiene had no influence on the damage to the kidney but the reduction of tissue content of non-protein sulphydryl markedly potentiated such damage (Hook *et al.*, 1982; Berndt & Mehendale, 1979).

This confusing situation has been resolved by the finding that the cysteine derivative (CyS-[1,1,2,3,4-pentachloro-1,3-butadiene]) is nephrotoxic. The current view is that the parent hexachloro-1,3-butadiene is converted in the liver to a glutathione adduct which leaves the liver and reaches the kidney where it is converted by the normal pathways to the mercapturic acid derivative and then by the action of an enzyme β-lyase is cleaved to form a reactive intermediate containing sulphur and the chlorinated moiety (Nash *et al.*, 1984; Jaffe *et al.*, 1983; Elfarra & Anders, 1984; Dekant *et al.*, 1988).

The bioactivation pathway of hexachloro-1,3-butadiene involves several steps and enzyme systems in several organs. Reviews on the enzymology and biological function of β-lyase are available (Dekant *et al.*, 1992; Cooper & Anders, 1990).

6.3.6 *Metrifonate*

Metrifonate is an organophosphorus compound which has been extensively used for the treatment of *Schistosoma haematobium* infections in humans and two World Health Organization trials have been carried out (Davis & Bailey, 1969; Plestina *et al.*, 1972; Holmstedt *et al.*, 1978).

Metrifonate is a phosphonate which rearranges to the phosphate, dichlorvos, a well-known insecticide and a direct inhibitor of acetylcholinesterase (Figure 6.4). The best evidence (Reiner *et al.*, 1975) for activation is that pure metrifonate is not an inhibitor and that all of the inhibition of cholinesterase is due to another compound produced from it. Direct chemical proof was provided when it was shown using gas chromatography and mass fragmentation methods that equitoxic doses to mice of dichlorvos and metrifonate lead to similar concentrations in the blood (Nordgren *et al.*, 1978). As shown in Figure 6.4 the production of dichlorvos from metrifonate is a chemical reaction influenced by the composition of the medium (e.g. pH) but not catalysed by an enzyme (i.e. activated but not bioactivated).

6.4 Cytochrome P_{450}s

From the description of the oxidative activities involved in detoxification and bioactivation it is clear that the mixed function oxidases play a decisive role in the expression of toxicity and can influence markedly our appreciation and interpretation of dose–response and structure–activity relationships.

The haemoproteins, the cytochrome P_{450}s, probably exist in all living organisms and have been found in bacteria, yeast, plants, insects, fish and mammals. They are distributed within mammalian cells associated with subcellular organelles – nuclear envelope, mitochondria and reticular endothelium (microsomal fraction) – and are identified by the formation of a complex with carbon monoxide with an absorption maximum at 450 nm.

The mixed function oxidases function in a cyclical reaction in which after the substrate becomes attached to the Fe^{3+} form which is then reduced via the NADPH reductase to the Fe^{2+} form. An oxygen molecule combines at this point, followed by further reduction utilising NADPH (and less efficiently NADH) to yield a highly reactive oxygen species which attacks the substrate, inserting an oxygen atom while the the other atom is reduced to water with the regeneration of the Fe^{3+} haemoprotein (Figure 6.5).

The haem of the cytochromes is synthesised by a pathway beginning with succinyl-CoA and glycine to form aminolaevulinic acid (ALA synthetase). Two molecules of ALA combine to form porphobilinogen. Four molecules of porphobilinogen condense and successively form uroporphyrinogen I, uroporphyrinogen III, coproporphyrinogen III, protoporphyrinogen, protoporphyrin and, with the insertion of the iron atom, protohaem. The last step is the attachment of the protohaem to the different apoproteins. In liver the first and last steps from ALA and protohaem are located within the mitochondria while the rest take place in the cell sap or, for the final attachment to the apoprotein perhaps, in the peroxisomes. This somewhat complicated biosynthetic pathway is subject to control by feedback mechanisms in which the inhibition of the first step, ALA synthetase by soluble haem, is a major mechanism. All the steps are potentially susceptible to inhibitors but the first and last step haems are particularly susceptible to metals. Other xenobiotics such as phenobarbitone and polychlorinated biphenyls stimulate the synthesis of cytochromes in the liver and other organs.

The classification of these enzymes was based on substrate specificity which was apparently very broad. However, in recent years the isolation and purification of the known xenobiotic metabolising cytochrome P_{450}s has become possible; their characterisation by cDNA cloning techniques and sequencing has and is allowing them to be sorted into families and subfamilies. The situation is proving to be very complex: for

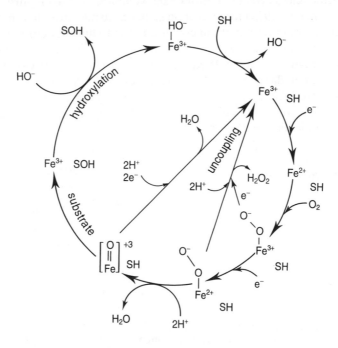

Figure 6.5 The reaction cycle of the cytochrome P_{450} enzyme systems. SH and SOH represent substrate and oxidised substrate. The uncoupling reaction, producing hydrogen peroxide/ 'excess water', competes with substrate hydroxylation. (*Source*: Raag & Poulos, 1991)

example, at least nineteen forms of human xenobiotic metabolising cytochrome P_{450}s have been identified, each with a distinct though overlapping substrate specificity (Gonzalez, 1992). Analysis of substrate specificities and expression of human P_{450}s has revealed differences from the rodent enzymes.

With the new techniques available the presence of xenobiotic metabolising cytochrome P_{450}s in many different tissues is being established (e.g. nasal tissue, Dahl & Hadley, 1991; Kaminsky & Fasco, 1992; nervous tissue, Mesnil *et al.*, 1985: Friedberg *et al.*, 1990; Volk *et al.*, 1991; Minn *et al.*, 1991). It is to be expected that these cytochromes will be found in particular cell types within an organ which may be expressed by exposure to different xenobiotics. The importance of these developments cannot be overemphasised, for instance in providing rational explanations of species differences in the response to intoxicants (extent and capacity). High-risk individuals may also be identified, e.g. those susceptible to lung cancer as a result of smoking tobacco (McLemore *et al.*, 1990; Shimada *et al.*, 1992; Bartsch *et al.*, 1992; see also Chapter 11). It must not, however, be assumed that the P_{450} cytochromes are the only enzymes capable of oxidising xenobiotics; xanthine oxidase (Zeigler, 1993), catalase and prostaglandin H synthase (Eling *et al.*, 1990) are among those implicated.

In addition to those P_{450}s active in oxidising exogenous chemicals there are others concerned with the oxidation of the endogenous steroids (Table 6.3). This is a fast-moving field and further discussion is beyond the scope of this book. It is a huge task to evaluate their distribution in cells within organs, their substrate specificity and inducibility across species. The results as they emerge will be important in the design of drugs (Cholerton *et al.*, 1992); i.e. in designing out undesirable properties of chemicals, selection of human populations with differing abilities in xenobiotic metabolism and extrapolation from animals to the human situation. The old concept of enzymes with very wide substrate specificity may require qualification and it may be possible more easily to modify the structure of chemicals so that they are more or less attacked by a particular isozyme.

The following reviews provide the background and give a perspective of this rapidly

Table 6.3   Mammalian cytochrome P_{450} families

P_{450}	No. of subfamilies	No. of forms	Reactions
CYP1	1	2	Xenobiotic metabolism
CYP2	8	57	Xenobiotic and steroid metabolism
CYP3	2	10[a]	Xenobiotic and steroid metabolism
CYP4	2	10[b]	Fatty acid ω and ω-1 hydroxylations
CYP7	1	1	Cholesterol 7α-hydroxylase
CYP11	2	3	Steroid 11β-hydroxylase
CYP17	1	1	Steroid 17β-hydroxylase
CYP19	1	1	Aromatase
CYP21	1	1	Steroid 21-hydroxylase
CYP27	1	1	Cholesterol 27-hydroxylase

[a] This is the total number of P_{450}s in the CYP3 family identified in rat, mouse, rabbit, hamster, dog and human, excluding five known pseudogenes.
[b] This is the total number of P_{450}s in this family identified in rat, rabbit, monkey, hamster and human.
Source: Gonzalez, 1992. For an update see Nelson *et al.*, 1993.

moving field: Gonzalez, 1989, 1992; Ioannides & Parke, 1990; De Matteis & Aldridge, 1978; Porter & Coon, 1991; Guengerich, 1990, 1991; Raag & Poulos, 1991; Lindamood, 1991; Nelson *et al.*, 1993; Gibson & Skett, 1994.

6.5 Active Transport of Intoxicants

Sometimes a rational explanation of toxicity selective to a particular organ is that the concentration of intoxicant is higher than in other tissues. This view contrasts to another hypothesis that a particular vulnerability of a cell within an organ is due to its function or biochemical make-up. Two examples of biological systems increasing the concentration of intoxicants in particular organs and/or cells are given below.

6.5.1 *Paraquat*

Two bipyridylium herbicides, paraquat (1,1'-dimethyl-4,4'-bipyridilium) and diquat (1,1'-ethylene-2,2'-bipyridilium), are toxic to mammals but not to the same organ. Paraquat causes damage to the lung and kidney, and animals and humans die due to respiratory insufficiency; many species present a similar pathology (Clark *et al.*, 1966). Diquat, in contrast, produces little or no change in the lung but causes necrosis in the proximal convoluted tubule of the kidney. After administration of the same amount of paraquat or diquat to rats, the concentration of paraquat rises in the lung and kidney and of diquat in the kidney only. In these experiments (Rose *et al.*, 1976) the concen-

Table 6.4 The concentration of paraquat and diquat in rat tissues after the oral administration of 680 μmol/kg body weight

Compounds and tissues	Hours after dosing			
	2	4	18	30
	(nmol/g tissue)			
Paraquat				
Brain	7	1	1	3
Lung	16	17	30	87
Liver	21	9	12	20
Kidney	75	55	58	108
Adrenal glands	13	30	16	26
Muscle	5	5	5	11
Plasma	14	7	8	14
Diquat				
Brain	1	1	1	1
Lung	4	6	6	6
Liver	6	8	14	10
Kidney	24	59	48	54
Adrenal glands	7	14	13	16
Muscle	1	3	2	5
Plasma	5	5	6	7

Source: Data taken from Rose *et al.*, 1976.

tration of paraquat in the lung 30 hours after dosing was 15 times that of diquat (Table 6.4).

Rat lung slices when incubated *in vitro* accumulate paraquat continuously. Over a period of 2 hours the ratio (slice/medium) increased with paraquat from 0.5 to 8.0, whereas with diquat it stayed within 0.5 and 0.8. The uptake of paraquat was prevented by a mixture of metabolic inhibitors, a low temperature and under nitrogen (Rose *et al.*, 1974). The kinetic constants for uptake indicate a K_m of 80 μM and a V_{max} of 300 nmol/g.tissue/h. (Figure 6.6). Paraquat within the lung is not bound and seems to be in solution within the tissue. For slices of other tissues (kidney cortex, skeletal muscle, liver, skin, heart, spleen and brain cortex) the rate of uptake was always less than 10% of the rate for lung slices.

When an energy-dependent system is demonstrated for an exogenous chemical the question should always be asked whether it is a system normally used for the transport of endogenous substances. From experiments showing that a variety of diamines and polyamines inhibited the uptake of paraquat, competition between putrescine and paraquat and direct measurements of the uptake of putrescine, it was concluded that paraquat and putrescine are taken up by rat lung by the same system. The kinetic constants for the uptake of putrescine are K_m 7 μM and V_{max} 300 nmol/g.tissue/h, i.e. concentrations of paraquat (K_m = 80 μM) ten times higher than putrescine are required to give the same rate of uptake (Smith & Wyatt, 1981).

The reason that paraquat selectively damages the lung is that the chemical utilises an energy-dependent system normally involved in diamine and/or polyamine uptake; concentrations of paraquat in lung increase with time and are many times those in plasma and other tissues. The high concentrations achieved *in vivo* and in the *in vitro* slice experiments are average concentrations in the whole tissue. However, the damage is not uniform in all cells and the morphological changes begin in the types 1 and 2

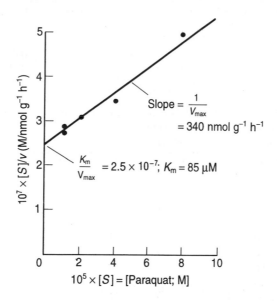

Figure 6.6 Evidence for a carrier-mediated uptake of paraquat into rat lung slices. The results presented have been recalculated from Rose *et al.*, 1974. The experiments were carried out at 37°C

epithelial cells. It is now known that these cells possess the transport system for both paraquat and putrescine. Since these cells are a small proportion of the total lung cell population the concentration of paraquat in these cells will be correspondingly higher.

Thus paraquat has a chemical similarity to diamines/polyamines which is paralleled by a biological similarity in their affinity for a carrier in a transport system for di- and polyamines in particular cells in the lung. These similarities ensure that paraquat, a substance which is toxic to many mammals, is concentrated in these cells thus initiating intoxication leading to cell death, lung dysfunction and death of the organism (see Chapter 7, section 7.4).

6.5.2 Beryllium

The intravenous injection of soluble beryllium salts into several species of animal results in a preferential concentration of beryllium in the liver and to a lesser extent in the spleen (Table 6.5), and within 3–4 days death due to liver necrosis. The concentration of beryllium in the liver follows the formation in blood of insoluble colloidal beryllium

Table 6.5 The distribution in tissues of the rat and the relationship between dose and the amount in the liver after intravenous injection of soluble beryllium salts

Intravenous dose of 83 μmol/kg body weight to 200 g rats

Time after injection (h)	Beryllium (μmol/g. tissue)[a]			
	Blood	Liver	Spleen	Kidney
Immediately	1.0	0.14	0.04	0.12
2	0.79	0.20	0.15	0.08
4	0.61	0.32	0.21	0.12
8	0.29	0.52	0.37	0.09
12	0.25	0.70	0.32	0.09
24	0.04	1.02	0.33	0.07

Beryllium in liver at 24 h after different doses

Dose (μmol/kg)	Beryllium in liver (% of dose)
111	25–33
83	32–50
49	40–52
28	29–30
7	24–32
1.74	5–6
0.84	2.5–10
0.084	2–3

[a] At 4 h and 24 h, 20% and 50%, respectively, of the dose was in the liver. At 24 h the heart, lung, brain, duodenum and skeletal muscle contained less than 0.08 μmol/g. tissue
Source: Both sets of data are taken from Witschi and Aldridge, 1968.

phosphate which circulates and is subsequently taken up by the reticulo-endothelial system in the liver (Kupffer cells) and spleen. Beryllium stays in the liver and cannot be removed by perfusion *in vitro*. The proportion of the administered dose in the liver is dependent upon the dose (Table 6.5). The availability of carrier free-emitting [^{7}Be] has allowed the concentration of beryllium to be measured down to very low doses. Doses of 7–110 μmol/kg result in approximately 30% of the dose being found in the liver. Below and down to 0.08 μmol/kg much less beryllium is found. It seems probable that this is due to little or no particulate beryllium phosphate being formed, the beryllium circulating as a soluble complex probably with an organic acid.

The presence of beryllium in the Kupffer cells has been shown histologically by a histochemical method for beryllium (Cheng, 1956), by a reduced phagocytic function (ability to remove injected colloidal carbon from the blood) of the liver (Stoner, 1961) and directly by separation of the different cell types in the liver (Skilleter & Price, 1978). A slow migration of beryllium from the Kupffer cells to the parenchymal cells takes place and the beryllium is taken up by the lysosomes and nuclei. The mechanism of cell necrosis by beryllium is not known; it seems possible that it may interfere with calcium distribution and/or function resulting in an activation of endonuclease as in programmed cell death (see Chapter 7, sections 7.11 and 7.13).

After inhalation of insoluble or slightly soluble particulate material, uptake by phagocytic cells ensure that depots of toxic material remain in the lung for a long time.

6.6   Biliary Excretion and Enterohepatic Circulation

Many substances appear in the bile and the main factors which influence such excretion are molecular weight, charge and species of animal. The molecular weight below which substances are almost excluded from the bile varies with species and is approximately 325 for the rat up to 500 for humans. The substances excreted include a wide range of properties and can be bases, acids and some neutral compounds but the system is geared to large ionised compounds. Conjugates such as glucuronides and particularly glutathione derivatives are good substrates for this excretion system which is a carrier system requiring energy.

There is no doubt that removal of an intoxicant from the internal circulation via the biliary system is an excretory process, for bile duct ligation or canulation increases toxicity. However, in some cases the intoxicant, e.g. methylmercury, which is excreted in the bile bound to thiol-containing compounds (probably glutathione), is reabsorbed from the gastro-intestinal tract thus prolonging its stay in the animal. In others, e.g. hexachloro-1,3-butadiene, nephrotoxicity is prevented by bile duct ligation. The mechanism involves the formation of the glutathione conjugate in the liver, the conjugate's almost exclusive excretion via the bile, breakdown in the bile canuliculi and in the gastrointestinal tract by pancreatic secretions and the intestinal flora and reabsorption of the cysteine derivative followed by acetylation to the mercapturic acid which is then taken up by the kidney (see section 6.3.5).

Thus excretion into the bile may increase toxicity, decrease toxicity or, even though it occurs, make little change or increase the residence time of an intoxicant. The following reviews on the physiology of bile formation and its influence on the disposition of xenobiotics are available: Klaassen *et al.* (1981); Klaassen & Watkins (1984). For the metabolic capabilities of the gut microflora consult Scheline (1980) and Rowland *et al.* (1985).

6.7 Methods to Establish if *In Vivo* Bioactivation Occurs

It is often difficult to decide if a chemical to which an organism is exposed is the chemical which is causing the toxicity, i.e. whether it is bioactivated. Sometimes bioactivation converts one toxic substance to another, e.g. phenylmercury has the lipophilic properties to penetrate the brain and cause neurotoxicity but because it is converted rather rapidly to inorganic mercury the predominant lesion is in the kidney (Gage, 1964). When the mechanism of toxicity is established or even if only some of the effects *in vivo* are defined it is relatively easy to devise comparative techniques to establish that others are being bioactivated.

Knowledge of bioactivation mechanisms allow informed judgements if bioactivation of a particular class of chemicals will take place. For example, there was much argument whether tetraethyllead is biologically active or has to be converted to the proximal intoxicant, triethyllead. Experiments to establish the truth of the latter were initially set up because the same neurological lesion was produced by the tetra- and triethyltin species and it seemed likely from the chemistry of the tetra compound that it would be biologically inactive. It is now known that pure tetra-methyl and -ethylleads and tins are biologically inert and intoxication only occurs after they are metabolised *in vivo* to the tri- species. First, judgement whether bioactivation might be occurring is a very tentative hypothesis whether the compound administered is likely to be directly active.

Many bioactivation mechanisms yield electrophilic species which react with nucleophiles such as bases in nucleic acids (adducts of RNA and DNA), thiol, histidine and lysine in proteins, the thiol of glutathione or sometimes inhibit the activity of enzymes. Thus, if after a compound is administered to an animal symptoms expected from acetylcholinesterase inhibition appear and erythrocyte acetylcholinesterase is depressed, but *in vitro* red cell cholinesterase is not affected, then bioactivation has taken place.

Even though the target for the initiation of toxicity is known to be acetylcholinesterase, decisions on whether bioactivation has taken place can be made by a comparison of inhibition of other esterases not directly involved in the toxicity, e.g. plasma cholinesterase or plasma or liver carboxylesterase. It is now known that organophosphorus pesticides containing the phosphorothionate group ($P = S$) are inert and that toxicity is due to conversion to the $P = O$ species. Similar considerations apply to other reactions *in vivo*. For example, liver glutathione may be depressed *in vivo* but the compound to which the animal has been exposed does not react with glutathione *in vitro*. When radiolabelled compounds are available it can be shown that after administration the radiolabelled compound is bound to proteins and nucleic acids, i.e. bound in the sense that it cannot be removed by denaturation by protein precipitating agents such as trichloracetic acid followed by further extraction with solvents to remove lipids. If the compound does not produce labelled protein or nucleic acid when incubated *in vitro* then the compound has been bioactivated to an electrophilic species *in vivo*.

The activity of the cytochrome P_{450} xenobiotic metabolising systems may be manipulated by the administration of other substances prior to or at the same time as the chemical being investigated. Phenobarbitone increases the activity of one family and methylcholanthrene or polychlorinated biphenyls another. If toxicity of a chemical is increased by these procedures then it is likely that the chemical is bioactivated. If toxicity decreases then detoxification pathways have been induced. Since other metabolising systems are also affected by these treatments, interpretation may be uncertain and especially so when the toxicity does not occur in the main metabolising organ. Other treatments such as by piperonylbutoxide or trimethyl phosphorothionate decrease the activity of P_{450} cytochrome systems; decrease of the toxicity of a chemical after such treatments leads to the hypothesis that the chemical may be bioactivated in untreated animals.

Experiments can also be done with the range of subcellular fractions, isolated cells, tissue slices and perfused organs where binding to macromolecules, preferably using radiolabelled intoxicant, may be shown to be decreased either by inhibitors of the metabolising systems added *in vitro* or, in the case of isolated microsomal fractions, by the omission of the essential cofactor NADPH, or may be shown to be changed when the tissues or cells have been taken from animals pretreated in various ways. In all of these studies it is essential to work with chemically pure intoxicants but it is especially important for *in vitro* studies. It is quite common for intoxicants to contain small amounts of highly active impurities.

The ultimate proof is the isolation of the metabolite, its chemical identification, synthesis and the demonstration that its administration to animals causes, often at a lower dose, the same form of toxicity. This is an ideal situation but often the species produced is so reactive that it cannot be isolated for identification. In these cases special methods may be devised to trap the reagent by binding to an added nucleophile (in the *in vitro* situation) or the intoxicant has to be postulated from the identification of the products of its reaction with macromolecules *in vivo*.

The above summary of ways to establish that an intoxicant is bioactivated may be compared with the examples discussed in section 6.3. A furthur example is the production of lung damage produced by trimethyl- and triethyl phosphorothiates. Although the bioactivated species has not been identified it has been concluded that these compounds are not directly toxic to the lung but require to be bioactivated probably in the lung itself; the liver appears to be mainly a means of detoxification (Aldridge *et al.*, 1987; Nemery & Aldridge, 1988a,b).

6.8 Discussion

The many reactions discussed in Chapter 5 and 6 influence the delivery of the intoxicant to which the organism has been exposed or of the bioactivated species to its site of action. Some reactions decrease the concentration of circulating free intoxicant by partition, binding or by modifying its chemistry to make it less toxic. Other reactions increase the concentration of intoxicant by their transport into particular cell types or toxicity is increased by metabolism to more active species. Sometimes one intoxicant is metabolised into another and the distribution of the damage is changed. Sometimes the bioactivated species is so reactive that all the damage occurs in the cell or organ where the metabolism takes place, but with more stable metabolites damage may occur in other organs.

Whatever philosophical view is held about the evolutionary reason or physiological basis for the enzymes which metabolise xenobiotics to which the animal has been and is exposed in its normal environment (diet, water, air) it is not possible to apply these principles to the metabolism of synthetic xenobiotics. Such chemicals, if absorbed make contact with the physiological milieu; if their structure is such that they gain access to and 'fit' to particular sites or catalytic centres, they will partition, bind or be chemically modified. The same applies to bioactivated species. It is not surprising that the xenobiotics metabolising systems with their wide specificity interact with new synthetic chemicals. Sometimes the result is detoxification and sometimes bioactivation. To state the obvious, what happens depends on the chemical structure of the intoxicant and its complementariness to the catalytic centres of the metabolising enzymes; if this results in metabolism then the type and/or extent of intoxication will depend on the chemical properties of the product.

By the ground-rule for xenobiotic metabolism it is usually assumed that the compound is made more hydrophilic (phase 1) and more able to be conjugated with a variety of groups (phase 2) to water-soluble products on their way to the kidney for excretion. Increasing knowledge of the chemistry of metabolism indicates that this ground-rule is becoming less a rule and more like 'what sometimes happens'.

Until relatively recently glutathione (Reed, 1990) was regarded only as a major protectant of biological material from all sorts of reactive species (Figure 5.5). So it is, but over the past few years a growing number of glutathione adducts have been shown to be toxic and/or are often bioactivated by other enzymes (see section 6.3.5 on hexa-chloro-1,3-butadiene; Van Bladeren, 1988). It has recently been shown that acrolein ($CH_2 = CH\ CHO$), which reacts rapidly with glutathione non-enzymically, produces an adduct which is nephrotoxic (Horvath *et al.*, 1992). To be nephrotoxic this adduct must be metabolised through to the first step of the renal mercapturic acid synthesis pathway. The aldehyde group seems to be essential since the S-propyl glutathione adduct is not nephrotoxic. Therefore, depending on the nature of the glutathione adduct, they may be toxic or non-toxic; in some cases the glutathione adduct even disso-ciates to reform the parent reactant, e.g. isothiocyanates (Bruggeman *et al.*, 1986; Van Bladeren, 1988).

There is a growing literature on the conversion of xenobiotics to more lipophilic rather than to more hydrophilic compounds. A variety of xenobiotic carboxylic acids are metabolised to xenobiotic lipids (mostly triacylglycerol analogues or cholesterol esters). Generally the biological/toxicological significance of such lipids is not yet clear (Fears, 1985; Hutson, 1982; Dodds, 1991; Moorhouse *et al.*, 1990, 1991). Xeno-biotic carboxylic acids enter the normal lipid metabolic pathways of breakdown or synthesis; some are toxic (see discussion on hypoglycin, the active principle from the ackee fruit causing vomiting sickness, and pent-4-enoic acid; Sherratt & Osmundsen, 1976).

Whether a xenobiotic chemical will be metabolised depends on its chemical struc-ture and whether it can form a complex with the enzyme (an enzyme–substrate complex). The rate of metabolism will depend on the structure of the chemical and the molecular structure and catalytic properties of the various enzymes. Whether a chem-ical is detoxified or bioactivated depends on the chemical properties of the products. Xenobiotic metabolising systems vary considerably across species and toxicity may also be influenced by such differences.

Although not all differences seen in the responses of animals and/or humans to chem-ical toxicants are due to differences in the routes and rates of metabolism of the admin-istered chemical, it is a general principle that if differences are found then the first hypothesis should be that this is so. The enhancement of computational power in the past thirty or so years has enabled complex differential equations to be solved and account taken that some of the systems may be saturated with substrate, i.e. be oper-ating at their maximum rate. Thus the delivery of the dose of active intoxicant to the target in particular cells will depend on a variety of constants some of which will be determined by Michaelis–Menton principles, e.g. K_m, V_{max}, K_{Aff} and k (rate constants) of the various systems involved. Compartmental pharmacokinetic (PK) models have been useful in determining the consequences of tissue dosimetry. However, the use of such PK models beyond the immediate test situation is limited and the compartments are derived from the data and are in essence mathematical concepts.

Physiologically based pharmacokinetic modelling (PB–PK) is more suited to determining relevant pathways, the consequence of distribution of intoxicant *in vivo* and tissue dosimetry: calculation of tissue doses of chemicals and their metabolites over a range of exposure conditions in different species becomes possible. This process entails at least four types of extrapolation: from high to low doses, between experimental animals and humans, from one route of administration to others, and from constant concentration dosing regimes in animal studies to discontinuous exposure. This is a fast-moving field; the reader can extend his knowledge of the mathematical and PB–PK modelling techniques and uses of the conclusions from the following reviews: Bischoff & Brown, 1966 (general approaches); Gehring *et al.*, 1978 (vinyl chloride); Clarke *et al.*, 1993 (2-methoxyethanol and 2-methoxyacetic acid); Tardif *et al.*, 1993 (toluene and *m*-xylene); Kedderis *et al.*, 1993 (tetrabromodibenzo-*p*-dioxin); Farris *et al.*, 1993 (methylmercury); Andersen *et al.*, 1987 (methylene chloride); Clewell & Andersen, 1989; Conolly & Andersen, 1991.

6.9 Summary

1 Many exogenous chemicals, once absorbed, are metabolised to products which have a greater biological activity than the original compound, i.e. they are bioactivated.

2 Bioactivation often takes place by oxidation by the cytochrome P_{450} xenobiotic metabolising systems and often leads to electrophilic compounds which react directly with nucleophilic centres in proteins, nucleic acids and small molecular weight compounds such as glutathione.

3 Bioactivation can lead to compounds causing a different type of toxicity, toxicity in an organ away from the organ where it was metabolised or to compounds of such high reactivity that they do not escape from the metabolising organ.

4 Glutathione, through reaction with its thiol group, is a powerful protectant against many forms of toxic insult. However, examples are known of glutathione adducts which are directly toxic or are furthur metabolised to toxic products.

5 Bioactivated products may be metabolised by the detoxification systems described in Chapter 5.

6 Cytochrome P_{450} enzymes are being characterised into families, some important in xenobiotic metabolism and others in the oxidation of endogenous steroids.

7 Cytochrome P_{450} enzymes are present in many tissues and in individual tissues are restricted to certain cell types.

8 Initial experiments to establish if a chemical is bioactivated depend on a variety of techniques to compare their *in vitro* and *in vivo* activities.

9 Transport systems can increase the concentration of intoxicants in particular cell types, thus causing selective toxicity in that or neighbouring cells.

10 Excretion of intoxicants via the bile can increase or decrease the chemicals' toxicity.

11   The view that phase 1 and phase 2 systems for xenobiotic metabolism are to render intoxicants more soluble and available for conjugation prior to excretion (a detoxification pathway) is not now generally acceptable.

12   Many xenobiotics are made more biologically active by oxidation and/or conjugation and some are made more lipophilic.

13   Whether a chemical is metabolised depends on its chemistry in relation to available enzymes. Whether a product of such metabolism is toxic depends on its delivery in sufficient concentration to target cells.

7

Initiating Reactions with Targets

7.1 Introduction

Reactions of intoxicants with biological targets initiate the processes leading to toxicity (stage 3, Figure 7.1). In previous chapters the large range of factors, passage through membranes, binding, partition into lipids and metabolism to less and more toxic chemicals have been discussed. Intoxicant, whether exogenous or generated *in vivo*, is delivered to many cells of different types and cause toxicity to only a few. Sometimes particular cells are affected because they acquire a higher concentration of the intoxicant. Others are affected because of their particular biological make-up or because of the particular level of activity at which they function, e.g. have a higher requirement for energy.

This part of the toxic process is its centre and defines primary events which are followed by early biological changes in stage 4 and clinical signs or symptoms of poisoning in stage 5 (Figure 7.1). In stage 3, dose–response and structure–activity relationships have a meaning unaffected by any of the other processes involved in delivery (phases 1 and 2; see Chapter 8).

Initiating reactions are with targets. A target is a cell, a subcellular organelle or a cell component which, when modified by a chemical, often leads to biological change(s) causing dysfunction and toxicity. For many toxic processes the cell involved has been identified but the detail of many in terms of reactions with particular cell macromolecules remain to be elucidated. This central concept can be stated as follows:

Defined clinical signs, symptoms and/or biological events (selective toxicity; see Chapter 10) result from specific interaction of a chemical with specific molecular component(s) of particular cells (targets).

'Selective' is used to denote changes down to the cell level (e.g. specify an organ or cell) and 'specific' to denote events within the cell and its macromolecular constituents (reaction with, for example, membranes, nucleus, mitochondria, enzyme or protein). Selective toxicity has been and is used with other meanings (see Chapter 10).

A complicated set of symptoms and signs of poisoning (syndrome) can arise from one initiating interaction with a target. However, it is entirely possible that for a given chem-

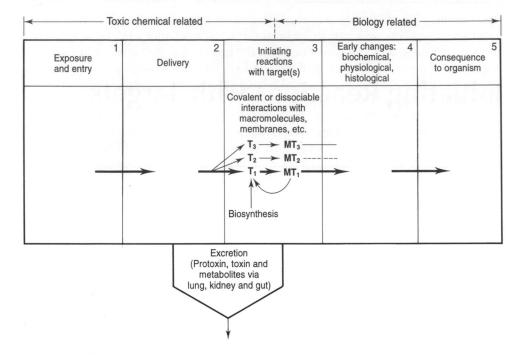

Figure 7.1 Reactions with biological targets which initiate toxicity (stage 3; see legend from Figure 2.1)

ical more than one form of toxicity may occur together, each dependent on interaction with different macromolecular components, i.e. the signs of toxicity are a summation of those from two or more intoxications. The existence of such multiple syndromes often becomes apparent when the toxicity of a series of homologues or structurally related compounds is examined, i.e. discontinuities in the structure–activity relationships appear.

In Figure 7.1, reaction with T_1 is the target which is involved in the development of toxicity. Reaction with target T_2 induces biological change which is not normally considered to be toxicity. Another target (T_3) introduced in Figure 7.1 is a target only in the sense that it reacts with the chemical toxicant but induces no biological change. In Chapters 5 and 6 such reactions have been classified as one way in which the concentration of circulating intoxicant might be reduced, thus affecting the delivery of the intoxicant to its site of action; this function is not further considered here. However, T_3 has been included in stage 3 because reaction to a very small extent with some macromolecules have led to dose monitoring techniques of great sophistication and sensitivity (see Chapter 11).

The chemical interaction may be reversible or covalent (see Chapter 3, Figure 3.1). For reversible interactions the persistence of toxicity will depend on the persistence of the intoxicant. For covalent if the intoxicant persists then more interaction takes place and the signs of intoxication become more severe; if the intoxicant is removed then recovery may still be slow awaiting the synthesis of new target or may not occur (as in mutation).

Stages 3 and 4 as shown in Figure 7.1 differ fundamentally. In stage 3, reaction is dependent on the properties, structure and/or reactivity of the chemical intoxicant, whereas stage 4 is the response of the biological system to the chemical insult. Stages 3 and 4 are therefore toxic agent (intoxicant) related and biology related respectively. However, in stage 3 the modified target is the initiator of the subsequent biological response(s) and can legitimately be considered as part of the biological response; therefore the border between toxic chemical related and biology related events is shown as the middle of stage 3 (Figure 7.1).

The toxicity of the chosen intoxicants illustrate cell selectivity and the types of chemical interaction with components of cells which initiate toxicity. In all cases the intoxicant enters the cell and causes the toxicity. Sometimes the chemical to which the organism has been exposed is bioactivated to the intoxicant; the initiating reactions with targets may be in the cell where the bioactivation occurs or in other cells (see Chapter 6).

The examples discussed in the following sections will cover a wide range of chemicals, tissues and types of attack. The biological consequences of a chemical reaction with a target can be very different:

1 Reaction with a cellular component which can be resynthesised or perhaps reformed by reversibility or reactivation. Except when the dose of chemical is overwhelming, reversible and functional change occurs in the biology of the cell.

2 Reactions with targets which lead to cell death. Although the initiating attack may be brought about by reaction of a wide variety of intoxicants with one of many targets attacked, the pathway to cell necrosis may have many common features. During or after removal of cell debris mitosis occurs in many tissues to replace the cells lost.

3 Reactions with targets which lead to death of cells which have no capacity in the adult to mitose. The central nervous tissue is the best example and, in some instances, even if the neurone does not die the capacity of the cell to replace damaged processes may be inherently deficient.

4 Reactions with genetic material of target cells. Mitosis before repair can result in modified DNA in the cell line (mutation), the consequences of which to the host can range from zero to the first step to the formation of a cancer cell.

7.2 Intoxicants which Affect Oxidative Energy Conservation (Many Tissues)

The toxicity of cyanide and carbon monoxide is due to interaction with cytochrome oxidase (section 4.2) and haemoglobin (section 4.3) respectively. Such interactions interrupt by different mechanisms the ability of cells to use oxygen for the oxidation of substrates necessary for energy conservation, i.e. the energy released by such oxidations through the generation of a H^+/OH^- membrane gradient necessary for the synthesis of ATP by the ATP synthase reaction in mitochondria (ADP + P_i → ATP). Reaction of cyanide with the copper containing cytochrome oxidase prevents the final stage of electron transport and, because of a decrease of oxygen utilisation, the concentration of oxygen in the cell, and consequently the oxygen content of the venous blood, is higher than normal. Reaction of carbon monoxide with haemoglobin prevents the delivery of oxygen to cells.

It might be thought that exposure to carbon monoxide and a low oxygen tension might have the same effects. Qualitatively this is so, but humans in an atmosphere of reduced oxygen tension so that the circulating haemoglobin is 50% reduced and 50% oxygenated are not in the same clinical state as those in a carbon-monoxide-containing atmosphere with the blood containing 50% carboxyhaemoglobin and 50% oxygenated. At rest, the former are hardly affected whereas the latter are near collapse. When one molecule of oxygen combines with one subunit of the haemoglobin tetramer (two α- and 2 β-subunits), the affinity of oxygen for the next subunit is increased and so on until all the subunits are oxygenated. In situations of high oxygen tension, as in the lung, this is physiologically advantageous leading to rapid oxygenation of the haemoglobin. When the blood reaches rapidly metabolising cells with a large oxygen demand the process goes into reverse, leading to the quick release of oxygen (even from 50% saturated haemoglobin). Carbon monoxide simulates oxygen not only in its affinity for haemoglobin but also in its influence on the affinity of oxygen attached to the other subunits. Thus release of oxygen for metabolic purposes from 50% CO/50% O_2 haemoglobin is very difficult. Therefore the biochemical lesion is the increased affinity of oxygen owing to

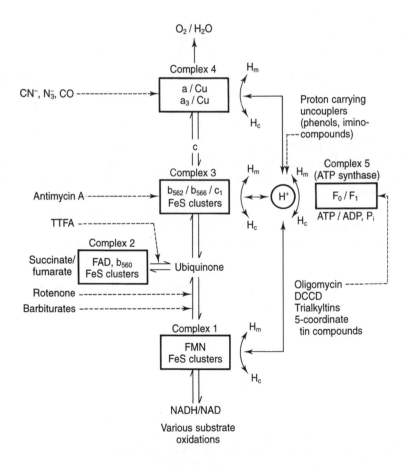

Figure 7.2 The specificity of various chemicals for different parts of the energy conservation system. a, b = several cytochromes; FMN = flavin mononucleotide; FAD = flavin dinucleotide; NAD and NADH = oxidised and reduced forms of nicotinadenine dinucleotide respectively; TTFA = thenoyltrifluoroacetone; DCCD = NN'-dicyclohexylcarbodiimide. The solid lines indicate reaction pathways in the system and broken lines indicate the approximate point where various chemicals act to perturb the system. Adapted from Hatefi, 1985

the formation of the carbon monoxide/haemoglobin complex so that the release of oxygen to the tissues is greatly reduced.

Although the oxygen consumption of many tissues will be reduced by poisoning by cyanide or carbon monoxide or in low oxygen tension, the symptoms originate from the central nervous system because of the high oxygen demand in different areas of this tissue; metabolism in these areas changes rapidly in response to many external stimuli (noise, light, speech, etc.). Modern techniques of positron emission tomography and magnetic resonance imaging can detect and now visualise such rapid changes (Cunningham & Cremer, 1985).

Energy conservation is a complex integrated system involving many different dehydrogenases at the substrate level, a series of steps in the electron transport chain to carry reducing equivalents to oxygen and three areas of the chain linked to the maintenance of a proton gradient which is the source of energy for the synthesis of ATP from ADP and inorganic phosphate. The ATP synthase system is remarkably similar throughout various species from bacteria to humans. In mammals and other species the system is contained within mitochondria. In plants the synthesis of ATP in chloroplasts occurs by similar mechanisms and thus, the mechanism of conservation of energy released by oxidation as ATP is the same in all living cells (Senior, 1988; Hatefi, 1985). Inhibitors (toxic chemicals) have played a great part in the detection, characterisation and integration of separate steps to form the whole process of energy conservation. The action of inhibitors on mitochondrial oxidative metabolism illustrates the exquisite specificity of different chemicals for the molecular components of the different steps in the system (Figure 7.2). The nature of the interaction of chemicals with specific steps in the whole system of oxidative phosphorylation has provided insights into the molecular mechanisms of individual steps; although the essential framework for oxidative phosphorylation is known, the molecular mechanisms involved in some steps, and particularly the final ATP synthase reaction, are not known in detail. This key enzyme is often called the F_1F_0-ATPase. In mitochondria the F_1 part has five subunits and the F_0 part may consist of up to twelve. This complexity accounts for the difficulties of establishing the details of the molecular mechanism; however, many different steps have been identified by the inhibitory (or sometimes the stimulatory) action of chemical inhibitors. Extensive research on the effects of such inhibitors on energy conservation illustrate the concept that specific macromolecular structures bring about specific reactions and each integrated step is potentially vulnerable to perturbation by different chemicals.

7.3 Pyrethroids (Nervous System)

The insecticidal properties of pyrethrum, the dry powder from two species of chrysanthemum, have been known for many years. The active constituents are six closely related esters of cyclopropanecarboxylic acid with alcohols of the cyclopentenolone series. Since the elucidation of the biologically active structures in natural pryrethrum, synthetic research has lead to the development of pyrethroids with much enhanced biological activity against insects, light stability and a high and low toxicity to insects and mammals respectively. Permethrin and deltamethrin (Figure 7.3a) contain several asymmetric centres and the different enantiomers differ in their toxicity, the *trans* isomer being much less toxic than the *cis* to mammals and to insects. Permethrin and deltamethrin also differ in that the latter possesses a cyano group on the α-carbon of the alcohol moeity. The symptoms caused in rats by permethrin and deltamethrin are different and

(a)

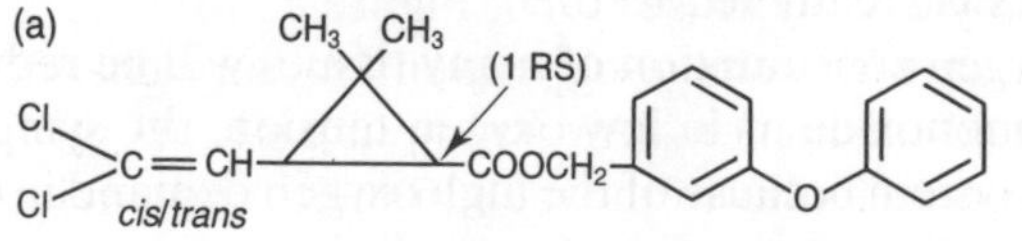

Permethrin (4 isomers; *cis/trans*, 1 RS)
Cis-permethrin (2 isomers; *cis*, 1 RS)

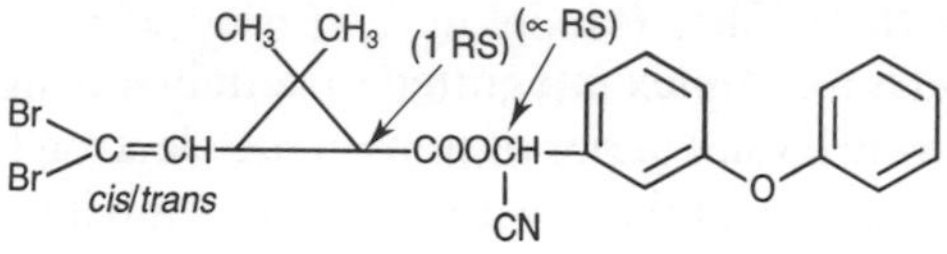

Deltamethrin (1 isomer; *cis*, 1 R, S)

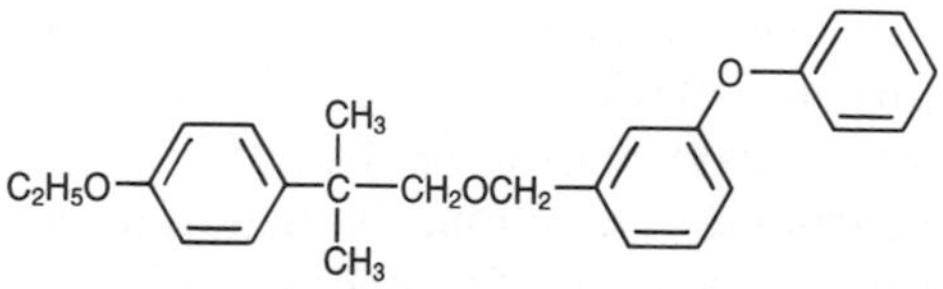

Etofenprox

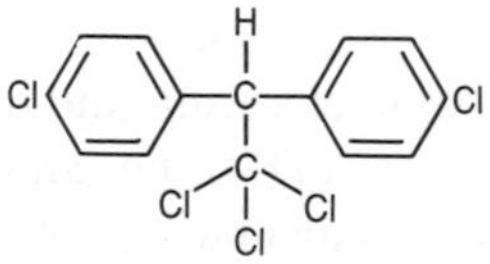

DDT

(b)

T (tremor) syndrome	CS (Choreoanthetosis: salivation) syndrome
Aggressive sparring	Pawing and burrowing
Sensitivity to external stimuli	Salivation
Fine tremor	Coarse whole body tremor
Coarse whole body tremor	Sinuous writhing
Prostration, raised temperature	Clonic seizures

(c)

Pyrethroid	Structural configuration	Time constant (ms)	Syndrome of poisoning
Without cyano group			
Phenothrin	(1R)*trans*	13	T
Cismethrin	(1R)*cis*	21	T
Permethrin	(1R)*cis*	28	T
Fenfluthrin	(1R)*cis*	105	–
S-5655	Mixture	150	T(S)
NAK-1963	Mixture	150	–
With α-cyano group			
Cyphenothrin	(1R)*cis* (α-S)	385	CS
Fenvalerate	(2RS) (α-S)	545	CS
Cypermethrin	(1R)*cis* (α-S)	1115	CS
Deltamethrin	(1R)*cis*	1770	CS

Figure 7.3 Pyrethroids: (a) chemical structure, (b) syndromes of poisoning and (c) action on sodium channels. The time constant quantifies the prolongation of the sodium tail current at the end of the nerve action potential. (*Sources*: (b) from Verschoyle & Aldridge, 1980; (c) data from Vijerberg & Van den Bercken, 1990, and Verschoyle & Aldridge, 1980)

pyrethroids may be separated into two classes showing either the T- or the CS-syndrome respectively (Verschoyle & Aldridge, 1980: Figure 7.3b).

Pyrethroids interact with voltage-dependent sodium channels involved in nerve impulse generation and conduction. A nerve impulse is brought about by a rapid temporary increase in the permeability of the membrane to sodium ions, resulting in a transient inward sodium current followed by an increase in potassium permeability causing an outward potassium current. The ionic currents cause a short-lived local reversal of the membrane potential from negative to positive and a nerve impulse occurs which is conducted along the nerve fibre (Hodgkin & Huxley, 1952). Pyrethroids delay the closing of the sodium channel activation gate and this results in a prolongation of the sodium tail current. The prolongation is characterised by time constants which quantify the delay (Figure 7.3c). The time constants range from 13 ms with phenothrin to 1,700 ms for deltamethrin. A correlation has been made between the time constant and the syndrome seen in rats: from 13 to 105 ms the T-syndrome and above 385 ms the CS-syndrome is produced and between the two a mixed syndrome may be seen. The results in Figure 7.3c also show that the time constant obtained varies with the structure of the pyrethroid. Although all toxic pyrethroids increase the time constant, the possession of an α-cyano group has a major influence on the size of the time constant; other aspects of structure also influence its magnitude. Target–chemical interactions usually lead to an on–off result, e.g. a molecule of an enzyme is either active or, when combined with a chemical, inactive. In contrast, the target–pyrethroid complex has quantitatively different properties depending on the structure of the pyrethroid.

Although the correlation between the two syndromes and the time constant of the sodium tail current is clear, the abruptness of the change from the T-syndrome to the CS-syndrome is surprising. A question to be answered is whether both syndromes are a result of the same action on the sodium channel and the difference is due to differing sensitivities of areas of the nervous system to the increasing time constants or whether the CS-syndrome is the summation of two syndromes. Recent research showing the high activity of deltamethrin on voltage-dependent chloride channels may indicate the possibility of another target (Forshaw *et al.*, 1993).

The wide range of highly lipophilic structures which bring about similar syndromes and influence the activity of voltage-dependent sodium channels is interesting. Many pyrethroids have been synthesised with considerable modification of the basic structure of permethrin and deltamethrin and many are now in commercial use. Structural and optical isomers show different toxicity and activity on sodium channels. DDT produces the T-syndrome and it seems likely that a whole range of diaryl compounds will do the same (Holan, 1971). Until recently all pyrethroids contained an ester group but a new class of compound with an ether rather than an ester linkage is awaiting approval (etofenprox; Figure 7.3a). Clearly such a wide range of compounds which have to be accommodated in a common mechanism indicate unusual molecular properties in the target which will allow the reversible interaction responsible for their biological activity.

7.4 Paraquat (Lung)

Paraquat has been used as a contact herbicide since 1963 and, although safe in application for this purpose, it is toxic to humans and animals when ingested. Experience indicates that the ingestion of >3 g per adult (>40 mg/kg bodyweight) is usually fatal.

As in man, the lung is most severely affected in rats, mice, dogs, monkeys and rabbits all at approximately the same dose; its toxicity is therefore a general phenomenon across species (Murray & Gibson, 1972).

Paraquat is a quaternary compound; uptake from the gastro-intestinal tract is facilitated and uptake against a concentration gradient into the type 1 and type 2 alveolar epithelial cells is via an energy-requiring polyamine uptake system (Smith & Wyatt, 1981; see section 6.5.1). Within a day after an approximate LD_{50} these epithelial cells are damaged and in the following days the destruction continues so that large areas of the alveolar epithelium is non-functional, oedema develops and there is an invasion by inflammatory cells. In surviving rats extensive proliferation of fibroblasts develops which on top of the primary damage results in later anoxic death (see section 8.5).

The paraquat cation is reduced to a free radical which is rapidly reoxidised by oxygen to generate superoxide anion. The reducing equivalent is NADPH and the reaction is catalysed by NADPH-cytochrome c reductase present in the endoplasmic reticulum (Gage, 1968; Farrington *et al.*, 1973). This diversion of energy-yielding equivalents from NADPH in the cytosol is also linked to the NADH oxidation of the energy conservation system in mitochondria (Figure 7.4a). Two mechanisms for cell damage are possible:

1 Depletion of energy sources so that the cell is unable to maintain itself.
2 Generation of superoxide anion and other oxygen species followed by a destructive action on membranes.

At an early stage before morphological changes can be detected, associated with the paraquat-induced cycling of the reduction and oxidation of NADP and NADPH respectively, is an activation of the pentose phosphate pathway and a corresponding inhibition of the incorporation of acetate into fatty acids (Figure 7.4b; Keeling *et al.*, 1982). Regulation of glucose 6-phosphate dehydrogenase occurs by the formation of a disulphide between a small molecular weight thiol (probably glutathione) and a thiol in the enzyme protein. An increase in protein disulphide has been demonstrated after paraquat perhaps due to oxidation by reactive oxygen species (Figure 7.4c; Bus *et al.*, 1976).

The primary target is type 1 and type 2 alveolar epithelial cells in which the cycling of the NADPH-reductase/paraquat couple takes place; these cells are affected while others are not because they contain more paraquat. The ultimate cause of death may well include deleterious effects of superoxide anion and other reactive oxygen species, all of which follow from the perturbation of the primary target (Figure 7.4a). Paraquat is ten times more toxic to rats in an atmosphere of 85% oxygen instead of air (Keeling *et al.*, 1981) and the cells affected are the same in both conditions. Since oxygen toxicity is caused by an attack on the lung endothelial cells it is clear that oxygen has potentiated the toxicity of paraquat and not the reverse. This phenomenon amplifies and supports the hypothesis that cell death may be due to an attack by several chemical species (see Figure 7.4a): oxygen should therefore not be given to treat respiratory insufficiency caused by paraquat.

Cyclical reduction and oxidation induced by paraquat is brought about by NADPH-cytochrome c reductase from lung, liver and kidney (Baldwin *et al.*, 1975) and its herbicidal action appears to be initiated by a similar system. Paraquat is a general intoxicant for many if not all mammalian cells and the selectivity for the alveolar type 1 and type 2 cells is due to the high dose presented to these cells. The lung is an organ designed for gaseous exchange, weighs only 0.5–1.7% of the body weight of mammals and yet in humans presents an alveolar surface of over 250 square metres on the gas side; a

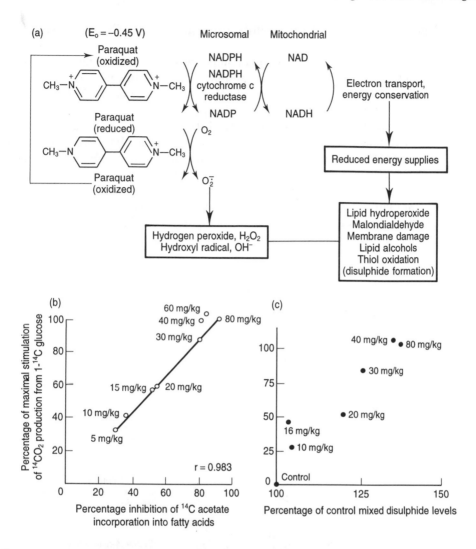

Figure 7.4 Paraquat: (a) oxidation–reduction of NADPH–NADP, potential by-products and deleterious consequences. Lung slices from rats exposed to paraquat were used to determine (b) effects on the pentose phosphate pathway and fatty acid synthesis and (c) increases in pentose phosphate pathway and mixed disulphide concentration. The pentose phosphate pathway was determined by the release of $^{14}CO_2$ from $[1-^{14}C]$-glucose and the synthesis of fatty acids by the incorporation of $[^{14}C]$-acetate. (*Source*: data from Keeling *et al.*, 1982)

corresponding large area of capillaries is required to transport gas to and from the diffusion site. This outer surface is vulnerable to chemical attack by reactive gases such as ozone, nitrogen dioxide, chlorine, phosgene, methylisocyanate, etc. Injury due to systemic circulation of chemicals following entry by other routes may be selective to either epithelial (paraquat, trialkyl phosphorothioates, bleomycin, nitrofurantoin) or endothelial cells (pyrollizidine alkaloids, α-naphthylthiourea, high concentrations of oxygen; Smith *et al.*, 1986).

7.5 Organophosphorus Compounds and Carbamates (Nervous System)

The acute toxicity of organophosphorus compounds and carbamates is due to the prevention of the hydrolysis of the neurotransmitter acetylcholine by the enzyme acetylcholinesterase. This enzyme is an essential component of the acetylcholine–receptor system in which after combination of acetylcholine with the receptor it is hydrolysed to biologically inactive products. The toxicity of the carbamate, eserine or physostigmine, is a constituent of the calabar bean and has been used in pharmacological studies of cholinergic systems and also as a treatment of myasthenia gravis. Organophosphorus compounds were first synthesised in Germany prior to the Second World War and their volatility and high toxicity led to their development as potential chemical warfare agents. After the war many new structures were synthesised and developed for use as insecticides. The range of possible structures is large (Figure 7.5); all the acidic groups of the phosphorus acid must be substituted and one of these groups must be hydrolysable,

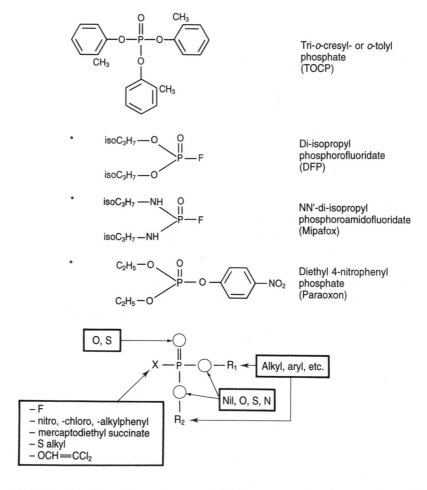

Tri-*o*-cresyl- or *o*-tolyl phosphate (TOCP)

Di-isopropyl phosphorofluoridate (DFP)

NN'-di-isopropyl phosphoroamidofluoridate (Mipafox)

Diethyl 4-nitrophenyl phosphate (Paraoxon)

Figure 7.5 Diversity of structures of esterase-inhibiting organophosphorus compounds and * formulae of these compounds used in the assay of neuropathy target esterase (NTE) (see Figure 7.9)

i.e P–X in Figure 7.5. All directly acting inhibitors of acetylcholinesterase and other esterases are in the oxon form (i.e. contain P = O). There are many pesticides in commercial use which contain a P = S group; these are metabolised and bioactivated *in vivo* to the oxon form (see Chapter 6). The toxicity of this class of compounds extends from the extreme of the chemical warfare agents to insecticides with a high safety record. Until recently it was thought that esterase-inhibiting organophosphorus compounds

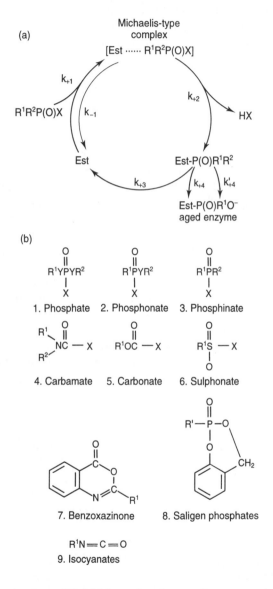

Figure 7.6 The mechanism of inhibition of serine or B-esterases by organophosphorus compounds and the chemical structures of inhibitors. (a) The reaction steps indicated by k_1, k_2 and k_3 are analogous to the esterase–substrate reaction. The step(s) indicated by k_4 are aging reactions (see Figure 7.7). (b) The different chemical structures which take part in the substrate-like reaction. Only phosphates and phosphonates can take part in the aging reaction. (*Source*: Aldridge, 1989)

were wholly synthetic and that there was no equivalent in the natural world. However, an acetylcholinesterase inhibiting organophosphorus compound, anatoxin-a(S),with a toxicity of approximately 10 μg/kg has been isolated from the algae cyanobacteria (see Table 1.1: Hyde & Carmichael, 1991).

The mechanism of the reaction of organophosphorus compounds and carbamates with esterases is analogous to enzyme–substrate reactions. It has been established that all organophosphorus compounds form an acylated enzyme intermediate: phosphorylated, carbamylated or acylated (when acetylcholine is the substrate acetylcholinesterase is acetylated). Using organophosphorus compounds labelled with [^{32}P] the labelled intermediate may be isolated and the phosphorus shown to be attached to one serine per molecule of enzyme. This one serine is unique in its reactivity and is part of the catalytic centre of the enzyme. The acetylated and carbamylated acetylcholinesterases have never been isolated because they are too unstable and therefore the mechanism of the reactions has been established by comparisons of the properties of the reactions of the three classes of compounds. In Figure 7.6a the whole process is shown as a cyclical system, the first step (k_1) being the combination of esterase with organophosphorus compound to form a Michaelis-like complex. This complex decomposes (k_2) to release the leaving group X leaving the phosphorus moeity attached to the serine by a covalent bond. Phosphorylated esterases are rather stable but when a substrate is being hydrolysed the acylated intermediate is very unstable. Thus the acetylated acetylcholinesterase is hydrolysed approximately 300,000 mol/min/mol enzyme. In contrast dimethylphosphoryl acetylcholinesterase is 4×10^7 times slower at a rate of 0.0085 mol/min/mol enzyme. Therefore although the reactions are mechanistically the same, organophosphorus compounds are inhibitors and carboxylic acid esters are substrates. Whether a compound is a substrate or an inhibitor depends mainly on the stability of the phosphorylated, carbamylated or acylated enzyme. There is a continuous spectrum from good substrate through poorly hydrolysed substrate and poor inhibitor to powerful inhibitor. Figure 7.6b shows chemical structures which react with esterases in the above way. Inhibitors which behave as substrates are different from many other active-site-directed inhibitors. For the latter, affinity for the catalytic site is required and an added reactive group in the molecule then reacts with groups in the

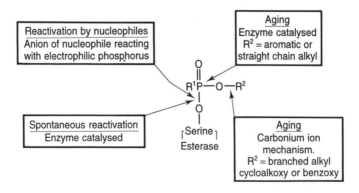

Figure 7.7   The properties of phosphylated esterases. Phosphylation is a generic term for attachment of phosphorus derived from organophosphates, phosphonates and phosphinates (see Figure 7.6)

88

neighbourhood of the catalytic centre. The resulting inhibited enzyme does not proceed through the normal catalytic mechanism (Sandler, 1980; Sandler & Smith, 1989).

Two reactions (k_4) are not part of the cyclical process (Figure 7.6a). These are possible because in the phosphylated esterases there are other groups attached to the phosphorus which, in the environment of the catalytic centre, can be released by two different time- and temperature-dependent processes called aging which lead to an enzyme derivative with a negatively charged phosphorus attached to the serine (Figure 7.7). The resulting P–O$^-$derivatives attached to one serine group in the enzyme are extremely stable and, when formed *in vivo*, return of activity can only take place by the resynthesis of new enzyme. In Figures 7.7 and 7.8 reactivation of phosphylated cholinesterases by nucleophiles has been included. By analogy with the formation of acethydroxamic acid from acetylcholine and hydroxylamine in the presence of cholinesterase (via the acetylated cholinesterase intermediate) phosphylated cholinesterases react slowly with hydroxylamine and rather faster with oximes reforming

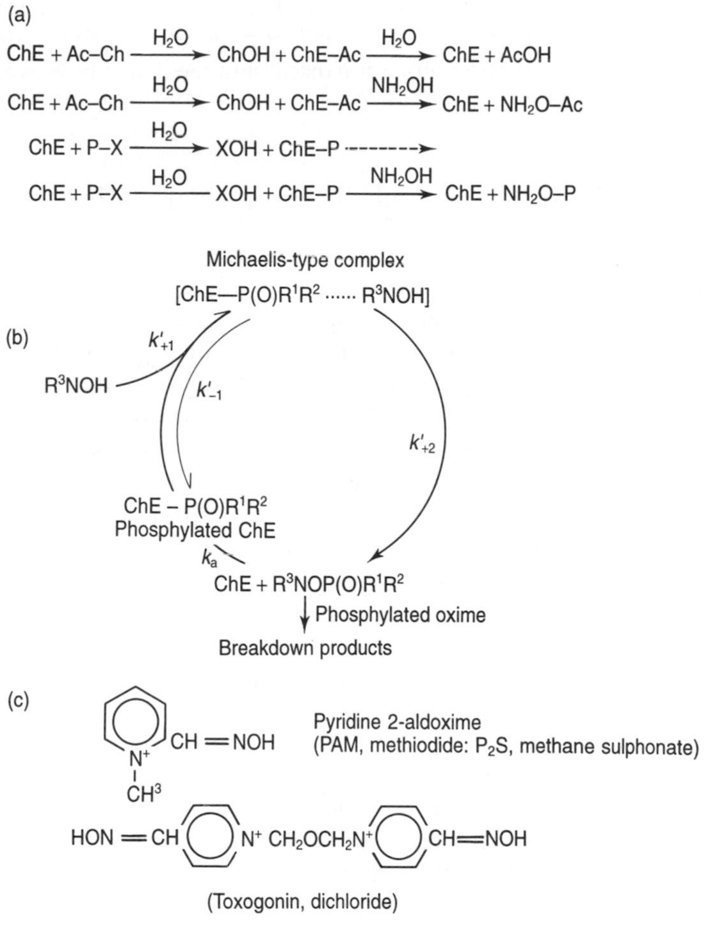

(a)

$$\text{ChE} + \text{Ac–Ch} \xrightarrow{\text{H}_2\text{O}} \text{ChOH} + \text{ChE–Ac} \xrightarrow{\text{H}_2\text{O}} \text{ChE} + \text{AcOH}$$

$$\text{ChE} + \text{Ac–Ch} \xrightarrow{\text{H}_2\text{O}} \text{ChOH} + \text{ChE–Ac} \xrightarrow{\text{NH}_2\text{OH}} \text{ChE} + \text{NH}_2\text{O–Ac}$$

$$\text{ChE} + \text{P–X} \xrightarrow{\text{H}_2\text{O}} \text{XOH} + \text{ChE–P} \dashrightarrow$$

$$\text{ChE} + \text{P–X} \xrightarrow{\text{H}_2\text{O}} \text{XOH} + \text{ChE–P} \xrightarrow{\text{NH}_2\text{OH}} \text{ChE} + \text{NH}_2\text{O–P}$$

Michaelis-type complex

[ChE—P(O)R^{1}R^2 ...... R^{3}NOH]

(b)

k'_{+1}

R^{3}NOH

k'_{-1}

k'_{+2}

ChE – P(O)R^{1}R^2
Phosphylated ChE

k_a

ChE + R^{3}NOP(O)R^{1}R^2

Phosphylated oxime

Breakdown products

(c)

Pyridine 2-aldoxime
(PAM, methiodide: P$_2$S, methane sulphonate)

(Toxogonin, dichloride)

Figure 7.8 Mechanism of reactivation of phosphylated cholinesterases by nucleophilic oximes. (a) Reaction of cholinesterase with substrates and organophosphorus compounds with and without hydroxylamine. ChE = cholinesterase; Ac-Ch = acetylcholine; P-X = organophosphorus compound. (b) Mechanism of reactivation. (c) Examples of oximes used therapeutically (see Chapter 8)

89

active enzyme (Figure 7.8a,b). The other product of the reaction, the oxime-phosphorus derivative is an inhibitor of the cholinesterase but cannot reinhibit because its concentration is rapidly reduced by dilution and instability. Reactivation is only possible with non-aged enzyme. Oximes used for the treatment of organophosphorus compound poisoning are one of the few examples of the rational development of therapeutic agents for chemical toxicity (Figure 7.8c; Chapter 8).

The reactions illustrated in Figures 7.6–7.8 apply to many acylating inhibitors and to all esterases with serine in the catalytic centre. If an esterase is inhibited in a progressive temperature- and pH-dependent reaction it is diagnostic that the esterase acts through a serine mechanism. Also, as complicated biological systems are found to be inhibited by organophosphorus compounds a reasonable hypothesis is that a serine-esterase (or protease) is involved.

Inhibitory powers are often expressed as the concentration required to cause 50% inhibition. This is adequate for reversible interactions described by affinity or dissociation constants. Covalent interactions are time-, temperature- and pH-dependent and are described by rate constants (see Chapter 3). If sufficient results are not available to derive the bimolecular rate constant then inhibitory power must be qualified by the time and temperature of incubation. For a full discussion see Aldridge & Reiner (1972) and Chapter 3.

7.6 Organophosphorus Compounds (Delayed Neuropathy; Axonopathy)

In 1930 in the USA an epidemic of neuropathy called ginger paralysis affected many people (Smith & Elvove, 1930; see section 6.3.3). It was established that the disease was caused by the contamination of ginger extract with triesters of phosphoric acid and cresols, mainly *o*-cresol (2-methylphenol). From that time until 1953 there was no advance in understanding of the mechanism of this disease except for the exclusion of some enzymes. In 1953 a similar neuropathy was reported (Bidstrup *et al.*, 1953) in three workers engaged in pilot plant production of a prospective organophosphate pesticide Mipafox and administration to hens caused the same signs and histopathology of the peripheral and long axons of the central nervous system (Barnes & Denz, 1953); DFP also caused the same lesions (for chemical structures see Figure 7.5). These observations were a decisive step forward since, although TOCP was a rather inert compound, both Mipafox and DFP were acutely toxic and were direct inhibitors of esterases including the cholinesterases. Subsequently, tri *o*-cresylphosphate was shown to be bioactivated to the directly acting saligenin phosphate (see section 6.3.3). Equally important was the positive finding that several other compounds which were acutely toxic did not lead to lameness and paralysis in hens 2–3 weeks after dosing, i.e. not all inhibitors of acetylcholinesterase caused delayed neuropathy. In paralysed hens the histopathological finding was initially classified as demyelination but it is now known that the primary lesion is damage to the axons, i.e. an axonopathy (Cavanagh, 1964).

Organophosphates are rather selective inhibitors; this led to the hypothesis that delayed neuropathy might be initiated by reaction with an esterase. If this were true then an esterase (later called neuropathy target esterase, NTE) must exist which is inhibited by those organophosphorus compounds which cause delayed neuropathy and not inhibited by those that do not. The general principles of the reaction of organophosphorus compounds with esterases are discussed in section 7.5 and in Chapter 3. The procedure developed for the analytical determination of such an enzyme is shown in

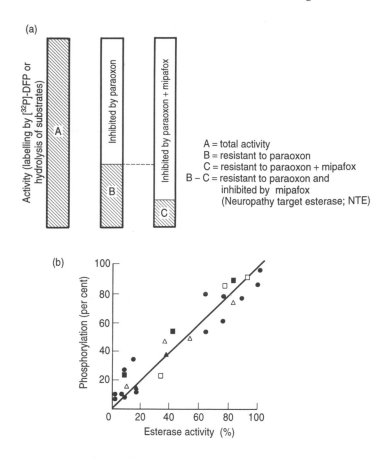

Figure 7.9 The development of the assay for neuropathy target esterase, NTE. (a) The shaded areas indicate activity measured by labelling with [^{32}P]-DFP or by hydrolysis of the carboxylic acid ester substrates, phenyl phenylacetate or phenyl valerate. (b) The linear relationship shown between results (B–C) obtained by labelling with [^{32}P]-DFP or hydrolysis of phenyl phenylacetate

Figure 7.9. The quantity B−C is a measure of protein phosphorylated by DFP or of substrate hydrolysis and indicates that an esterase is present in the nervous system; since it is sensitive to the neuropathic Mipafox and not inhibited by the inactive Paraoxon (Figures 7.9a,b) NTE has the credentials for a target in organophosphorus delayed neuropathy. Using this analytical technique for NTE, organophosphorus compounds which cause delayed neuropathy 2–3 weeks later also reduce by 70–80% in 1 day NTE activity in brain and spinal cord. Those hens treated with other compounds which caused less inhibition showed no signs of toxicity. This 'NTE/70–80% inhibition' hypothesis held for many compounds (Johnson, 1975a,b, 1982) but it was later found that some compounds (phosphinates, sulphonyl fluorides, carbamates) did react with NTE and after 70–80% inhibition in hens no later signs of delayed neuropathy appeared. The difference between these compounds and others was that there was no possibility of aging (see group B in Figure 7.10a). Not only were these compounds unable to cause the disease but pretreatment of hens rendered them resistant to active compounds. If after pretreatment the hens were left for different times before a later challenge with DFP, no delayed neuropathy developed until sufficient NTE activity had been

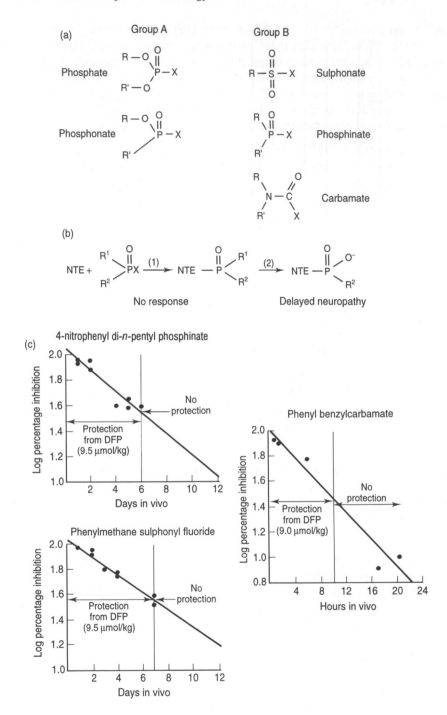

Figure 7.10 Development of the 'NTE/70–80% inhibition/aging' hypothesis. (a) Group A organophosphorus compounds inhibit NTE, age and cause delayed neuropathy. Group B inhibit NTE, cannot age and do not cause delayed neuropathy and when administered before, prevent delayed neuropathy by group A compounds. (b) The NTE/70–80% inhibition/aging hypothesis. (c) After inhibition by compounds of group B, protection is provided until biosynthesis or reactivation has made 70–80% NTE available for inhibition by a later challenge dose of DFP (from group A)

biosynthesised *in vivo* for 70–80% inhibition by DFP to be possible (Figure 7.10c). The principle, therefore, was that those agents which inhibited NTE but could not age protected hens against a subsequent dose of an active compound; this is powerful evidence for the involvement of NTE. Based on substantial evidence using many organophosphorus compounds the initiating reaction for organophosphorus delayed neuropathy was defined as the 'NTE/70–80% inhibition/aging' hypothesis.

However, recent observations indicate that other factors are involved:

1 Those compounds which are protectors when given before a dose of an active organophosphorus compound but when given after are also promoters and delayed neuropathy may be induced with only 30–40% inhibition of NTE (Lotti *et al.*, 1991).

2 Phosphoroamidates such as Mipafox and hexylmethamidophos [R(S) isomer] cause delayed neuropathy but apparently do not age since the inhibited NTE can be reactivated by treatment with potassium fluoride – a test that aging has not taken place (Johnson & Safi, 1993; Milatovic & Johnson, 1993).

3 Young hens are insensitive to delayed neuropathy. Rats have always been thought to be totally insensitive but it has recently been shown that this is a question of age – old rats develop delayed neuropathy and young rats with promoters after the dose of organophosphorus compound also develop the disease. Thus there are biological factors which influence the development of the lesions in the nerves of young rats and these factors can be suppressed by promoters (Moretto *et al.*, 1991).

Although the NTE/70–80% inhibition/aging hypothesis is now not generally applicable, the evidence that NTE is an important target in the mechanism of delayed neuropathy is very strong. NTE has unusual properties: it is tightly bound to membranes and has so far not been isolated in an active form, it ages very rapidly for a wide variety of chemical R-groups in the P-O-R, the group R when released during the aging reaction becomes attached to (presumably) neighbouring protein, and since it can be inhibited by protectors with no signs of toxicity its biological function is not known. The biological events during the 2–3 weeks after dosing are unknown; recent reviews are Lotti (1992), Johnson (1993), Lotti *et al.* (1993) and Aldridge (1993).

7.7 Acrylamide (Nervous System; Axonopathy)

Acrylamide is a water-soluble substance used in its polymerised form as a water flocculator to remove solids and particularly as a grouting agent to render earthworks in mining and tunnel construction strong and waterproof. Very large quantities are manufactured and poisoning in humans has occurred during its manufacture and use. It is very water soluble and soluble in some solvents so that absorption occurs not only by mouth and into the lung but also via the skin.

In humans the symptoms consist of trunchal ataxia with relatively high acute exposure which may be cerebellar in origin and peripheral neuropathy in which both motor and sensory nerve fibres are involved in the distal parts of the limbs. Difficulty in walking is due to weakness of feet and legs, and clumsiness of hands and loss of tendon reflexes develop early. Sensory symptoms are numbness of the feet and hands. Excessive sweating occurs, predominantly at the extremities of feet and fingers known as cold, dripping extremities. Diagnostic signs and symptoms are trunchal ataxia, predominantly motor peripheral neuropathy together with excessive sweating and redness and peeling of the skin of hands and feet.

Nerve conduction velocities in both motor and sensory nerves are usually normal although nerve action potential may be abnormal. Sensory nerve action potential is the most sensitive electrophysiological test even though from clinical examination motor nerves may appear to be more affected than sensory nerves. Provided the patients are not too severely affected, recovery from a short or prolonged exposure is usually complete. For those severely affected residual abnormalities of ataxia, distal weakness, reflex loss or sensory disturbance may remain.

Acrylamide has been shown to produce peripheral neuropathy in many animal species (Miller & Spencer, 1985). In the earliest detailed study both central effects at the highest dose were reported as well as entirely peripheral effects at lower doses (Kuperman, 1958). When the acrylamide was given in a range of small repeated amounts or as the same amount at longer time intervals, the effects appeared to be cumulative (see section 9.5).

The damage in the peripheral nervous system is to the medium and large nerves and is a primary axonopathy followed by a secondary demyelination. Degeneration occurs in the distal regions of the long sensory and, later, motor peripheral nerve fibres and also, but to a much lesser extent, in the distal regions of long axons in the spinal cord. Degeneration of Purkinje cells of the cerebellum may occur early in intoxication with large amounts. The earliest change shown by electron microscopy is the accumulation

(a)

Compound	Neurotoxicity (potency %)	Reaction with glutathione ($l.mol^{-1} min^{-1}$)
Acrylamide	+(100%)	0.91
N-hydroxymethylacrylamide	+(30%)	0.91
NN'-diethylacrylamide	+(13%)	0.058
N-methylacrylamide	+(4%)	0.058
Ethylcrotonate	–	0.24
Methylmethacrylate	–	0.17
Methylene bisacrylamide	–	0.54
NN'-pentamethylene acrylamide	–	ND
NN'-bis acrylamide acetic acid	–	ND
33'-iminopropionamide	–	ND
S-B-propionamido glutathione	–	ND

(b)

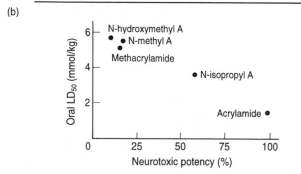

Figure 7.11 Neurotoxic potency of acrylamide and various related compounds in the rat compared with the oral LD_{50} and the rate of reaction with glutathione *in vitro*. ND = not determined. (*Sources*: (a) data from Hashimoto & Aldridge, 1970; Edwards, 1975; (b) data from Hashimoto *et al.*, 1988)

of neurofilaments in the distal regions of many axons of the peripheral nervous system (Prineas, 1969; Schaumburg *et al.*, 1974; Fullerton & Barnes, 1966).

The mechanism of the interference of acrylamide with the function of long axons of particularly long peripheral nerves is unknown. Acrylamide itself is a reactive molecule and reacts readily with soluble thiols and those in macromolecules. The structure–activity relationships are not understood for their reactivity with thiols does not follow their ability to cause peripheral neuropathy (Figure 7.11a). It is not certain that acrylamide is the intoxicant; one possibility is that the epoxide formed from acrylamide might be the aetiological agent (Bergmark *et al.*, 1991).

Most of the early experimental studies have concentrated on the peripheral nervous system but acrylamide causes a variety of toxic effects: cerebellar Purkinje cell necrosis, cancer, testicular toxicity and developmental toxicity. The mechanisms are unknown and explanations are required for the relative biological activity of acrylamide and its derivatives to cause not only peripheral neuropathy but also the above effects (Dearfield *et al.*, 1988). Toxicity and neurotoxic potential in the rat have been correlated (Figure 7.11b).

7.8 2,5-Hexanedione (Nervous System; Peripheral and Central Axonopathy)

The initial structure–response relationships indicated that *n*-hexane and methyl *n*-butylketone and 2,5-hexanedione (Figure 7.12) all produced the same clinical picture and morphological changes in the long axons in peripheral nerve and to a lesser extent in the central nervous system (central–peripheral axonopathy). This was explained by the finding that 2,5-hexanedione, a γ-diketone, was the proximal intoxicant for all three compounds. Previous experience with methyl iso-butylketone which gave no problems in use is also consistent with this hypothesis since it cannot be oxidised to a diketone with the keto groups two carbon atoms apart. The structure–response relationships have been expanded to many compounds (Figure 9.5) and the γ-diketone hypothesis is confirmed. Dose–response relationships also indicate that the circulating concentrations of 2,5-hexanedione are inversely related to the time taken for the clinical signs to appear, i.e the higher the concentration the shorter the time (Table 9.1).

Histological examination of peripheral nerves after treatment with compounds which are metabolised to 2,5-hexanedione show focal axonal swelling associated with an increase in neurofilaments (Krasavage *et al.*, 1980). Thus this diketone produces a specific lesion in the nerves which almost certainly is due to a disturbance of neuronal function. For most compounds the swellings are distal but for the more reactive compound 3,4-dimethyl-2,5-hexanedione the lesions are more proximal (Graham *et al.*, 1984).

The precise mechanism involved has not yet been agreed. The structure–response relationships imply that pyrrole formation is involved in any reaction with protein. Two hypotheses have been proposed: (1) interference with some energy-yielding process in the neurone so that neurofilament formation, maintenance and/or turnover is defective, and (2) direct reaction with neurofilament protein (DeCaprio, 1985). Two variants have been postulated for the latter; either the formation of a pyrrole following reaction with the ε-nitrogen of lysine (Figure 7.12) increasing lipophilicity or, in an additional oxidative reaction of the pyrrole with the same or a neighbouring neurofilament, to cause cross linking (Graham, 1980). 3,3-Dimethyl-2,5-hexanedione, a compound

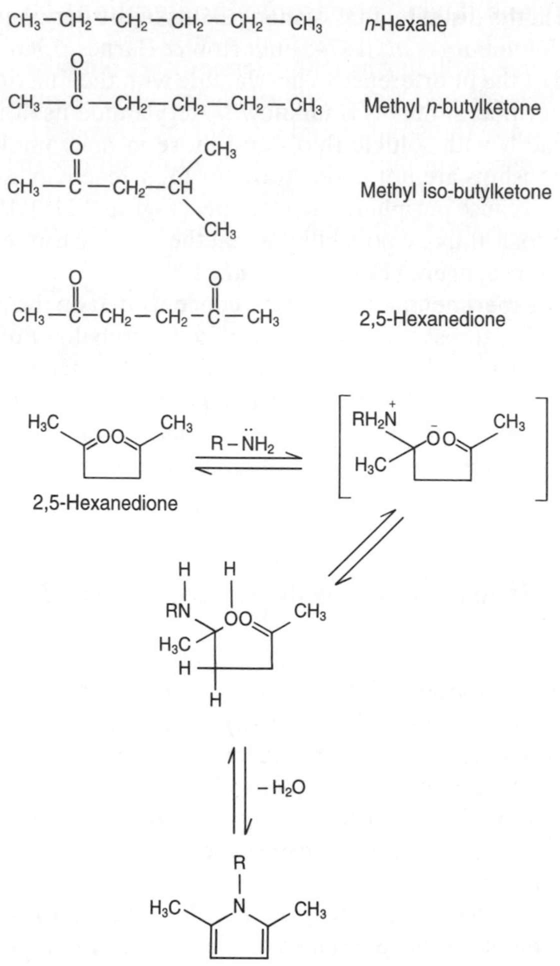

Figure 7.12 Chemical structures of compounds metabolised *in vivo* to the γ-diketone 2,5-hexanedione and its reaction with the ε-amine group of lysine in proteins

which can react with lysine but cannot form a pyrrole, does not cause the specific type of 2,5-hexanedione axonopathy (Sayre *et al.*, 1986). Also 3-acetyl-2,5-hexanedione, which forms a stable pyrrole but cannot take part in an oxidative cross-linking reaction (DeCaprio & O'Neill, 1985; Genter St.Clair *et al.*, 1988), does not cause the typical axonopathy. These observations tend to support the 'direct reaction with lysine in neurofilaments followed by cross-linking' hypothesis. For additional reviews see DeCaprio (1985, 1987) and Couri & Milks (1982).

2,5-Hexanedione also causes testicular atrophy initiated by early damage to the supporting Sertoli cells. The nurturing, transport and structural roles of the Sertoli cells are dependent upon microtubule integrity. Evidence has been produced to support the view that the 2,5-hexanedione disrupts the normal functioning of these tubular assemblies by reactions similar to those postulated for neurofilaments (Boekelheide, 1987, 1988; Boekelheide & Eveleth, 1988).

7.9 Trichlorethylene (Liver Peroxisome Proliferation)

A variety of compounds including hypolipidaemic drugs, phthalate esters used as plasticisers and some halogenated hydrocarbon solvents when administered to mice and rats cause an increase in the number and size of peroxisomes in the liver. The active compounds form a diverse group and the only unifying hypothesis for their structure–response relationships seems to be that they all possess or are metabolised to a compound with an acidic function (Table 7.1). This acidic function need not be carboxyl

Table 7.1 Structure and common names of compounds which cause peroxisome proliferation in the liver

Structure	Name
	Trichloroacetic acid
	Mono-ethylhexyl phthalate
	Ethylhexanoic acid
$HOOC - (CH_2)_{14} - COOH$	Hexadeca-1, 16-dioic acid
	Clofibrate
	Wy-14643
	4-THA

For reviews consult Reddy & Lalwani, 1983; Cohen & Grasso, 1981; Hawkins *et al.* 1987; Elcombe, 1985; Rao & Reddy, 1987; Lock *et al.* 1989.

since a sulphonamide and compounds with an acidic NH in a tetrazole moeity (compound 4-THA) are active.

Trichlorethylene is not directly active but must be oxidised and rearranged to trichloracetic acid thus fulfilling the requirements for an acidic function. Of the other metabolites, dichloracetic acid and trichlorethanol, only dichloracetic acid is active (DeAngelo *et al.*, 1989; Prout *et al.*, 1985; Larson & Bull, 1992). Trichlorethylene causes extensive peroxisome proliferation in the mouse but much less in the rat; this difference seems mainly to be explained by pharmacokinetic factors in metabolism to the tri-and dichloracetic acids; both of these acids are active if administered directly to both species.

Peroxisomes are present in many tissues of animals and can be demonstrated by electron microscopy and by cytochemical reactions for catalase. Liver peroxisomes are larger and possess an array of enzymes in addition to catalase. These include urate oxidase (often seen as a crystalloid core), hydrogen peroxide producing flavine oxidases, carnitine acyltransferases and many enzymes involved in β-oxidation of fatty acids (C_8–C_{22}) which are different from those involved in β-oxidation of fatty acids in the mitochondrial system, e.g in the peroxisome system each removal of two carbons results in the formation of one molecule of hydrogen peroxide. There is no requirement for carnitine and no inhibition by cyanide (Lazarow, 1978; DeDuve & Baudhuin, 1966; Tolbert, 1981; Lock *et al.*, 1989; Reddy & Kumar, 1977). A bifunctional protein (molecular weight 80,000) possesses the activities of two enzymes in the β-oxidation pathway in peroxisomes: enoyl-CoA hydratase and 3-hydroxy acyl-CoA dehydrogenase. It is a good marker for peroxisomes since after proliferation it may become the most abundant protein in a liver homogenate (Watanabe *et al.*, 1985); in normal liver cells peroxisomes occupy <2% of the cytoplasmic volume which can be increased to 25%. Large increases in messenger RNA's encoding for some of the enzymes have been isolated during the rapid increase in synthesis of protein during peroxisome proliferation.

When peroxisomes are induced by many compounds including metabolites of trichlorethylene, proliferation of endoplasmic reticulum is also seen. There is an increase in a cytochrome of the P_{450} class, first designated P_{452} and now $P_{450}IVA1$, which brings about ω-hydroxylation of lauric acid: these changes in microsomal metabolism may be linked to changes in peroxisomal metabolism (Lake *et al.*, 1984; Sharma *et al.*, 1988). Formation of new peroxisomes may be by division of existing peroxisomes (Lazarow & Fujiki, 1985).

Therefore trichloracetic and dichloracetic acids cause an increase in the number and size of a pre-existing organelle and the increase in the array of enzymes for β-oxidation is proportional to the peroxisomal volume density. These changes are also associated with changes in the endoplasmic reticulum. The target for tri- and dichloracetic acid which initiates this 'physiological activation' is still a subject of much research. Two hypotheses are being considered: (1) activation of specific genes either directly or via combination with a receptor (Reddy & Lalwani, 1983), and (2) perturbation of lipid metabolism so that there is 'substrate overload' and a product of this perturbation may result in feedback control or control by mechanism 1 (Lock *et al.*, 1989). Recent research has provided evidence that a nuclear hormone receptor (R) binds peroxisome proliferators (PP) to form a complex PPAR (activated receptor) which recognises specific DNA sequences and activates specific gene transcriptions. In this research carnitine acyltransferase was the marker enzyme studied and it was shown that the order of the *in vivo* structure–activity profile was approximately followed by activity in the experimental system (Green *et al.*, 1992; see Figure 7.13). It is not certain whether

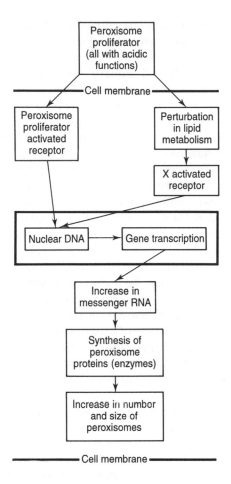

Figure 7.13 Current hypothesis for the mechanism of induction of peroxisome proliferation

mechanisms (1) or (2) are involved but other observations suggest that it may be (1); see Price *et al.*, 1985 and Wysynski *et al.*, 1993.

If further research confirms that all biological effects of peroxisome proliferators are receptor-mediated whether, directly or by proxy, and that dose–response and structure–activity relationships are compatible with the known values for *in vivo* potency it will have important implications for the quantitative assessment of risk of exposure of humans to trichlorethylene. Both peroxisome proliferation and cancer induction by trichloroethylene may be linked and both vary with the species exposed (Rao & Reddy, 1987). The interpretation of these experimental observations in animals in relation to the negative epidemiological surveys in humans (Axelson *et al.*, 1978; Paddle, 1983) will be much easier when the mechanisms are understood (Ashby *et al.*, 1994).

7.10 Glycol Ethers (Testis, Embryonic and Foetal Development)

Testicular function is spermatogenesis which is a unique process involving various timed stages of differentiation, the whole cycle taking thirteen days in the rat and sixteen days in humans. The seminiferous tubules contain germ cells at different stages of differentiation, beginning with the spermatogonia which exist as two types: one to generate other spermatogonia and the other destined to become mature sperm. First the spermatogomia mitose to become diploid primary spermatocytes and then by meiosis to form secondary spermatocytes containing half the normal complement of chromosomes (haploid). The next stage to spermatids is followed by several stages of transformation leading to mature sperm. The many stages in the formation of mature sperm are called B-type spermatogonia, leptotene, zygotene, pachytene, diplotene spermatocytes, Golgi and cap spermatids; they have also been characterised into fourteen stages (Leblond & Clermont, 1952). The seminiferous tubules also contain Sertoli cells. The junctions between these elongated cells form the blood–testis barrier that partitions the seminiferous epithelium into two tubular compartments, one for spermatogonia and early spermatocytes and the other for more differentiated and more fully developed spermatogenic cells. These two compartments possess unique chemical milieu. The Sertoli cells are vital for spermatogeneis – they provide support for the attached spermatids, protection and probably nutrition until the spermatids become germ cells. The Leydig cells exist in the interstitium and are the main site of synthesis of testosterone which is distributed via the blood vessels and lymphatic space. The product of the testis is immature sperm which continue to mature on their way down the efferent ducts, a network of channels served by a variety of accessory organs such as the epididymides, prostrate, seminal vesicles and other glands. The process of spermatogenesis is therefore highly organised ensuring the continuous supply of mature sperm through a variety of discrete stages, no doubt at each stage involving changes in the sperm's molecular biology.

In the female, two stages of meiotic division of the primary oocyte occur to produce one large haploid ovum which at conception is fertilised by the entry of the sperm. Foetal development which follows is also a highly organised pattern of growth and differentiation (see section 7.14). Thus the whole process from the production of sperm and receptive ovum to the birth of the foetus is organised into a series of controlled mitoses and at specific times differentiation to yield new morphological structures with different biochemical and molecular biological properties. These stages therefore present the potentiality of specific perturbation by chemicals. Such a potentiality has been realised in humans by the unexpected limb malformations in the offspring of mothers who had been prescribed thalidomide during pregnancy (1959–1961) and the sterility of male factory workers (1977) after occupational exposure to the soil fumigant 1,2-dibromo-3-chloropropane. In these examples the effects on the embryo and the testis occurred at exposures which caused no ill health. At the time there was no experimental animal model for the teratogenicity of thalidomide, but exposure to low concentrations of the halopropane had been shown to impair the reproductive function of male rats (Torkelson *et al.*, 1961). In addition to the problem of devising and interpreting testing methods, a major problem is the assessment of the relevance of the research to human exposure when the background of failure of conception, foetal death, spontaneous abortions and developmental defects is so high.

The ethers of ethylene and propylene glycols are solvents used in lacquers, varnishes, printing inks, textile dyes and as additives to brake fluids and gasoline. They are uncharged, lipid- and water-miscible and are readily absorbed by many routes including the skin. Ethylene glycol monomethylether (2-methoxyethanol) causes degeneration of the testicular germinal epithelium, testicular atrophy and infertility in several species. In rats killed at different times after a single exposure to 2-methoxy- or 2-ethoxyethanol, the meoitic spermatocytes (pachytene stage) were found to be the most susceptible (Chapin *et al.*, 1984; Creasey & Foster, 1984) and the earlier and later stages were damaged only after exposure to higher amounts or over a longer period. Decreased fertility was found at the time after exposure that meoitic spermatocytes would be expected to have matured (Chapin *et al.*, 1985). Damage to spermatocytes at this stage has been demonstrated *in vitro* (Gray *et al.*, 1985). Other compounds such as 2-propoxy- and 2-butoxyethanol are inactive, as are ethers of 2-propanol, but the acetates of the active compounds are also active because they are hydrolysed *in vivo*.

Oxidation of the hydroxy group via aldehyde to carboxyl by alcohol dehydrogenase and aldehyde oxidase respectively, i.e. to methoxy- and ethoxyacetic acids, is necessary for activity (Moss *et al.*, 1985). The inactive 1-methoxy-2-propanol is a poor substrate for alcohol dehydrogenase and is extensively metabolised to carbon dioxide (Miller *et al.*, 1983). The propoxy- and butoxyacetic acids are inactive in Sertoli–germ cell cultures up to 10 mM (Gray *et al.*, 1985; Gray, 1986). 2-Methoxyacetic acid is converted to a coenzyme A derivative and thus enters intermediary metabolism pathways (Mebus *et al.*, 1992); the significance of this finding to the compounds' testicular toxicity is as yet unknown.

Glycol ethers also affect embryonic and foetal development. The effects include increased incidence of various malformations, increased foetal death and decreased foetal growth at exposures which cause no maternal toxicity. The type of defect is dependent on the time during gestation when exposure occurs. The structure–response relationship is the same as in testicular toxicity, i.e. 2-methoxy- and 2-ethoxyethanol are active and the higher oxy derivatives of ethanol and all ethers of 2-propanol are inactive (Horton *et al.*, 1984; Nelson *et al.*, 1984). Metabolism to the corresponding acetic acids is necessary for activity and when these are applied to rat embryos in culture the same pattern of activity is seen (Yonemoto *et al.*, 1984; Rawlings *et al.*, 1985).

In summary, 2-methoxy- and 2-ethoxyethanol affect the testis and the embryo. Metabolism to the corresponding acetic acids is necessary for toxicity. Toxicity in the testis is at the meiotic stage of spermatocyte development and in the embryo causes various malformations depending on the time during gestation of exposure. Effects are therefore cell-specific and depend on exposure when differentiation is taking place. The

Table 7.2 Stage-specific toxicity to the testis and effects on embryonic and foetal development caused by various chemicals

Compound	Male spermatogenesis (stage affected)	Ref.	Female embryonic and foetal development	Ref.
2-Methoxyethanol ⎤ 2-Ethoxyethanol ⎦	Meiotic spermatocytes (pachytene stage)	1	M, D, G	6
Dipentylphthalate	Sertoli cells	2	F	2
2,5-Hexanedione	Sertoli cells	3		
Acrylamide	Spermatids (Golgi stage)	4	No effect	7
1,3-Dinitrobenzene	Sertoli cells	5		

M = malformations; D = foetal death; G = slow foetal growth; F = decreased fertility due to effects in female, all at doses which do not cause maternal toxicity.
References: (1) Creasey and Foster, 1984; Heindel *et al.*, 1989; (3) Hall *et al.*, 1992; (4) Sakamoto *et al.*, 1988; (5) Blackburn *et al.*, 1988; (6) Horton *et al.*, 1984; (7) Field *et al.*, 1990.

molecular mechanisms are unknown. Many chemicals affect the testis and some also affect embryonic and foetal development (Table 7.2). 2-Methoxyethanol, 2,5-hexane-dione and 1,3-dinitrobenzene cause changes in Sertoli cell morphology and function but it seems likely that these changes result from different mechanisms.

7.11 Beryllium and the Rare Earths (Liver, Reticulo-endothelial System)

Beryllium and some of the rare earths cause hepatotoxicity; parenchymal cell necrosis by beryllium and predominantly fatty liver by the rare earths (Evans, 1990); the mechanisms whereby these are produced is not known. All are poorly absorbed from the gastro-intestinal tract but have a high intrinsic toxicity – for experimental purposes the intravenous route is the best. Intravenous injection causes toxicity to few tissues except the liver and spleen. The chemical properties which lead to this pattern of toxicity is that all the rare earths and beryllium form insoluble hydroxides and phosphate in physiological medium at neutral pH. After intravenous injection of soluble salts beryllium circulates as small, insoluble particles probably loosely attached to plasma proteins. Although beryllium does enter the parenchymal cells the particulate form becomes localised in the reticulo-endothelial cells (Kupffer cells in the liver).

The proportion of beryllium taken up by the liver and the rate of excretion from the rat depends upon the dose administered. At the higher doses the retention is probably associated with the low solubility of the colloidal material; at low doses it is excreted as a soluble complex e.g. citrate (Scott *et al.*, 1950; Witschi & Aldridge, 1968; see section 6.52) Similar findings are suggested for yttrium (Hirano *et al.*, 1993) and the principle probably applies to most of the rare earths since all, after intravenous injection, result in circulating insoluble phosphates/hydroxides.

Beryllium is toxic to the Kupffer cells, their phagocitising function decreases markedly by quite low doses (Skilleter & Price, 1981) and this is followed by damage which results in transfer of the beryllium to the circulation and uptake by the spleen (Skilleter & Price, 1978; Dinsdale *et al.*, 1981). Similar responses are caused by rare earths (Evans, 1990). The uptake of beryllium by liver cells is closely associated with its appearance in lysosomes (Witschi & Aldridge, 1968; Skilleter & Price, 1979) and movement of beryllium into the nucleus may well be due to the increase in solubility of beryllium in the more acidic milieu of the lysosomal cytosol.

Thus the ability of beryllium and the rare earths to form circulating colloidal forms after intravenous injection ensures their uptake by the liver. The mechanism whereby they cause the death of these cells is not known. Beryllium causes parenchymal cell necrosis with no increase in triglycerides; the rare earths lanthanum, cerium, praseodymium, neodymium and samarium, in contrast, show hepatotoxicity with release of enzymes into the plasma and a large rise in triglycerides (fatty liver) while these responses do not occur with gadolinium, dysprosium, holmium, lutetium and yttrium. It appears that gadolinium causes a selective depletion of Kupffer cells with little or no toxic response in parenchymal cells (Bouma & Smit, 1989). This response to gadolinium is sufficiently specific to be used as an experimental tool in research on the involvement of Kupffer cells on the hepatotoxicity of carbon tetrachloride (Edwards *et al.*, 1993). Current research illustrates that there is much cooperation between neighbouring cells within tissues. Further experimental studies of the complex mechanism of distribution of beryllium and the rare earths will surely enhance our knowledge of mechanisms of liver injury. The affinity of beryllium for a component(s) of the nucleus

(Witschi & Aldridge, 1968) raises the question whether subsequent cell death is programmed or not (see section 7.13). Reviews for beryllium are to be found in Skilleter (1989) and for rare earths in Evans (1990).

7.12 Triorganotins (Nervous System; Intramyelinic Vacuoles and Neuronal Necrosis)

The triorganotins were synthesised and developed as industrial and agricultural fungicides and as antifouling paints for ships but they are toxic to most forms of life, i.e. are generally biocidal. A poisoning episode in France (Alajouanine *et al.*, 1958) caused the death of one hundred people when they ingested an over-the-counter medicant diethyltin diiodide. The signs and symptoms of poisoning in humans and animals confirm that an impurity, triethyltin, was the offending agent.

Tin as a metal or as its salts has a very low toxicity. Although some have made a case for tin as an essential element no conclusive evidence is available. Successive alkylation of tin produces monoalkyltins of low toxicity, dialkyltins toxic to the liver and trialkyltins toxic to the nervous system. Thus the biological activity of these tin derivatives cannot be predicted from the properties of the parent metal. Different salts of both dialkyltins and trialkyltins have different physical properties, e.g. the nitrates or sulphates will be much more hydrophilic than the lipophilic halides or hydroxides. Trialkyltins in physiological fluids form the chloride and hydroxide, and whatever compound is administered these are the main forms which will circulate *in vivo* and pass through or partition into biological membranes. Triorganotins bind to very few proteins. From a comparison of the chemical and biological properties of triethyltin and a 5-coordinate organotin compound (A in Table 7.3) it has been concluded that there are two forms of attachment to macromolecules. In 5-coordinate binding two ligands are involved, whereas in 4-coordinate binding one ligand only is involved with affinity probably increased by its location in a hydrophobic pocket, thus reducing competition from hydroxyl (Aldridge *et al.*, 1981).

Signs of poisoning by triethyltin in rats are muscular weakness, paresis and paralysis accompanied by a decrease in body temperature. There is an increase in brain water and by light microscopy and EM the water is associated with ballooning of the myelin surrounding the nerve axons (intramyelinic vacuoles). By EM examination a few vacuoles may be detected as early as 1–2 hours after dosing but a significant increase by weight in brain water cannot be detected for 9–12 hours. However, if the fall in body temperature is prevented by increasing the environmental temperature, an increase in brain water begins immediately. The extra water contains chloride and sodium, characteristics of extracellular fluid, and is present around both central and peripheral nerves. The signs of poisoning originate from the intracranial pressure and, if exposure ceases, the lesions are reversible with no residual pathology. Therefore the lesions produced by triethyltin are highly selective with a primary increase in water in one place only (intramyelinic vacuoles). It is as though triethyltin affects an energy-requiring biological system designed to prevent accumulation of fluid between the myelin sheaths while keeping them wet with extracellular fluid (Aldridge, 1995).

The signs of poisoning by trimethyltin are quite different. Animals and humans develop marked functional disturbances including tremors, hyperexcitability, aggression and seizures. The later histopathological changes are irreversible damage in the limbic region of the hippocampus, amygdaloid nucleus and the pyriform and olfactory

Table 7.3 The properties of trimethyltin, triethyltin and a 5-coordinate tin compound

(Compound A)

Binding and biological activity				Ref.
Macromolecules				
Haemoglobin (rat and cat only)	+	+	−	1,2
Enzymes				
Hexokinase (yeast)	+	+	+	3
Glutathione S-transferase (ligandin)	+	+	+	4
Mitochondrial ATP synthase	+	+	+	5
Physical effects				
Chloride/hydroxyl exchange	+	+	−	6
Toxicity				
Neuronal necrosis	+	−	?	7
Intramyelinic vacuoles	−	+	−	8,9

Types of interaction

The chemical name for the 5-coordinate tin compound is 2[(dimethylamino)methyl] diethyltin bromide.

References: (1) Elliott *et al.*, 1979; (2) Taketa *et al.*, 1980; (3) Siebenlist & Taketa, 1983; (4) Tipping *et al.*, 1979; (5) Aldridge, 1976; (6) Selwyn, 1976; (7) Brown *et al.*, 1979; (8) Aldridge and Brown, 1988; (9) Verschoyle & Aldridge, unpublished; see Aldridge, 1995.

cortices. If animals or humans survive, severe memory deficits may be detected. There is no evidence that the selective damage is due to selective distribution of trimethyltin.

No molecular explanations are available for either the intramyelinic vacuoles caused by triethyltin or the neuronal necrosis by trimethyltin nor is there an explanation for the absolute difference between the toxicological properties between these two compounds (Table 7.3; see Chapter 9 for a discussion of structure–activity relationships). Whatever are the explanations, the different responses to these two compounds are produced in the brains of many mammals; the physiological systems affected must therefore be common to many species. For a detailed comparison of the toxicity of triethyltin and trimethyltin see Aldridge & Brown (1988).

7.13   Cell Death (Necrosis and Apoptosis)

The balance between cell populations in an organism is controlled by regulating the rate of cell division, differentiation and death of particular cells. Since the early days of cellular pathology cell death has been thought to be an entirely degenerative phenomenon produced by injury (necrosis) but a new concept – apoptosis – involving a more positive mechanism for a biologically and genetically programmed cell death is also now accepted (Wyllie *et al.*, 1980, 1984; Wyllie, 1992). There are two distinctive patterns of morphological change when a cell dies. One consists of swelling before rupture of plasma and organelle membranes, dissolution of organised structure, an early loss of soluble proteins such as lactic dehydrogenase from the cytoplasm with the loss of cell viability shown by the passage of vital dyes into the cell. This is cell injury in which vital metabolic systems are disrupted, e.g. loss of available ATP, and has been termed coagulative necrosis and typically affects groups rather than single cells and evokes inflammatory processes. The other morphological pattern involves condensation of the cell (shrinkage) with maintenance of cell integrity and the formation of surface protuberances (blebbing). These blebs separate as membrane-bound globules which are rapidly phagocytosed and digested by neighbouring cells without inflammation. This type of cell death was first called shrinkage necrosis but is now, with its wider involvement in normal processes of health, called apoptosis. The significance of apoptosis is much wider than cell death caused by exposure to chemicals and involves many physiological processes including differentiation, immune systems, metamorphosis and carcinogenesis (Collins & Rivas, 1993; Cohen *et al.*, 1995).

Perturbation of calcium (Ca^{2+}) homeostasis is a key and perhaps common event in cytotoxicity. It has long been known that calcium accumulates in necrotic tissue and that early disruption of intracellular $[Ca^{2+}]$ is frequently associated with cell injury and death (Carafoli, 1987; Orrenius *et al.*, 1989, 1992; Schanne *et al.*, 1979; Komulainen & Bondy, 1988). Current thinking is that apoptosis involves the target cell being active in its own destruction, a form of cell suicide. The most compelling evidence for this hypothesis is that in certain cells such as thymocytes apoptosis requires the biosynthesis of macromolecules; an early paper provided evidence that cell death is delayed or prevented by inhibitors of protein or messenger RNA synthesis (Lieberman *et al.*, 1970; Farber, 1971). This view may be summarised:

> It appears that cell damage induced in the intestinal crypt epithelium by these three agents (cytosine arabinoside, nitrogen mustard, X-irradiation) is an active, rather than passive, process and is due to a metabolic reaction of the cells to some preceding biochemical lesion and not to the biochemical lesion *per se*. Their reaction would appear to be dependent upon new protein formation and perhaps akin to enzyme induction.

Many aspects of the process are as yet unclear but the currently accepted working hypothesis is shown in Figure 7.14. The biosynthesis of the protein induced by the stimulus is thought to be involved in a controlled rise in intracellular Ca^{2+} which activates a Ca^{2+}-dependent endonuclease. This enzyme cleaves DNA into fragments of 180–200 base pairs which may be separated on agarose gel electrophoresis to show a characteristic 'DNA ladder' (Cohen & Duke, 1984).

Calcium is an activator of many enzymes (proteases, phospholipase) and which can disrupt normal cell function. Current research is examining the necessity of each step in the order shown in Figure 7.14: it has not yet been established how far this will explain

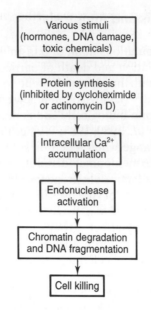

Figure 7.14   Current hypothesis for the pathway of programmed cell death (apoptosis)

chemically induced injuries and death in many different cells though there seems little doubt that some involve the programmed system (McConkey *et al.*, 1988; 1989; Orrenius *et al.*, 1992). Current questions under investigation are:

1   Is this scheme applicable to many chemicals which cause cell death *in vivo*?
2   Is this scheme limited to certain cell types?
3   Which intoxicants induce the synthesis of macromolecules?
4   What is the relevance of experimental findings on cells *in vitro* to *in vivo* toxicity?

Some recent papers are beginning to explore these questions (Shen *et al.*, 1992; Raffray *et al.*, 1993; Corcoran *et al.*, 1994).

7.14   Mutation and Carcinogenesis

Mutation is a permanent transmissible change in the genetic material, usually in a single gene, while cancer is a local, uncontrolled cell division. These simple definitions hide the complexity of the mechanisms whereby cancer is caused by chemicals.

   At the moment of human conception the twenty-three chromosomes of the ovum fuse with the twenty-three donated by a single sperm. The genetic material of this primary cell, the zygote, consists of the forty-six chromosomes comprising the double stranded helical polymer DNA. This DNA contains all the information necessary to ensure growth, differentiation, control of growth and function of the cells which make up the whole organism. After five divisions, the resultant thirty-two cells divide and the process of differentiation begins as the DNA of the differing cells are switched on to produce many different proteins. These embryonic tissues contain cells which will not only perform different functions but will be able, at differing times (in the foetus, neonate and later) to switch off or suppress the further division of some cells. Each cell in the body possesses the whole genome and by the adult stage almost all of the genome is suppressed. Thus we have a finely tuned internal mechanism to ensure that the number of cells within many tissues will remain constant. This cell 'steady state' is regulated by growth factors. The rate at which cells carry out their functions may be up- or down-regulated by messages carried from one tissue to another by hormones.

In chemical carcinogenesis stimuli from outside the organism affect these finely controlled systems so as to allow uncontrolled growth, i.e. mitosis after cell transformation. The tumours may be located in particular tissues and may start from one cell; the tumours may cover a huge range of properties ranging from slow-growing and self-contained (benign) to rapidly growing and invasive in the original tissue and in other parts of the body (malignant). Thus any mechanism of carcinogenesis must take account of many possible influences on the processes involved in the complex homeostasis of the organism which might be changed by modification of DNA.

DNA is the target for most carcinogens. After many years of research and particularly studies on the nitrosamines it is now accepted that compounds which are electrophilic or are bioactivated to electrophilic reagents interact with the many nucleophiles in biological tissues including DNA. Reaction occurs at a variety of bases in different positions in the genome; the most frequent modified base is at the N^7-position of guanine although better correlations with an ability to induce cancer in mammals is reaction in the O^6-position. Such modified bases may be repaired but if the cell divides before repair or if an error occurs in the repair process then a change in the genome is fixed, i.e. a mutation. Many mutations are lethal and some are biologically irrelevant, but others become a cell line which develops into a tumour or neoplasm. The concept that such reactions of electrophiles with DNA may initiate mutation(s) which are the starting point for the development of cancer is the basis for the Ames *in vitro* test (see Chapter 10, section 10.5).

There are a significant number of chemicals which are not mutagenic in the Ames test or in other short-term tests which, nevertheless, are carcinogenic in rodents. It seems possible that these substances influence systems within the biological cascade leading from DNA modification to mutation to neoplasm. For DNA modification to occur the electrophilic chemical must enter the cell which subsequently mutates, for non-genotoxic carcinogenesis the chemical may not be in the mutating cell but be an inducer in cells of other tissues which influence the behaviour of the mutated cell. Thus while 'complete' and active electrophilic carcinogens are relatively easy to detect and are almost certainly a hazard to humans, such decisions about non-genotoxic chemicals carcinogenic to rodents are difficult to make: they may have quite different dose–response relationships and also be species specific (Purchase, 1994; Ashby & Paton, 1993). Thus the relevance of positive results from rodent studies to human hazard is as yet unresolved. In Table 7.4 are listed thirty agents carcinogenic to humans (see Vainio *et al.*, 1991; Doll & Peto, 1981), the target organs and a 'structural alert'. This alert is based on chemical structure–activity (ability to react with DNA or be bioactivated to an active chemical) relationships built up by years of experience and particularly with the substrate pattern of bioactivating systems in mammals (see Chapter 6; Tennant & Ashby, 1991). In retrospect, of the thirty compounds twenty-two could have been recognised by the structural alert system. The eight remaining non-alerting chemicals are five oestrogen/contraceptive regimes, diethylstilboestrol and cyclosporin; the carcinogenicity of benzene remains a problem (Ashby & Paton, 1993). The latter compounds, neglecting benzene, act in the hormone field with the exception of cyclosporin which is an immunosuppressant. While these results are reassuring for electrophilic reagents the mechanism of non-genotoxic carcinogens is an urgent problem.

Carcinogenesis is a rare cellular event (Berenblum, 1974). In this context there are many unanswered questions about the primary mutation caused by the modification of DNA, e.g. how many different 'potentially carcinogenic mutations' take place, does

Table 7.4 Established human carcinogens, their target organ and relationship to a structural alert

Carcinogenic agent	Target organ (suspected) in humans	Structural alert (+ or −)
Aflatoxins	Liver (lung)	+
4-Aminobiphenyl	Bladder	+
Arsenic, arsenicals	Lung, skin	+
Azathioprine	Lymphatic system, mesenchyma, hepatobiliary system, skin	+
Benzene	Haematopoietic system	−
Benzidine	Bladder	+
N,N-bis(2-chlorethyl) -2-naphthylamine (chlornaphazine)	Bladder	+
Bis(chloromethyl)ether and chloromethyl methyl ether	Lung	+
1,4-butanediol dimethane sulphonate (myleran)	Haematopoietic system	+
Chlorambucil	Haematopoietic system	+
1-(2-chloroethyl)-3-(4-methylcyclohexyl) -1-nitrosourea	Haematopoietic system	+
Chromium(VI) compounds	Lung (nasal cavity)	+
Cyclosporin	Lymphatic system	−
Cyclophosphamide	Bladder, haematopoietic system	+
Diethylstilboestrol	Cervix/vagina, breast,testis (uterus)	−
Melphalan	Haematopoietic system	+
8-Methoxypsoralen (methoxsalen) plus UV	Skin	+
Combined chemotherapy with alkylating agents	Haematopoietic system	+
Sulphur mustard gas	Pharynx, larynx, lung	+
2-Naphthylamine	Bladder, (liver)	+
Nickel compounds	Nasal cavity, lung	+
Oestrogen replacement therapy	Uterus (breast)	−
Oestrogens(non-steroidal)	Cervix/vagina, breast, testis (uterus)	−
Oestrogens (steroidal)	Uterus (breast)	−
Oral contraceptives (combined)	Liver	−
Oral contraceptives (sequential)	Uterus	−
Radon and its decay products	Lung	+
Thiotepa	Haematopoietic system	+
Treosulphan	Haematopoietic system	+
Vinyl chloride	Liver, blood vessels (brain, lung, lymphatic system)	+

Note: The first two columns are taken from Vainio *et al.*, 1991 and are a summary from International Agency for Research in Cancer (IARC) databases. Included in the list are defined chemicals but others less defined have been omitted, e.g. alcoholic beverages, furniture and cabinet-making, asbestos, etc. The structural alert data are taken from Ashby & Paton 1993.

the reaction with bases in DNA take place at particular reactive hotspots or does a 'fruitful' reaction occur as a statistical event in a few cells out of many? Current research on activated oncogenes may supply some of the answers (Bishop, 1991; Cohen & Ellwein, 1991).

It would be expected that if changes in DNA were fixed in the sperm after exposure to chemicals or in the developing ovum then changes might be seen in the progeny after conception. Experimental evidence is accumulating that male-mediated abnormalities in the progeny can be found (Anderson, 1990) as well as increases in tumour incidence in subsequent generations. Less work has been done on female-mediated abnormalities due to chemicals although epidemiological findings suggest that they do occur.

Dose–response relationships, *in vitro* tests for carcinogenic potential and bio-monitoring for exposure to carcinogens are considered in Chapters 8, 9, 10 and 11 respectively.

7.15   Immunotoxicity

The function of the adaptive immune system which has evolved in vertebrates is to recognise and subsequently destroy foreign and potentially harmful antigens. This confers the ability to resist infections and probably to interfere in pathways leading to malignancy. Various congenital defects in the immune system and the use of immuno-suppressive drugs result in an increased susceptibility to infection and a higher risk of some forms of cancer. It follows that the potential exists for selective perturbation by chemicals of one or more steps in the immune system and this may result in primary or secondary consequences leading to ill health. The immune system exists and has evolved to ensure homeostasis. Whatever is the response to intoxicants it is not for the benefit of the organism, and natural exogenous and synthetic chemicals interact with components of the immune system if they are 'complementary' in the sense that they can interact with one another.

Natural and non-specific defence mechanisms such as phagocytic cells exist to promote resistance to disease. The important features of the adaptive immune system are memory, specificity and capacity to distinguish between self and non-self; lymphocytes play a central role. Lymphocytes are clonally distributed and each clone possesses a unique membrane receptor for antigen (memory). Recognition of an antigen induces cell division resulting in expansion of the clone. A proportion of such lymphocytes differentiate into effector cells to eliminate the antigen, and the remainder provide an increased pool of specific antigen-sensitive lymphocytes that can bring about a quicker and more aggressive response following exposure to the same antigen.

In addition to the complexity of the clonal distribution there are two classes of lymphocytes: T- and B-cells. B-cells differentiate in lymphoid organs (spleen, lymph nodes, lymphoid tissue in the intestinal, respiratory and urogenital tracts) into plasma cells which produce large amounts of antibody with a molecular specificity identical to the membrane antigen receptor expressed in the stimulated lymphocyte. These antibodies are important in host resistance to external bacterial infections.

Antigen is recognised by T-lymphocytes only if it is presented on the surface of another cell; they are then stimulated to divide in the thymus into cells able to recognise and lyse infected host cells. Other T-cells can be induced which promote (T helper/inducer) and regulate (T killer/suppressor) immune responses. The adaptive immune system is therefore highly complex and stable owing to a variety of checks and balances.

When considering the relevance of this system to interactions with exogenous chemicals the concept of self and non-self is crucial. Interaction of chemicals with soluble and membrane macromolecules (often protein) may convert accepted-as-self (no response) to a modified constituent recognised-as-foreign (antigen). After recognition there are three main types of response with undesirable consequences to the host (Figure 7.15):

1 Allergic (hypersensitivity).
2 Autoimmunity (disposal of normal and essential components).
3 Immunosuppression (decrease of resistance to invading pathogens).

In allergy the adverse response is restricted to the offending exogenous chemical agent, whereas in chemical-induced autoimmunity the adverse response is not so restricted but involves responses directed at self antigens also. In both cases there are strong influences of genetic factors predisposing to specific responses to a chemical (via an antigen derived from it). Sometimes the antigen formed by reaction of the chemical with a normal constituent is the direct cause of the disease or malfunction (immune toxicity) and sometimes the immune response is secondary to the primary damage caused by the chemical (immune pathology). In the latter case the primary damage may be to the whole population but then genetic factors will determine whether the secondary response occurs in one subpopulation. Immunosuppression (as required for tissue transplantation) can be brought about by a variety of mechanisms but that most frequently studied involves toxic effects in the thymus with little influence of genetic factors. When immunosuppression occurs an important factor to incorporate into

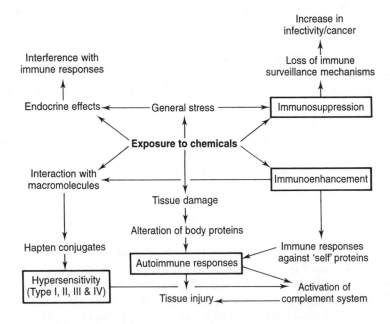

Figure 7.15 Responses of the immune system to exposure to some chemicals. (*Source*: Zelikoff *et al.*, 1994)

predictions of its relevance to human health is the normal capacity of the system, i.e. its immunological reserve.

The reactions of chemicals with the immune system obey the normal rules for many of the stages in toxicity, e.g. exposure, delivery and especially reactions which detoxify or bioactivate. Covalent interaction with macromolecules is common but not exclusively involved in the formation of antigen.

It is beyond the scope of this volume to elaborate on the clinical consequences following recognition of an antigen (in the context of exposure to chemicals, a conversion of a self protein to a non-self or abnormal protein). The clinical consequences range from the nuisance of some mild skin reactions to some serious diseases (autoimmune) such as systemic lupus erythematosus (SLE), mysthenia gravis and so on. The above short account of the properties of the main components of the immune system and the clinical consequences and classification of its abnormal action or inaction should be supplemented by other texts (Roitt *et al.*, 1989; Gleichmann *et al.*, 1989; Dean *et al.*, 1986).

Many substances cause hypersensitivity of the lung, skin and gastro-intestinal tract (Luster & Dean, 1982; Baer *et al.*, 1973) and others induce autoimmune reactions (Ahlstedt *et al.*, 1980; Gleichmann *et al.*, 1989). All originate from exposure of self-protein to a chemical or its bioactivated metabolite (hapten); the modified protein is then recognised as different by a proportion of the population of humans or animals. The relation between the chemical nature of the hapten and the subsequent immunogenicity of the modified protein or the immunogenicity of different proteins modified by the same hapten is not known. The site of reaction must be important, i.e. is it on the surface and are products of reactions ignored when the modified group such as a catalytic centre is buried within the protein structure?

Often it is thought that allergic and autoimmune responses show no dose–response relationships. Dose–response studies reveal the existence of two populations, one sensitive and one resistant. The subsequently highly sensitive population will be less sensitive on the first exposure and have a dose–response for the induction process. The induced expansion of the lymphocyte clone leads to an enhanced response on subsequent exposure which will also have a dose–response relationship to a range of much reduced concentrations.

Immunosuppression is brought about by chemical toxicity to an essential component of immune system (Luster *et al.*, 1987; Gleichmann *et al.*, 1989). Dialkyltin compounds cause thymus atrophy in rats. Administration by mouth in the diet or by injection causes a decrease in thymus weight and in other 'immune organs' such as the spleen, popliteal lymph node, etc. (Seinen & Willems, 1976; Seinen *et al.*, 1977a; Figure 7.16). After a single dose the thymus loses weight but then recovers rather rapidly. The most active compounds are di-*n*-octyl and di-*n*-butyltin. However, lyphoid atrophy did not occur in mice, guinea pigs or Japanese quail fed with these compounds (Seinen *et al.*, 1977a). Incubation of rat thymocytes with di-*n*-butyltin caused a marked decrease in their viability, but mouse, guinea pig and human thymocytes were unaffected by higher concentrations. Dialkyltins are therefore selectively cytotoxic to thymocytes and other T-cell-dependent lymphoid tissue and, as a consequence, cause a suppression of several indicators of thymus-dependent immunity (Seinen *et al.*, 1977b). T-cell maturation (thymocyte differentiation) proceeds through several stages which are characterised by various CD (cell differentiation) markers. Recent studies have established that di-*n*-butyltin exerts a specific antiproliferative effect on a subset of immature thymoblasts (Pieters *et al.*, 1992; Snoeij *et al.*, 1988). The relevance of these observations to exposure

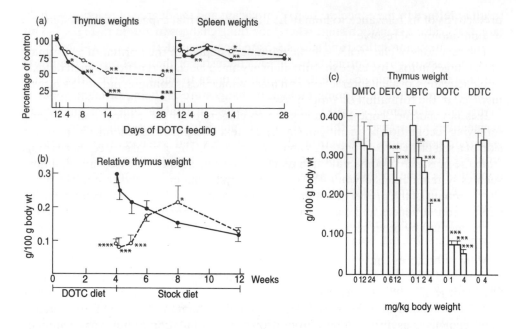

Figure 7.16 The influence of dialkyltin compounds on thymus weight. The tin dichlorides are: DMTC, dimethyl; DETC, diethyl; DBTC, di *n*-butyl; DOTC, di *n*-octyl. DDTB is di *n*-dodecyl tin dibromide. For (a) ---○---, 50 ppm; —●—, 150 ppm. For (b) —●—, diet only; ---○---, 150 ppm. For (c) Each mg/kg body weight was injected intravenously each day for five days. For statistical significance, * P<0.05, ** P<0.01, *** P<0.001 (*Sources*: Seinen & Willems, 1976, and Seinen *et al.*, 1977a)

of humans to dialkyltins is not clear. In addition to their as yet unknown sensitivity is the unknown immunological reserve of humans which may differ in different age groups.

Both TCDD (2,3,7,8-tetrachlorodibenzo-*p*-dioxin; McConkey & Orrenius, 1989; McConkey *et al.*, 1988; Pohjanvirta *et al.*, 1989; Pohjanvirta & Tuomisto, 1994) and the metabolites of 2-methoxyethanol, 2-methoxyacetaldehyde and 2-methoxyacetic acid also cause thymus atrophy (Smialowicz *et al.*, 1991, 1993; Exon *et al.*, 1991). In view of the very different chemical structures of TCDD, 2-methoxyacetic acid and di-*n*-butyltin it seems probable that the respective mechanisms are not the same.

7.16   Discussion

Different types of toxicity in mammals classified by clinical diagnosis, morphological change or changes in physiological function are mediated by different chemically induced interactions in the target cells. Although the details of the molecular events taking place with targets in these cells, i.e. the initiating reactions, are in many cases unknown, there is little doubt that they will be found to be highly specific.

This statement is the central concept of mechanistic toxicology. The chemical events which are the initiating reactions leading to toxicity constitute the central stage in the processes from exposure to clinical signs and symptoms, and whether intoxication will result is defined by the concentration of intoxicant and the degree of reaction with the target. It is also a transition stage where one thing changes to another: stages 1–3 are chemical-intoxicant-defined and stages 3–5 are the biology-defined events (Figure 7.1). This emphasis on and contrast between the chemistry of the reactions of the intoxicant and the later biological events must not be taken to imply that the latter are not chemical events; the developing biological changes are all being brought about by changes in cell chemistry resulting from a decrease in catalytic functions, membrane permeability and transport, the steady state of physiological metabolites, etc.

Certain conclusions follow from this. If an intoxicant interacts with a chemical grouping in a macromolecule and causes a particular type of intoxication then reaction with the same grouping by another chemical will cause the same form of toxicity. However, a particular form of toxicity, e.g. peripheral axonopathy, cell death, may also be initiated by several intoxicants each reacting with a different macromolecule. Thus in the pathway from initiating reactions with targets to intoxication there can be part which is common, e.g. the same signs and symptoms of peripheral neuropathy can be produced by a variety of chemicals with different reactivities and probably reacting with different targets. It is also clear that most of the reactions of intoxicants with macromolecules do not initiate toxicity.

It is possible that sometimes more than one interaction by the same chemical is required to cause toxicity (Aldridge, 1995). These could be interactions with more than one component of one cell or possibly with a component from a different cell. In the text some examples have been mentioned when the data available indicate this possibility. A consequence of this hypothesis is that the chemical would have to have unusual properties; the probability of a comparable degree of reaction with two different components in one or two cells being caused by the same concentration of intoxicant is rather low. Such a two-target mechanism is likely to result in discontinuities in structure–response and structure–activity relationships. Carcinogenesis is a form of toxicity which probably needs several changes for a tumour to result. If we accept that tumours can originate from one cell then to accumulate several changes (?mutations) would be statistically unlikely. Accepting this view, complete carcinogens would be those which by their reactivity could cause all the necessary events to happen in one cell.

Sometimes an unexpected structure–response relationship may by further study be revealed to be a superimposition of one form of toxicity on another with discontinuities appearing when new structures are examined.

Intoxication initiated by chemical interaction with one component is analogous to a genetically inherited disease. Direct evidence that a human mutation produces an alteration in the primary structure of protein was the demonstration that haemoglobin from people with sickle cell anaemia migrated in an electric field at a different rate from normal haemoglobin (Pauling *et al.*, 1949). Later the electrophoretic abnormality was shown to arise from the substitution of glutamate by valine at a particular point in the molecule of glutamic acid in normal haemoglobin. The general ground-rules have been stated very clearly (Tatum, 1959):

1 All biochemical processes in all organisms are under genetic control.
2 These biochemical processes are resolvable into individual stepwise reactions.
3 Each biochemical reaction is under the ultimate control of a single gene.
4 Mutation of a single gene results only in an effect on the ability of the cell to carry out a single primary reaction.

When this general statement is applied to proteins other than enzymes then the analogy between mutations and the specific actions of chemicals is complete. Spontaneous mutations, besides having deleterious consequences, can also be harmless. Many substitutions of amino acids will have minimal effects on the functions of proteins. It has been stated (Galjaard, 1986) that 10–20% of congenital disorders are due to a single gene mutation and at present more than 3,400 different syndromes have been identified to be inherited according to Mendelian pattern (Stanbury *et al.*, 1983). Disease can be a consequence of mutation and can be caused by chemical intoxicants, but in both cases many of the interactions will have no direct effect on the health of the organism. However, just as some mutations are silent until the organism is challenged by some external agent (drug, chemical) so primary attacks of chemicals may cause a silent change which may potentiate the response to another chemical stimulus (see Chapter 11). Current epidemiological developments also suggest that genetic factors carry an enhanced susceptibility to cancer after initiation by DNA-damaging agents.

7.17 Summary

1   Selective toxicity denotes changes down to the cell level; specific toxicity denotes the interaction with components of the cell; dose is the internal amount or concentration of intoxicant; the dose initiating toxicity is that within the target cell.

2   Defined clinical signs or symptoms and/or biological events (selective toxicity) result from specific interaction of an intoxicant with specific molecular component(s) of particular cells (target).

3   Cell selective toxicity can be caused in several ways: (a) accumulation of chemical, directly active or only after bioactivation; (b) reaction of intoxicant with a subcellular component unique to the cell; (c) reaction of intoxicant with a component of many cells resulting in toxicity in cells vital to immediate life of the organism.

4   Specific interaction with subcellular components (targets) depend on their mutual chemistry.

5   Some types of toxicity result from secondary events after the cell-specific and primary reaction with the intoxicant.

6   Initiation of cell toxicity may need interaction with more than one target.

7   *In vivo* toxicity is determined by exposure leading to an effective target dose. *In vitro*, higher concentrations can be used and reaction with components other than the target can occur; the relevance of any *in vitro* response to the *in vivo* situation must be established.

8   An intoxicant which interacts with only one particular component at all concentrations, i.e. it is completely specific, is analogous to a genetically inherited disease.

8

Biological Consequences of Initiating Reactions with Targets

8.1   Introduction

From initiating reactions as described in Chapter 7 follow many biological consequences. These consequences may be immediate and short-lived, take some time to develop or may last a short or long time or be permanent. Some of these possibilities have been discussed in relation to clinical effects in Chapter 4 (acute or chronic intoxication).

In contrast to stages 1–3, stage 4 consists of biological events not influenced by the nature of the chemical, i.e. they are biology rather than chemical related (Figure 8.1). For example, if acetylcholinesterase activity is reduced by a wide range of chemical structures of organophosphorus compounds or carbamates then the biological consequences result from the change in the activity of the enzyme and not the particular chemical causing the change. Also, although the chemistry of a reaction with a particular target may be dissimilar, initiation of/in the same biological pathway will result in the same defined signs of poisoning and causes of death. Another example is that although beryllium, acetaminophen, carbon tetrachloride and pyrrolizidine may initiate liver necrosis by different mechanisms the consequences to the animal are the same – the loss of liver function indicated by loss of liver glycogen, changes in carbohydrate metabolism and an inability to detoxify neurotoxic ammonia by-product by conversion to urea.

New problems in toxicology often arise from the recognition that exposure leads to an unexpected pattern of clinical signs; nowadays this usually arises after administration to experimental animals in toxicity testing procedures. Sometimes, however, exposure of humans result in such an awareness. In a pilot plant using dimethylnitrosamine, cirrhosis of the liver was diagnosed in the few workers exposed. The medical practitioner who noticed this considered it unusual since the men were young and had no history of excessive consumption of alcohol. Follow-up by experimental research resulted in the discovery that dimethylnitrosamine causes not only liver necrosis but is also a potent carcinogen for the liver and kidney (Magee & Barnes, 1967).

Although for a given species it is possible to determine an exposure–response relationship (i.e orally administered chemical and defined clinical response), it is only when the relation between exposure delivery (dose) and primary interaction at the cell level

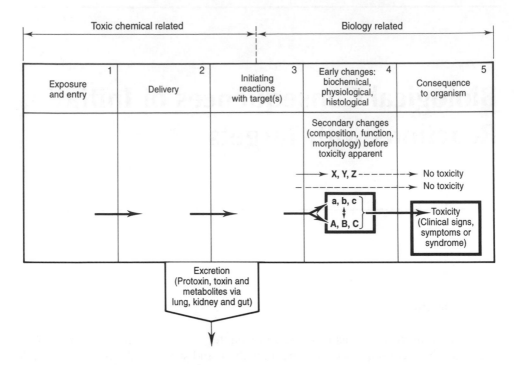

Figure 8.1 Diagrammatic representation of stages 4 and 5, the biological and clinical consequences of initiating reaction(s) with targets (stage 3; see legend to Figure 2.1)

is better understood that early indicators of biological change can be devised; often, then a more rational attempt to predict from animal to humans and to estimate the risk of exposure becomes possible.

In the examples to follow a range of different tissues and cell types and different types of toxicity are described together with recovery, repair and some therapeutic measures. In most cases of toxicity caused by chemicals recovery follows a predictable course; in some the first response is followed by other secondary events due often to recruitment of other cells into the damaged tissue. Stages 4 and 5 cover a huge area of biology, i.e. the perturbations of homeostatic mechanisms, recovery and repair mechanisms and the various responses in different tissues to functional deficits and cell death. The examples are chosen to illustrate some of the principles involved. For the histopathological methods, both technical and diagnostic, other sources must be consulted. The aim is to emphasise the continuum between initiating interactions and the final expression of toxicity and to show how, with the development of knowledge of the molecular composition of cells, measurements can be made to indicate the origin and extent of the perturbations.

8.2 Functional without Morphological Change: Perturbation of the Cellular Utilisation of Oxygen

Many substances influence the utilisation of oxygen for cellular metabolism and its associated energy conservation process (section 7.2 and Figure 7.2). Since the stages of electron transport are tightly coupled to the synthesis of ATP, similar responses follow intoxicants which interact with several targets in the energy conservation system. After exposure to cyanide in sufficient amount to inhibit cytochrome oxidase, the terminal step of electron transport, death is rapid and the diagnostic feature is that the venous blood contains unusually high concentrations of oxyhaemoglobin indicating a block in cellular utilisation of oxygen (see section 4.2). The tissues from which the signs of poisoning originate are those with a high oxygen uptake and performing a function immediately essential for life, i.e the heart and the brain. Cardiac irregularities are often seen but the main cause of death is respiratory arrest of central origin. For non-fatal and lower exposure the temperature of the animal falls. Most of the substances such as cyanide, azide, rotenone, oligomycin and 5-coordinate tin compounds form reversible complexes with the relevant components of the system and, as the compound is excreted or metabolised to less toxic compounds, recovery will be complete.

Treatment of cyanide poisoning is intended to reduce the concentration of circulating hydrocyanic acid and cyanide ion. Methaemoglobin has a higher affinity for cyanide than cytochrome oxidase and conversion of a proportion of the haemoglobin to this ferric form of haemoglobin by the injection of sodium nitrite produces a large concentration of alternative binding sites and reduces the concentration of circulating cyanide sufficiently to save life. Regeneration of haemoglobin takes place by erythrocyte reductase systems. Cyanide is also converted to the non-toxic thiocyanate by the enzyme rhodanese utilising thiosulphate as the sulphur donor. This enzyme is normally not fully saturated with thiosulphate but is sufficiently active to detoxify both endogenous cyanide and the low concentration absorbed from cigarette smoke. Injection of sodium thiosulphate increases the rate of detoxification of exogenous cyanide. Such treatments often work because the difference between a lethal concentration of cyanide in the blood and one compatible with survival is small; a small dissociation of the cytochrome oxidase/cyanide complex will save life.

Other substances such as the aromatic and acidic phenols uncouple the uptake of oxygen from the synthesis of ATP. These substances act as proton carriers discharging the proton gradient necessary for ATP synthesis (Mitchell's chemiosmotic theory). Thus the normal ratio of ATP synthesised to oxygen consumed (P/O ratio) in mitochondria is 3 whereas in the presence of, for example,the herbicide 2,4-dinitro-*o*-cresol, this ratio decreases in *in vitro* experiments with increasing concentrations to near zero. *In vivo*, the system is so tightly geared to the maintenance of the ATP content of the cell that oxygen utilisation increases and ATP concentrations are maintained even though synthesised with less efficiency; much of the energy of oxidation is dispersed as heat and the signs and symptoms are due to excessive heat production. After exposure of humans to dinitro-*o*-cresol the symptoms include nausea, gastric upset, restlessness, sensation of heat, flushed skin, sweating, rapid respiration, tachycardia, fever accompanied by a high temperature followed by cyanosis, collapse and death. Less but more prolonged exposure causes fatigue, restlessness, anxiety, excessive sweating and unusual thirst. In experimental animals mitochondria isolated from rats exposed to 2,4-dinitro-*o*-cresol are partially uncoupled, i.e. the P/O ratio is less than the controls. The signs indicate an increased metabolic rate and if heat production exceeds the capacity for heat loss then fatal hyperthermia can occur. No treatment is available to reduce the circulating concentration of dinitro-*o*-cresol; the only treatment for the biological effects are measures to reduce the temperature (ice baths) and to replace the excessive fluid loss due to sweating.

8.3   Functional without Morphological Change: Perturbation of the Cholinergic Transmitter System

The mechanism of reaction of organophosphorus compounds and esters of carbamic acids with the cholinesterases has been discussed (see section 7.5). The reduction of the ability of acetylcholinesterase to remove the released acetylcholine after a nerve impulse results in signs due to prolonged interaction of acetylcholine with muscurinic or nicotinic receptors. After exposure the concentration of acetylcholine rises in all parts of the nervous system and the effects seen are a consequence of this (Table 8.1). The organophosphorus compounds and carbamates in common use as pesticides are lipophilic and are not positively charged so that they penetrate to all parts of the nervous system. Some drugs such as the positively charged prostigmine have restricted access to the nervous system and the signs and symptoms reflect this. The best monitor of exposure relevant to toxicity is the erythrocyte cholinesterase (see section 11.6); 50% inhibition can be tolerated without overt signs of poisoning (latent poisoning). With 50–80% inhibition the patient can walk but complains of fatigue, headache, dizziness, nausea, numbness, sweating, tightness in the chest and salivation and sometimes vomiting, abdominal cramps, diarrhoea (mild poisoning). With 80–90% inhibition the patient cannot walk, is weak, has difficulty in talking, and muscle fasciculations and miosis are seen (moderate poisoning). With 90% or more inhibition the patient may become unconscious, have marked miosis, muscle fasciculations, flaccid paralysis, secretions from mouth and nose, and respiratory difficulties (severe poisoning).

Table 8.1   Cholinergic manifestations of organophosphorus poisoning

Anatomical site	Signs and symptoms
Muscarinic effects	
Bronchial tree	Tightness of chest, wheezing suggestive of bronchoconstriction, rhinitis, dyspnea, increased bronchial secretion. cough, pulmonary oedema, cyanosis
Gastro-intestinal	Nausea, vomiting, abdominal tightness and cramps, diarrhoea, faecal incontinence
Sweat glands	Increased sweating
Salivary glands	Increased salivation
Lacrimal glands	Increased lacrimation
Cardiovascular	Bradycardia, fall in blood pressure, ventricular tachycardia
Eyes	Miosis (contraction of pupils), blurring of vision
Bladder	Urinary incontinence
Nicotinic effects	
Striated muscle	Muscle twitching, fasciculation, cramp, weakness including muscles of respiration
Sympathetic ganglia	Pallor, tachycardia, elevation of blood pressure, hyperglycaemia

Central nervous effects

These are various and include giddiness, anxiety, excessive dreaming or nightmare, headache, tremor, apathy and depression, difficulty in concentrating, slurred speech and ataxia. With severe poisoning there may be a depression of the respiratory and circulatory centres with dyspnea and cyanosis

All stages of poisoning from mild to severe should receive medical treatment. For mild poisoning an anticholinergic such as atropine to antagonise the action of the raised concentration of acetylcholine should be adequate. For moderate to severe poisoning the use of therapeutic oximes is necessary to reactivate the inhibited cholinesterase (see section 7.5 and Figure 7.9). The dosage of atropine may have to be repeated and the patients continuously titrated to the disappearance of sweating and salivation. Other anticholinergics with better access to the central nervous system may be required. For some intoxicants in this class central convulsions occur; in such cases a benzodiazepine such as diazepam is useful, but in very severe cases artificial respiration may be required.

A special prophylactic procedure for protection against chemical warfare agents has been developed. Inhibition of acetylcholinesterase up to 50% can be tolerated. Predosage of a carbamate, prostigmine, to produce less than 50% carbamylated acetylcholinesterase will protect against a dose of organophosphorus agent which would normally be fatal. The mechanism is based on the fact that survival depends on possessing little more than 10% of normal acetylcholinesterase activity. Carbamylated enzyme is unstable and as soon as more enzyme is phosphorylated the steady state readjusts and some of the carbamylated cholinesterase spontaneously reactivates. At the same time the organophosphorus compound is rapidly detoxified (Aldridge, 1980, 1989; Ballantyne & Marrs, 1992; Leadbeater, 1988).

The actions of most organophosphorus compounds are explained by inhibition of either acetylcholinesterase or neuropathy target esterase (delayed neuropathy; see sections 7.6 and 8.4). Neither causes early cell death. In a recent report, soman (pinacolyl methyl phosphonofluoridate, a chemical warfare agent) has been shown to cause neuronal necrosis in selected areas of the central nervous system – bilateral symmetrical lesions in the piriform cortex, regions of the hippocampus, frontal cortex and dorsolateral thalamic nuclei (Kadar *et al.*, 1992). This must be regarded as an unusual property of soman because organophosphorus compounds do not usually cause persistent convulsions followed by a long period of irritability with recurrent epileptic episodes. More research is required on mechanisms so that we may understand not only why soman has this property but also why others do not.

Thus, in general, anticholinesterase compounds cause a wide-ranging syndrome of toxicological signs and symptoms of poisoning because of their influence on a biological controlling mechanism involving the neurotransmitter acetylcholine. In sublethal doses recovery is complete with no residual morphological changes.

8.4 Functional without Morphological Change: Perturbation of the Voltage-dependent Sodium Channels

The T- or CS-syndromes following pyrethroid poisoning in experimental animals have been described in section 7.3; they are similar in humans (He *et al.*, 1989). The components of the syndrome for the α-cyano pyrethroid deltamethrin (see Figure 7.3) may be experimentally subdivided and associated with the measured dose in the brain. If deltamethrin is injected intraperitoneally the rate of absorption is slow enough to allow a study of groups of rats with particular signs. The order of appearance of signs, as the concentration of deltamethrin rises in the brain is salivation, tremor and choreoathetosis (Figure 8.2a; Rickard & Brodie, 1985). The concentration reaches a peak and as it decreases the writhing convulsions cease. Cyclic guanosine monophosphate (cyclic GMP) is increased in the cerebellum but not in other areas of the brain after pyrethroids

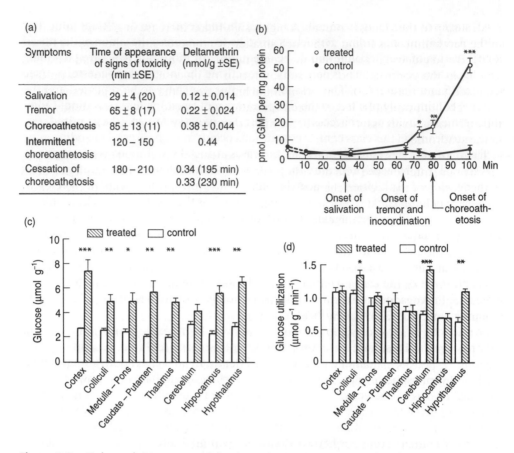

Figure 8.2 Deltamethrin concentration, signs of poisoning in rats and cyclic GMP levels in the cerebellum and the glucose content and utilisation in different areas of brain at the onset of choreoathetosis. (*Sources:* (a) and (b) from Brodie & Aldridge, 1982; levels of statistical significance: * $p < 0.01$, ** <0.005, *** <0.001. (c) and (d) from Cremer *et al.*, 1980; measurements were made at the onset of choreoathetosis after deltamethrin 40 mg/kg b.w. administered intraperitoneally; levels of statistical significance: * $p < 0.02$, ** <0.01, *** <0.001)

producing both the T- and CS-syndromes. If the above experimental procedure is used and the concentrations of cyclic GMP in the cerebellum is related to signs of poisoning, increases are only found a little before the onset of choreoathetosis and reaches a maximum of more than ten times the control (Figure 8.2b; Brodie & Aldridge, 1982). If the amount of deltamethrin administered by intraperitoneal injection is changed so that the time of appearance of the different signs of poisoning are changed then the increases in cyclic GMP are related to the appearance of choreoathetosis and not to the time. It has therefore been concluded that the increase in cyclic GMP is a secondary phenomenon with deltamethrin acting as a locomotor stimulant rather than as a convulsant acting in the central nervous system.

The glucose content of areas of rat brain changes after the administration of deltamethrin and at the onset of spontaneous writhing movements. Significant increases of glucose content occur in most areas with the exception of the cerebellum (Figure 8.2c; Cremer *et al.*, 1980). Glucose utilisation measured at the same time had an inverse relationship to the glucose content. A highly significant increase in glucose utilisation in the cerebellum was found with much smaller or no increase in other areas (Figure 8.2d). Blood glucose is also rather markedly raised: 13.28 μmol/g compared with 8.47 μmol/g in the controls. The high concentration of glucose in the blood would be expected to increase its concentration in the brain; this is the case for all areas except the cerebellum which, by its enhanced utilisation of glucose, lowers the steady state; the high utilisation is associated with the high concentration of cyclic GMP at this stage in the syndrome.

These experiments illustrate the complex consequences of perturbation of one activity in the brain. Interference with the voltage-dependent sodium channels result in a delay in the closing of the sodium channel activation gate and a prolongation of the sodium tail current (Figure 7.3). This causes, instead of a single nerve impulse, a long train of impulses in many nerves, the extent of which depends on the traffic in the particular areas. In terms of muscular activity, which is excessive in severe poisoning by both the T-class or the CS-class of pyrethroid, the utilisation of body energy sources becomes so high that the animals may become moribund through exhaustion. Rapid and quantitatively large changes of metabolism of different areas of the brain which normally occur depending on the external input to the sense organs may now be studied by positron emission tomography (PET) and magnetic resonance imaging techniques. Location of primary/secondary etc. sites of action of intoxicants on the brain may also become easier. Thus by the use of selective probes, a further understanding of the complex responses in the brain may be achieved. If this can be linked to dose–response relationships then animal data may be more easily used to predict the same relationships in humans.

8.5 Cell Death: Liver and Lung Damage and Fibrosis

Many chemicals cause necrosis of liver cells. The hepatocytes affected can be a small isolated group of parenchymal cells (focal necrosis), in zones (centrilobular, midzonal or periportal) or almost all cells in a lobule. There is significant heterogeneity in hepatocytes in different areas particularly in their content of drug processing systems (cytochrome P_{450}s, epoxide hydrolase, glutathione transferase, etc.). The extent of induction of cytochrome P_{450} isozymes by, for example, phenobarbitone and 3-methylcholanthrene also differ. These differences may be significant in explaining why different agents cause more or less damage at different sites. Research on mechanisms of necrosis has implicated many different processes: bioactivation, membrane damage, alterations in hepatic blood flow, haemorrhagic necrosis, lipid peroxidation, glutathione depletion and others. The many possibilities of metabolic transformation of intoxicants has made it rather difficult to establish the time sequence of the necrotic process. There are also many examples of potentiation of hepatotoxicity of one compound by another which adds another level of complexity. For a review of the literature on toxic responses in the liver see Plaa (1986).

Many hepatotoxins cause an accumulation of abnormal amounts of lipid (fatty liver). The increase in lipid, mainly triglyceride, results from an imbalance between the rate of synthesis and rate of release from the parenchymal cells. Although it is a common response to exposure to many intoxicants which cause hepatocyte necrosis, fatty liver is not an obligatory step, e.g. ethionine and cycloheximide cause fatty liver but no necrosis.

Administration of large amounts of intoxicants to animals and humans may cause massive necrosis followed by liver failure and death, but with lower exposures (e.g. to carbon tetrachloride, aflatoxin, dimethylnitrosamine and ethanol) a smaller number of cells will be affected. The remaining cells are stimulated to divide to replace those damaged but, in addition, the system concerned with structural elements of the liver are activated and by fibroblastic activity abnormal amounts of collagen are laid down. The different molecular forms of collagen normally present are all increased in concentration. Possibly in some cases there may be some deficiency in the rate of the repair systems (disposal of the damaged cells and cell division to form new cells) and fibroblasts take over. The replacement of cells by collagenous scar tissue reduces the metabolic capacity of the liver. Although the liver normally has a high biological reserve, in time with repeated non-lethal doses of liver intoxicants the functional capacity is so reduced that normal metabolism cannot be maintained (Lieber, 1990).

Lung fibrosis is a relatively common response to the inhalation of particles such as asbestos, coal dust, silica, beryllium oxide, etc. which are small enough to reach the alveolar region. It also occurs following paraquat reaching the lung by the systemic route (section 7.3). In humans, the respiratory effects of ingestion of solutions of paraquat may be quite mild for the first few days. However, within a week lung function becomes abnormal and over the next few days or weeks function deteriorates and the patient may die of anoxia. Postmortem reveals a lung heavier than normal and histological examination demonstrates extensive fibrosis often with complete obliteration of the normal architecture of the lung. Human lung seems to be particularly prone to this secondary effect following the primary damage to type 2 alveolar cells. The extent of collagen synthesis is different in different species: rats, mouse, dogs and monkeys can provide an experimental model for fibrosis following paraquat but the guinea pig and hamster are unsuitable (Murray & Gibson, 1972; Smith & Nemery, 1986). The mechanism of the excessive laying down of collagen and the reasons for the species differences in this response to pneumo-intoxicants which damage the alveolar cells are not understood. The view that the fibrosis is part of the reparative process which the lung undergoes as a consequence of extensive lung damage (Smith & Heath, 1976) is not an adequate explanation of the species differences; also lung damage caused by different intoxicants results in different levels of fibrosis. It has been suggested that the recruitment of fibroblasts and the subsequent synthesis of collagen in the interstitium requires two insults: the first to damage the alveolar cells and the second to slow down cell division of type 2 cells and thus their subsequent transformation to type 1 cells (Adamson *et al.*, 1977; Haschek & Witschi, 1979).

Fibrosis is, therefore, an abnormal deposition of collagen following tissue damage. Pulmonary fibrosis can be caused by a variety of toxic agents, both bloodborne and airborne. Although tissue damage is a prerequisite for fibrosis, little is known of the early events which progress to a fibrotic lesion instead of normal repair. Following acute lung injury fibrosis usually occurs when the initial lesion involves alveolar epithelial damage and the subsequent development of alveolitis. For chronic lung injury the mechanism of fibrosis is complex but a prolonged insult may be essential for both acute and chronic exposure (Smith *et al.*, 1986).

8.6 Cell Death: Neuronal Necrosis in Specific Areas of the Brain

After the administration of trimethyltin, histological examination shows that a pathological end-point is bilateral and symmetrical damage in neurones of the hippocampus, pyriform cortex, amygdaloid cortex, neocortex and the cerebellar Purkinje cells (Brown *et al.*, 1979, 1984). For a variety of exposure protocols of single or divided oral administration over periods of up to four weeks, the distribution of dead neurones in the hippocampus was not uniform and was most severe in the fascia dentata, less in other regions, and the Sommer sector was largely spared. In the neighbouring regions reactive astrocytes are seen as a response to the neuronal necrosis, and at late stages the areas where neurones were lost becomes shrunken. This distribution of lesions is very similar in the mouse (Chang *et al.*, 1982, 1983), rat (Brown *et al.*, 1979; Bouldin *et al.*, 1981) and in hamsters, gerbils and marmasets (Brown *et al.*, 1984). After an episode of poisoning (probably to a mixture of tetramethyltin, trimethyltin chloride and dimethyltin chloride) one of six men exposed died and neuronal necrosis was seen in the amygdaloid nuclei and in cerebellar Purkinje cells. These end-point pathology results define the cellular selectivity in the brain for a compound which does not appear to be selectively distributed.

The time course (pathokinetics) in the rat of the development of the lesions after administration of 10 mg/kg b.w. trimethyltin chloride by gastric intubation followed by electron microscopy in perfused fixed material indicates the following sequence (Brown *et al.*, 1979, 1984): (1) 1–5 h, no difference compared with control material; (2) 12 h, accumulation of condensed (?proteinacious) material between the smooth endoplasmic reticulum tubular cisterns possibly derived from newly synthesised protein; (3) 24 h, dense bodies in many regions often associated with rough endoplasmic reticulum, polyribosomes and Golgi formations containing vacuoles. The vacuolation of the Golgi apparatus in the hippocampus, cortical pyramidal neurons and in large sensory ganglion cells was intense in the plane of section and was transformed into a cluster of vacuoles; (4) 48 h, dense bodies and autophagosomes are the dominant feature in the hippocampus, neocortex, pyriform cortex and amygdaloid nucleus and are diffusely distributed throughout the cell extending into the dendrites. Rough endoplasmic reticulum and polyribosomes were lost or dispersed explaining the chromolytic appearance noted in light microscopic studies. At this stage clumping of nuclear chromatin is seen, one of the first signs indicative of cell death; (5) up to 10–20 days, the number of cells affected in the different areas of the brain increases.

The time sequence of symptoms (Brown *et al.*, 1979) is, first, tremor of the head and neck in some rats (1–2 days), aggressive sparring and convulsions (3 days) and generalised body tremor (4 days). The aggression and self-mutilation (3–4 days) became so intense that the animals had to be placed in separate cages. At 18 days they could be returned to communal cages and after a short bout of mild aggression, they became quiet and the few survivors behaved normally. The neurological syndrome in humans following the four episodes of occupational exposure included specific behavioural impairment (spontaneous seizures, disorientation, insomnia, anorexia, memory and learning impairments and attacks of rage and temper alternating with bouts of depression). Both surviving humans and rats showed memory deficits.

From a study using an *in vivo* technique in free-moving rats which allows continuous monitoring of extracellular neurochemical events, it has been concluded that one component of trimethyltin-induced neurotoxicity may be a consequence of local increases in the extracellular excitotoxic amino acid glutamate (Brodie *et al.*, 1990). However, there is at present no accepted view about the primary site of attack and the relationship among the timing of the signs of poisoning, the histopathological changes, neurochemical changes and the concentration of trimethyltin in the brain is not understood. Considerable loss of neurones in the hippocampus seems to be compatible with normal behaviour as judged by general clinical examination but more detailed tests reveal abnormalities.

8.7 Cell Death: External Stimuli and Neuronal Cell Necrosis

1,3-Dinitrobenzene causes symmetrical lesions in the rat brain stem with glial swelling, vacuolation in certain brain stem nuclei associated with arteriolar haemorrhages and secondary neuronal death (Philbert *et al.*, 1987). A single injection regime produces an excessive amount of methaemoglobin (MetHb) but a modified protocol of three smaller intraperitoneal injections of 10 mg/kg 1,3-dinitrobenzene at 0, 4 and 24 h reduces MetHb levels to only 20–30% of normal. With this experimental set-up, symmetrical lesions in the inferior collicoli (auditory reflex centres), pontine tegmentum and deep cerebellar nuclei were regularly obtained. Regional blood flow was generally increased but the highest increases were in those areas susceptible to later damage (Romero *et al.*, 1991). No petechial haemorrhages were detected up to 8 h but a few appeared at 12 h and they were well developed at 24 h in all susceptible areas. Using horseradish peroxidase to detect vascular damage the same time sequence was found, and with light and electron microscopy early swelling and retraction of astroglial processes were observed at 12 h. Thus the time sequence of morphological change seems to be similar to the increases in blood flow, petechial haemorrhages, leakage of protein through the vascular bed, oedematous areas and swollen astrocytes which were all limited to the ultimately susceptible areas.

1,3-Dinitrobenzene is lipid-soluble and will distribute rapidly and penetrate most cells. The nitro group can be reduced by enzymes with nitroreductase capability (xanthine oxidase, aldehyde oxidase, microsomal NADPH-cytochrome c reductase) to reactive intermediates which can form oxidation–reduction (redox) cycles by-passing the normal energy conservation system and generating reactive oxygen species (see section 7.4 and Figure 7.4 on paraquat). The increased blood flow may be a consequence of the demand for energy in the susceptible areas and, together with the generation of reactive oxygen species, reduction of protectants and depletion of energy stores, may be the cause of the cascade of morphological change leading to neuronal death. In this hypothesis the primary effect would be the redox cycling of 1,3-dinitrobenzene (through its metabolites) in the endothelial cells and astrocytes but the hypothesis does not account for the intoxicant's selectivity for particular areas of the brain. An insight into this problem has been gained by the observation that if noise input is restricted into one ear (say the left) of a rat exposed to 1,3-dinitrobenzene the lesions in the cochlear nucleus and inferior colliculus supplied by this ear were much less than in those supplied by the right ear, i.e. dinitrobenzene lesions in rats with one ear protected from noise are unsymmetrical, with hearing loss on the unprotected side (Ray *et al.*, 1992).

This mechanism leads to the concept of metabolic vulnerability as a facet of the selective vulnerability to chemicals of cells of the nervous system. The brain is therefore an active rather than a passive target for some toxic chemicals, i.e. the functional state of the brain even in the normal range can determine its sensitivity. The significance of this for a noisy working environment contaminated by some chemicals is obvious. Thus the mechanism of the selective neuronal loss caused by 1,3-dinitrobenzene is postulated to involve several steps and factors: (1) dose of 1,3-dinitrobenzene in endothelial cells and astrocytes; (2) metabolism of 1,3-dinitrobenzene; (3) involvement of a metabolite in redox cycling; (4) metabolic insufficiency/generation of reactive oxygen species; (5) endothelial and glial cell damage; (6) neuronal death. It has been suggested (Romero *et al.*, 1991; Ray *et al.*, 1992) that other intoxicants of the nervous system may follow the same pathogenetic pathway but not necessarily start with the same initiating reaction, e.g. mononitrobenzene (Morgan *et al.*, 1985), misonidazole (Griffin *et al.*, 1980), metronidazole (Rogulja *et al.*, 1973), 6-aminonicotinamide (Schneider & Cervós-Navarro, 1974), 6-chloro-6-deoxyglucose (Jacobs & Ford, 1981) and acute thiamine deficiency (Collins *et al.*, 1970; Watanabe *et al.*, 1981).

1,3-Dinitrobenzene also causes selective Sertoli cell damage in the testis. Sertoli cells play a key role in controlling the development and maintenance of spermatogenesis and constitute the main functional component of the blood–testis barrier (Russell, 1980). Cell damage is isomer-specific, the 1,2- and the 1,4- isomers being ineffective (Blackburn *et al.*, 1988); neither of these isomers appears to produce metabolites which take part in redox cycling.

8.8 Axonopathy: Primary Effects on the Nerve Axon

Some organophosphorus compounds cause a mixed central/peripheral neuropathy; there is substantial evidence that this is associated with the inhibition of an esterase (NTE, neuropathy target esterase) in the nervous system (see sections 7.6 and 9.7). After a single exposure to several compounds with a low anticholinesterase/high NTE potency no initial signs of poisoning are seen and it is 10–21 days before clinical and morphological signs of axonal degeneration are seen (Lotti *et al.*, 1984; Lotti, 1992). In humans, clinical characterisation is of a flaccid paralysis of the lower limbs although in the most severe cases the upper limbs are involved. The histopathological findings have led to the definition of the disease as a central/peripheral, distal sensory/motor axonopathy similar to other neuropathies (2,5-hexanedione, section 7.8; acrylamide, section 7.7) and is a common response in many species. The degenerative lesions in the central nervous system are mainly in the spinal cord and these, as in the peripheral nervous system, occur more in the distal portions of the large diameter and long fibres than in the small short ones (see later; also Bouldin & Cavanagh, 1979a,b; Cavanagh, 1973).

Clinical signs and recovery after exposure depend on the localisation of the lesion. The site of the lesions can be manipulated experimentally by intra-arterial injection of a direct and highly active compound which is rapidly detoxified by metabolism. Such an injection of DFP (see Figure 7.5) into one leg of a cat caused a unilateral neuropathy in the injected leg. A similar injection of DFP into hens caused the expected delayed abnormalities in gait but only in the injected leg. In other experiments, 24 hours after treatment the NTE was more than 80% inhibited in the sciatic nerve of the injected leg and only about 40% in the other leg (i.e. less than the 70–80% needed for the development of neuropathy (Table 8.2). If protection was provided by local intra-arterial injection of phenylmethane sulphonyl fluoride (PMSF; see Figure 7.10) and DFP injected subcutaneously for general distribution 24 hours after the first injection then the leg treated with PMSF was normal but gait impairment was seen in the other. Bilateral injection of PMSF by the intra-arterial route protected both the peripheral nerves from morphological change but the hens developed a spastic gait due to axonopathy in the spinal cord (Caroldi *et al.*, 1984). These experiments provide strong support for the NTE hypothesis and also suggest that the

Table 8.2 Intra-arterial injection of DFP and/or PMSF into the leg of a hen and the induction of unilateral neuropathy

Compound injected (mg/kg b.w.)		NTE (% inhibition)				Ataxia (graded 0–4)	
		Brain	Spinal	Sciatic nerve			
PMSF	DFP			Injected leg	Other leg	Injected leg	Other leg
–	0.25 (i.a.)	30	33	93	33	2,1,0	0,0,0
–	0.25 (i.v.)	38	33	34 (both legs)		0,0,0	
1.0 (i.a.)	–	16	13	42	8	0,0,0	
1.0 (i.a)	1.1 (sc)	–	–	–	–	0,0,1	2,4,4
1.0 (i.v)	1.1 (sc)	–	–	–	–	4,4	

DFP = di-isopropylphosphorofluoridate; PMSF = phenylmethane sulphonyl fluoride; NTE = neuropathy target esterase; i.a. = intra-arterial injection into one leg; i.v. = intravenous injection into the wing; sc = subcutaneous injection. DFP was injected 24 h after PMSF.
Source: Data from Caroldi *et al.*, 1984.

essential degree of reaction of DFP with NTE occurs in axons and not in cell bodies; consequently NTE is probably concerned with some axonal function. Signs of poisoning differ depending on the site of inhibition of NTE; this is important because although recovery from peripheral axonopathy in long axons occurs by growth from the end of the axons towards and to their end-organs, such recovery does not happen if the lesions are in the spinal cord. It may be deduced that those affected in the Ginger Jake episode (sections 6.3.3 and 7.6) must have had severe lesions in the spinal cord because many remained severely affected for the rest of their life.

Following axonopathy a secondary demyelination occurs. Enzymes are induced during the repair process; the β-glucuronidase and β-galactosidase are two such enzymes (Dewar & Moffatt, 1979). Sensitive methods are available for their determination and increases in activity indicate the extent of the previous damage to the nerves (Figure 8.3). Functional deficit and β-glucuronidase activity increased with increasing exposure to the neuropathic compounds methylmercury or acrylamide. However, significant increases in β-glucuronidase occurred only in the distal portion of the sciatic/posterior tibial nerve after acrylamide whereas after methylmercury the lesions were generally distributed throughout the nerve and increases in the enzyme were found in both the proximal and distal regions (Rose & Dewar, 1983). The axonopathy caused by misonidazole (Rose *et al.*, 1980) have also been examined by these techniques and the minor increases in β-glucuronidase found after pyrethroids have been found to be associated only with near lethal doses, i.e. probably caused as a secondary consequence of intense activity in the nervous system (Rose & Dewar, 1983; Aldridge, 1990).

Other proteins such as neurone-specific enolase and creatine kinase B/beta-S100 protein are specifically distributed in central neurone and glial cells respectively: all are present in whole peripheral nerves (Schmechel *et al.*, 1978; Cicero *et al.*, 1970; Huang *et al.*, 1992). Since immunoassay techniques of sufficient sensitivity exist to determine the presence of the proteins in different parts of the nervous system, they may become useful for the detection of the extent of site-specific damage.

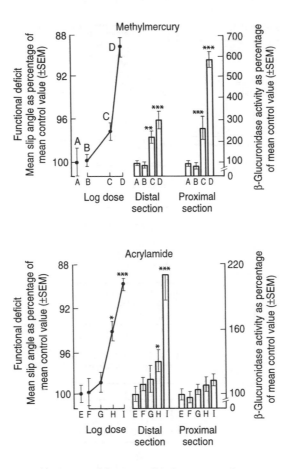

Figure 8.3 Distribution of lesions and functional deficit in rats after intoxication by methylmercury and acrylamide. Nerve section was of the sciatic/posterior tibial nerve. Oral dose schedules were: for methylmercury chloride, 1 dose per day for 7 days of, (A) solvent only, (B) 2.5 mg/kg, (C) 5.0 mg/kg, (D) 7.5 mg/kg; for acrylamide, 1 dose per day for 5 days of, (E) solvent only, (F) 6.3 mg/kg, (G) 12.5 mg/kg, (H) 25 mg/kg, (I) 50 mg/kg. For tests of significance: * $p < 0.05$, ** <0.01, *** <0.001. (*Source*: Adapted from Rose & Dewar, 1983)

8.9 Chemical Carcinogenesis: DNA Adduct to Tumour

Based on histopathological criteria the various stages in chemical carcinogenesis have been described as illustrated in Figure 8.4. This scheme, while indicating a number of morphological stages, gives no clue as to the number of molecular events required for the formation of a malignant tumour. For complete carcinogens, i.e. those which will produce tumours after one exposure, all the necessary adduct formation with DNA must occur within a few hours. For dimethylnitrosamine (DMN) most of the compound will have been metabolised within 24 hours whereas tumours may take 10 months to appear. This experimental situation, although complex, is much less complex than that when the animal is subjected to a life-time of exposure; the slope of the linear exposure–response relationship seems to indicate that probably at least three carcinogen-related events must take place (section 9.4). A complex interplay must occur between

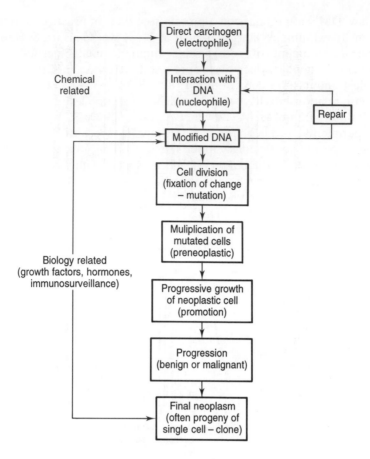

Figure 8.4 Diagrammatic representation of stages in chemical carcinogenesis from formation of DNA adduct to neoplasm. (*Source*: Adapted from Williams & Weisburger, 1986)

mutated cells and the normal control mechanisms to maintain balanced turnover and repair. The influence of diet on the outcome of long-term carcinogenicity experiments is profound (NRC/NAS, 1982; Reddy *et al.*, 1980) and genetic factors probably play a significant part in susceptibility to cancer in the human population. The use of pure strains of animal and the interpretation of the results of such experiments both for human risk purposes and for mechanistic understanding pose obvious difficulties. As yet there is no measurement (effect marker) which can indicate that some cells or particular cells will progress to become tumours (see Figure 12.1); activated oncogenes may eventually supply essential information to characterise cells destined to become neoplasms, and protein products of these transformed cells may become effect markers of specific tumours (i.e. originating from specific cells). Early nuclear enlargement is often associated with subsequent development of tumours but its mechanism is unknown (Ingram & Grasso, 1985, 1987).

Devising experimental protocols to elucidate this multi-stage and slow change of a normal to a neoplastic cell is a challenging problem. Many carcinogenic chemicals are bioactivated before reaction with DNA; the rates of these reactions may be manipulated for experimental purposes. If rats are given a single intraperitoneal injection of

40 mg/kg b.w. DMN after 3 days on a protein-free diet (in practice on pure sucrose) renal mesenchymal tumours start to appear at 12–16 weeks (Hard & Butler, 1970a). Before the development of recognisable tumours small foci of proliferating mesenchymal cells appear which may represent an early stage in the progression to recognisable tumours (Hard & Butler, 1970b). In a more recent study the exposure–response relationships have been established for early lesions and final tumours as well as for alkylation of DNA (Driver *et al.*, 1987; Figure 8.5). This was an advantageous experimental protocol for two reasons: (1) because renal mesenchymal tumours never occur spontaneously in the rat, and (2) because the cells of the small proliferating foci and of the tumour secrete mucin (stained with alcian blue) and express a trypsin-like proteolytic enzyme on their surface (stained by a fluorescent marker), they could be readily identified and counted.

After 20–24 months at 25 mg/kg DMN, renal mesenchymal tumours were usually found in one kidney but at higher exposures both kidneys were affected. Few tumours were present and even at the higher exposures rarely more than two tumours per kidney

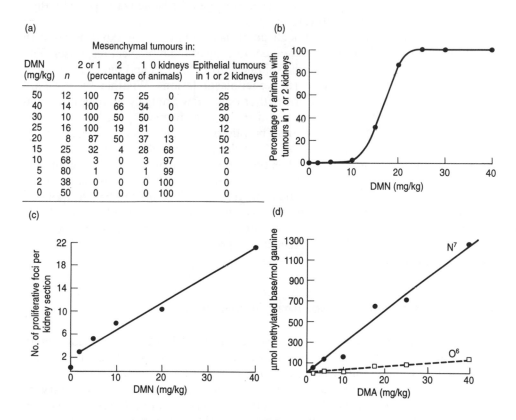

(a)

| DMN (mg/kg) | n | \multicolumn{4}{c}{Mesenchymal tumours in:} | Epithelial tumours in 1 or 2 kidneys |
| | | 2 or 1 | 2 | 1 | 0 kidneys | |
		\multicolumn{4}{c}{(percentage of animals)}	
50	12	100	75	25	0	25
40	14	100	66	34	0	28
30	10	100	50	50	0	30
25	16	100	19	81	0	12
20	8	87	50	37	13	50
15	25	32	4	28	68	12
10	68	3	0	3	97	0
5	80	1	0	1	99	0
2	38	0	0	0	100	0
0	50	0	0	0	100	0

Figure 8.5 Dimethylnitrosamine (DMN) and the induction of renal mesenchymal tumours in rats. (a) The number of rats with tumours 20–24 months after a single intraperitoneal injection of DMN. (b) The total percentage of rats with renal mesenchymal tumours 20–24 months after exposure to DMN. (c) Mesenchymal proliferative foci 3 weeks after exposure to DMN (at 3 weeks the number of recognisable foci was at a maximum). (d) N^7-methyl-guanine (●) and O^6-methyl-guanine (□) in kidney 18 hours after exposure to DMN (at 2 hours the values were slightly higher). (*Source*: Data from Driver *et al.*, 1987)

were found (Figure 8.5a). The total number of animals with tumours in relation to the exposure to DMN followed a sigmoid curve up to 100%, i.e. not linear (Figure 8.5b). This relationship was not shown for the number of epithelial tumours; above 15 mg/kg DMN it was unrelated to the exposure, and below 15 mg/kg no tumours were seen (Figure 8.5a). The number of proliferating foci were counted at 3 weeks when the number detected were at a maximum. In contrast to the sigmoid tumour/DMN exposure relationship, the number of proliferating foci showed a linear relationship down to the lowest exposure (Figure 8.5c). The amount of methylated guanine also was linear in relation to the DMN exposure with a ratio of $N^7 : O^6$ of approximately 8 : 1 (Figure 8.5d). Although the amount of methylated guanines in the liver was about six times the amount in the kidney no liver tumours were seen in these rats. The number of proliferating foci were counted in a single complete longitudinal section through each kidney and were located in the cortex. The total number per kidney is not known but it must be large. The determined methylated guanines were from the total extracted DNA from the whole kidney and their distribution within the kidney is unknown. However, the linear relation between methylation and amount of DMN seems to eliminate most of the potential pharmacokinetic problems associated with the bioactivation of dimethylnitrosamine to the proximal methylating agent.

This interesting experiment, although potentially simpler than experiments with continuous exposure, illustrates the great complexity of the biological responses. The morphological similarities between the spindle cells in the foci and the final tumours suggests that they may represent early preneoplastic lesions. Whether the cells are capable of progressing to tumours or whether only a few are truly preneoplastic and the rest are subject to host defence mechanisms or some form of spontaneous regression is not known. Many questions could be raised concerning the specificity of the chemical initiating interactions but also about the complex cellular responses occurring between the chemical attack which in this experimental protocol will be complete within 24 hours after exposure. Until many of these stages are defined and characterised it seems unlikely that experimental studies in animals will be able to be extrapolated with any certainty to human exposure. When considering possibilities for markers for cells programmed to become tumours, whether there is a close or distant relationship of the tumour cell (in morphology, biochemical properties, etc.) to its cell of origin is a permanent problem.

8.10 Inflammatory Response: Toxic Oil Syndrome

The epidemiological evidence that this disease was caused by the consumption of an oil sold for cooking purposes containing rape seed oil previously denatured with aniline but 'refined' to remove aniline is presented in section 12.5.

The disease began acutely with many thousands of patients admitted to hospital with respiratory symptoms (WHO, 1984). Many died at this stage but others entered intermediate and chronic stages extending for many months (Tables 8.3 and 8.4). The most frequent symptoms of the acute stage were pulmonary oedema, and peripheral eosinophilia was intense: 83% of the patients having >500 and 69% having >1,500 cells/mm^3. The pathology of the lung using biopsy material indicated that the primary lesion was in the endothelial cells, with cytoplasmic swelling, vacuolisation with proliferation and partial obliteration of the lumen (Martinéz-Tello *et al.*, 1982). An inflammatory infiltrate (lymphocytes and macrophages) with oedema of the subendothelial

Table 8.3 Frequency of major clinical signs in toxic oil syndrome

Acute phase (months 1–2)	%	Intermediate phase (months 2–4)	%	Chronic phase (month 4 onwards)	%
Eosinophilia	86	Eosinophilia	–	Eosinophilia (slowly disappears)	–
Pulmonary oedema	72	Pulmonary hypertension	3	Pulmonary hypertension	10
Myalgia	71	Myalgia	49	–	–
Fever	44	–	–	–	–
–	–	Weight loss	36	Muscle wasting	–
–	–	Liver pathology	21	Liver pathology	32
–	–	Sicca syndrome	20	Sicca syndrome	–
Rash	41	Skin oedema	14	Scleroderma	22
–	–	Sensory neuropathy	10	Peripheral neuropathy	37
–	–	Alopecia	9	–	–
–	–	Thromboembolism	1	–	–
–	–	–	–	Dysphagia	–

Source: Data taken from a study of 914 patients by Abaitua & Posada in WHO, 1992.

Table 8.4 Causes of death in toxic oil syndrome

Age/sex Acute phase	Cause of death (22 May–14 July 1981)	Age/sex Chronic phase	Cause of death (14 Oct.–30 Dec. 1981)
56/M	Respiratory failure	12/F	Sepsis
66/M	Respiratory failure	32/M	Pulmonary embolism
16/F	Respiratory failure	37/F	Cardiorespiratory failure
47/F	Hypovolaemic shock	17/F	Sepsis
47/M	Pulmonary infarct	45/F	Sepsis
20/F	Hypovolaemic shock	17/F	Sepsis cachexia
31/F	DIC; hypovolaemic shock	24/F	Internal haemorrhage
52/M	Pulmonary embolism	29/M	Sepsis cachexia
67/F	Hypovolaemic shock	10/F	Sepsis
28/F	Respiratory failure		
48/F	Respiratory failure		

Source: Data from Martinéz-Tello *et al.*, 1982.

space was seen, i.e. an endovasculitis. Medium-size arteries showed intimal thickening with fibroblast proliferation and lymphocyte infiltration. The acute phase was therefore characterised by a pulmonary (septal) oedema and interstitial infiltrate of mononuclear cells. Type 2 cells proliferated with a decrease of type 1 alveolar cells accompanied by some alveolar oedema containing desquamated type 2 cells. The current view is that the primary lesion leading to the clinical condition of respiratory insufficiency is in the endothelial cells.

The acute phase lasted for 1–2 months in many patients followed by an intermediate phase of 2–4 months in which there is a continuing severe myalgia and sensory neuropathy, some liver damage, skin oedema and sicca syndrome (dryness of the mouth). Weight loss was a frequent sign. In some patients this was followed by a chronic phase of indeterminate length depending on the severity of the disease. In this phase the most frequent signs and symptoms were peripheral neuropathy accompanied by muscle wasting, scleroderma and hepatopathy. Pulmonary hypertension has appeared in some patients in the intermediate phase and more frequently in the chronic phase. In many patients with physical rehabilitation there is much improvement but not cure and in some very serious disability persists to this day with hospitalisation. Many patients who recovered from the respiratory illness did not proceed to the chronic phase.

The cause of death changed as the disease progressed (Table 8.4). At the early stages respiratory failure is the most frequent cause of death whereas in the chronic phase (6–8 months) infection is the most usual (Martinéz-Tello *et al.*, 1982). The signs and symptoms are well documented (Abaitua & Posada in WHO, 1992). Toxic oil syndrome is a new disease with a multi-organ and complicated syndrome. A unifying hypothesis is that the basic lesion is endothelial injury which presents itself as a fairly acute response in the lung which is followed by a long-lasting non-necrotising vasculitis involving vessels of every type and size in nearly every organ (Martinéz-Tello & Téllez in WHO, 1992). This lesion is associated with many thrombotic phenomena and most of the late symptoms can be regarded as secondary to this basic lesion. For example, the neuropathy, scleroderma, liver damage and pulmonary hypertension could all result from a decrease of the capacity of the capillaries to supply adequate blood owing to the narrowing of the lumen by cell infiltration and fibrosis. Such final consequences of the non-necrotising vasculitis could explain the final course of the disease in some patients.

The presence of eosinophilia is suggestive of immunological involvement but it is not known whether it was present before the seriousness of the early pulmonary symptoms was appreciated and it is difficult to be sure if it is associated with the active disease during the chronic stage. It is still unknown whether the respiratory illness is an example of primary immunotoxicity or whether immunological involvement is only at the later stages as immune pathology. It is possible that the primary lesion is a toxic reaction which, provided sufficient oil was consumed, would affect everyone (section 12.5 and Figure 12.3).

In late 1989, a new disease appeared in the USA characterised by high peripheral eosinophilia and incapacitating muscle pain. Over 1,500 cases have been reported with 27 deaths. The symptomology of toxic oil syndrome and eosinophilia myalgia syndrome show many qualitative similarities (WHO, 1991, 1993; Kilbourne *et al.*, 1991) but the relative intensity of the symptoms occurring was different. Thus the early pneumonia in toxic oil syndrome with many deaths was not seen in eosinophilia myalgia syndrome although there were frequent complaints of respiratory problems. Epidemiological studies have established that the latter disease was associated with the consumption of a particular brand of l-tryptophan (Swygert *et al.*, 1990; Slutsker *et al.*, 1990). When compared with pure l-tryptophan the case-tryptophan has been shown to contain several impurities.

As yet the aetiological agents causing these two diseases have not been identified. The main reason for this is that no animal model for the disease has so far been found when case-associated oils or l-tryptophan are administered to a quite wide range of animals. Thus there is no bioassay system available and therefore the rational process of purification as a prelude to the identification and synthesis of the respective aetiological agents cannot be attempted (see Figure 9.3). Thus the occurrence within ten years of two major poisoning episodes presenting new diseases both with high peripheral eosinophilia and myalgia is a challenge to both toxicology and biological science.

8.11 Discussion

The consequence of an initiating reaction of an intoxicant with a biological component is like throwing a pebble into a pond. The ripples spread in many directions and some reach the edge giving rise to clinical signs of ill health, disease and sometimes death. Others ripples, although a direct consequence of the initiating event are less significant or may be irrelevant for the final disease. However, these may be important for dose and effect monitoring since they run in parallel to the toxic response. If the pebble (i.e. the dose) is small then the ripples do not reach the edge and are contained by the size of the pond (i.e. biological reserve). The biological reserve is the degree of interference with a biological system which can be tolerated without a demonstrable undesirable consequence and influences the threshold exposure and dose. As the exposure and dose are reduced then the normal repair and recovery systems play their part in reducing the response. Health is a steady state between the eventuality of damage and the repair of damage which includes the normal turnover of macromolecules and replacement of cells by division. With an increased rate of damage, normal repair processes may be overwhelmed and therapeutic measures or means to contain the disease long enough for repair to occur must be applied.

Although the usual signal for therapeutic measures is the appearance of signs of poisoning, methods to influence the outcome of exposure can exert their action in all five stages (Table 8.5). Aside from 'prevention is better than cure' (stage 1), opportunities for reduction in toxicity have been described in the text: section 8.2.1, cyanide poisoning by competitive binding on methaemoglobin or increased detoxification to thiocyanate (stage 2); section 8.2.2, organophosphorus poisoning by reactivation of inhibited acetylcholinesterase and prophylaxis by pretreatment with carbamates (stage 3), and atropine for competition with the increased concentration of acetylcholine and benzodiazopines for central convulsions (stages 4 and 5). The main objectives of treatment measures are: decreasing the dose of intoxicant to reach the target (stage 2), reactivation of the modified target (stage 3) and prevention of the consequences of initiation of toxicity (stages 4 and 5). The number of rational treatment measures is small; this is because the window of opportunity for most agents is small. To be useful, an agent should have a defined specificity, be tolerated well and not cause toxicity at the doses used, be stable and not rapidly removed from the circulation and, for those binding the intoxicant such as chelating agents for heavy metals and organometals, should not cause a redistribution of the intoxicant, e.g. 2,3-mercaptopropanol (BAL) forms an uncharged complex with mercuric mercury and although mobilising mercury from several tissues increases the concentration of mercury in the nervous system. The later dithiol agents, 2,2-dimercaptosuccinate and others containing negative charges, are less liable to this fault (Magos, 1976; Clarkson, 1981; Aposhian & Aposhian, 1990).

Many toxic substances exert their action by their own or a metabolites' electrophilic reactivity. Glutathione is an *in vivo* nucleophile which does protect but is easily depleted. *N*-Acetylcysteine has been devised and used for the treatment of patients poisoned by excessive ingestion of acetamidophen (paracetamol) which is metabolised to reactive intermediates (Hinsen, 1980; Vermeulen *et al.*, 1992). It has recently been shown in a controlled prospective trial to save life even if treatment is delayed for one day (Keays *et al.*, 1991). In principle *N*-acetylcysteine or other nucleophiles may well have a future in reducing the concentration of reactive intoxicants in acute cases of poisoning. The therapeutic oximes (sections 8.2.2 and 7.5) were directly devised from a knowledge of the mechanism of interaction of organophosphorus compounds with cholinesterases

Table 8.5   Methods for the prevention of prophylaxis and therapy for poisoning by chemicals

Stage 1	PHYSICAL REDUCTION OF EXPOSURE
	1 Industrial hygiene
	2 Protective clothing, masks, respirators, personal monitors
	3 Reduction of absorption from gastro-intestinal tract by kaolin, activated charcoal, etc.
Stage 2	PHYSICAL METHODS FOR REDUCING THE CONCENTRATION OF INTOXICANT
	1 Haemoperfusion
	REVERSIBLE BINDING TO MACROMOLECULES
	2 Reversible binding to macromolecules – antibodies
	3 Reversible binding to macromolecules – methaemoglobin for cyanide
	DETOXIFICATION BY ENZYMES
	4 Hydrolysis of organophosphorus compounds
	5 Conversion of cyanide to thiocyanate by rhodanese
	REVERSIBLE REACTION WITH SMALL MOLECULES
	6 Chelation of metals and organometals with dithiols
	COVALENT REACTION WITH SMALL MOLECULES
	7 Detoxification of electrophilic intoxicant with nucleophile *N*-acetylcysteine
Stage 3	COVALENT REACTION WITH ALTERNATE TARGET
	1 Reaction of organophosphorus compounds with esterase and serum cholinesterase
	REACTIVATION OF MODIFIED TARGET
	2 Oximes to reactivate phosphylated acetylcholinesterase
	PROPHYLAXIS BY PREFORMATION OF UNSTABLE MODIFIED TARGET
	3 Carbamylation of acetylcholinesterase
Stage 4	ANTAGONISTS
	1 Atropine against acetylcholine; naloxone against narcotics
	2 Benzodiazepines as anticonvulsants
Stage 5	TREATMENT OF SIGNS AND SYMPTOMS
	1 Maintain life while circulating intoxicant is detoxified or excreted, e.g. cooling when temperature rise is excessive, narcotics to reduce stress, artificial respiration to treat anoxia

(Ballantyne & Marrs, 1992). They are effective because the catalytic centre of the enzyme assists in the reactivation process; the opportunity to utilise such a mechanism for other therapeutic agents to reactivate modified targets is clearly limited. The same potential restriction applies to the prophylactic measure of partial preinhibition of a target to produce an unstable product (e.g. by preadministration of carbamates prior to exposure to organophosphorus compounds).

The emphasis in clinical practice is the treatment of the acutely poisoned patients. As knowledge of mechanisms of the more chronic cascades of biological events towards clinical toxicity increases so other possibilities may emerge, e.g. preventing fibrosis, apoptosis, etc.

8.12 Summary

1   The cascade of consequences resulting from chemical-induced initiating reactions are biological and not chemical related.

2   Intoxication can lead to functional changes both with no morphological change or with morphological changes leading to cell death.

3   In most tissues recovery from intoxication takes place by replacement of dead cells by division of unaffected cells. In the brain, adult neurones cannot divide so necrotic cells cannot be replaced.

4   Activation of repair systems can, in some circumstances, lead to permanent loss of function, e.g. fibrosis.

5   In the brain the site of neuronal loss caused by some intoxicants may be modified by different external stimuli.

6   Similar clinical signs and symptoms can result from different primary mechanisms.

7   Chemical carcinogenesis is a rare cellular event and the mechanisms from DNA adduct to tumour are not understood.

8   Some cell-specific intoxications can cause widespread and long-lasting changes in almost all tissues, e.g. intoxication of endothelial cells leading to general vasculitis.

9   Therapeutic measures can involve: (a) detoxification or reduction of the concentration of the intoxicant, (b) reactivation of the modified target, or (c) antagonism of early biological effects.

10 Prophylactic measures can involve: (a) pretreatment with a detoxifying system such as an enzyme or chemical reactant, (b) pretreatment with an agent capable of reactivation of the target, or (c) pretreatment with an agent leading to partial reaction with the target to yield an unstable product.

9

Exposure, Dose and Chemical Structure, Response and Activity, and Thresholds

9.1 Introduction

An exposure– or dose–response relationship defines the exposure or dose of a chemical causing a defined biological effect. In its most often used form in toxicology it is the relationship between that administered (e.g. by mouth, inhalation, etc.) and the death of the animals. The exposure causing the death of 50% of the animals exposed, LD_{50} (lethal dose = exposure) is a measure of the toxicity of the chemical and is widely used as a preliminary screen. The LD_{50} procedure has been much criticised for its large use of animals trying to produce a result of (usually) unnecessary statistical accuracy which is of limited utility. Sometimes it is used for bioassay purposes but usually only small numbers are required to obtain LD_{50} values of adequate accuracy (Weil, 1952). The experimental procedure is simple and the value obtained is operational but conceals much biological complexity. Many factors influence the delivery of the toxic chemical to its target and the amount to which the target is exposed is often only a fraction of that administered to the animal. Only the concentration of intoxicant causing interaction at the target and the first biological effect yields a value for dose–response uncomplicated by these other factors. Moving from primary interaction with target (stage 3 of Figure 2.1) through the later biological consequences (stage 4) to clinical signs of poisoning (stage 5), the dose–response will not remain the same. For example, although 50% reaction with the target (stage 3) may be sufficient to cause biochemical (e.g. enzyme leakage from cells, changes in the metabolism of cells or tissue) or physiological effects (e.g. changes in nerve conduction velocity, sweating, sensitivity to sound or light (stage 4)), 90% reaction may be required for clinically recognisable illness. In mechanistic terms, dose–response relationships are needed to establish cause and effect, i.e. to establish that the same degree of reaction with a target always causes the same biological effect.

Information valuable for the formulation of mechanistic hypotheses is obtained from experiments which show that a variety of chemical structures cause the same form of toxicity, i.e. a structure–response relationship. Such qualitative information can be very useful but structure–activity relationships are more valuable, i.e. different chemicals are ranked in order of their potency (derived from dose–response) in inducing the same

136

biological change. Thus the interpretation of structure–activity relationships determined using animals is difficult due to the many factors which influence exposure–response relationships. The definitive relationship is that which links chemical structure with the initiation of disease. If the chemical to which the organism is exposed is the toxic agent, binding to sites irrelevant from a toxicological viewpoint, then metabolism to less or non-toxic metabolites, various excretory mechanisms, etc., distort the structure–activity relationship at the target. Each of these processes will have distinct structure–activity relationships which will, almost inevitably, be different from that at the target. If the chemical administered has to be bioactivated to become toxic, another layer of distorting factors is interposed between exposure and reaction at the target. Thus structure–activity relationships determined for the whole animal, isolated physiological preparations or even subcellular organelles are 'apparent' constants only. Once the target involved in the initiation of toxicity is known, the relative contribution of the other competing factors may be established. Quantifying the factors which cause species differences enables more certain prediction from animal experimentation to risk of exposure of humans (see Chapters 10 and 15). In many instances the target is unknown in molecular terms but the cell affected can often be defined.

The importance of dose in therapy and toxicity has been known for many centuries:

> What is it that is not poison? All things are poisons and none that are not. Only the dose decides that a thing is not poisonous. (Paracelsus, 1538)

For Paracelsus, dose was that administered to the patient whereas in toxicology it should indicate what has entered the organism, and exposure is that outside (that inhaled, applied to the skin or administered by the oral route; see section 4.1). With modern techniques it is possible to determine the concentration of chemical delivered to the affected cells (dose); this, sometimes with the additional knowledge of the length of time it is present, determines whether a chemical will or will not cause toxicity. Thus for exposure and dose the correct terms are exposure–response and dose–response respectively. Structure–response data states whether a chemical does or does not cause a particular form of toxicity; structure–activity using exposure or dose incorporate exposure– response or dose–response respectively.

9.2 Essential and Toxic Compounds

The above famous statement by Paracelsus was made in reply to the criticism by academic medical men about his use of poisons to treat the sick. He illuminates a fundamental issue that the qualitative distinction between poisonous and non-poisonous substances is not real: increasing the dose can make a substance change from being non-poisonous (and sometimes beneficial) to poisonous. Many exogenous substances (drugs) can become toxic at doses above those that are beneficial, e.g. digitalis, beta-blockers for the treatment of hypertension, endogenous hormones such as insulin, vitamin D, thyroxine, etc. Some essential dietary elements such as copper, zinc, selenium, chromium, manganese, cobalt and iodine are toxic in large doses. The maintenance of normal function is achieved by metal-buffering systems which keep the circulating concentration of the element very low but in equilibrium with, for example, enzymes for which it is an essential cofactor.

Thus Paracelsus' statement is true for exogenous (drugs, vitamins) and endogenous (hormones) materials; sometimes toxicity is brought about by an intensification of their beneficial function leading to malfunction and sometimes essential substances become toxic at higher doses in ways which are unrelated to the mechanisms of their beneficial effects. All beneficial biological actions induced by chemicals are governed by their concentration; too little and the organism is deficient, too much and toxicity occurs. Toxicity does not occur if the dose is below the threshold. Exceptions are probably those chemicals which induce mutations following their reaction with genetic material.

9.3 Exposure–response for Bioassay: The Malathion Episode in Pakistan

From the early 1950s malathion had been used extensively as a non-systemic insecticide and had an excellent safety record. However, of 7,500 sprayers using it for mosquito control in a malaria eradication programme in Pakistan in 1976 2,800 became ill and 5 died. The symptoms were those expected for inhibition of acetylcholinesterase and the poisoning occurred after spraying preparations made from malathion 50% water dispersible powders (WDP) some of which contained greater than normal amounts of isomalathion (Baker *et al.*, 1978).

The administration of other organophosphorus compounds can increase the toxicity

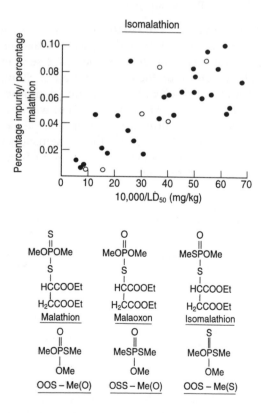

Figure 9.1 Influence of isomalathion content on the toxicity cf malathion. The toxicity (LD_{50}) of pure malathion to rats is 10,000 mg/kg. The chemical structures of compounds identified in technical and formulated malathion are shown (see Aldridge *et al.*, 1979). o and ● indicate that the results were obtained in two different laboratories

of malathion, i.e. potentiate its toxicity. A large number of specimens of malathion (WDP) manufactured by different firms and used and stored in different countries were tested for their toxicity to rats (Figure 9.1). Reported values for the toxicity of technical malathion varied from 100–8,000 mg/kg b.w. but pure malathion has a toxicity of only 10,700 mg/kg (confidence limits 9,300–12,300). In Figure 9.1 the horizontal axis is the ratio $10,000/LD_{50}$ of the specimen examined, i.e. on this scale pure malathion would have a value of 1. A range of values up to 70 were obtained indicating a maximum toxicity of approx 140 mg/kg. These studies established: (1) that the major cause of the increase in toxicity of malathion was its content of isomalathion (Aldridge *et al.*, 1979; Baker *et al.*, 1978); (2) that prolonged storage of the malathion (WDP) in the hot conditions in Pakistan caused the isomerisation of malathion to isomalathion, and (3) that both temperature and composition of the support material in the powders increased the rate of isomerisation. Thus the use of exposure–response relationships as a bioassay system established that impurities which could increase the toxicity of malathion to experimental animals also do so in humans (Aldridge *et al.*, 1979). Malathion in both insects and mammals is bioactivated to malaoxon, a powerful inhibitor of acetylcholinesterase. In mammals, carboxyl esterases remove one or both ethyl groups from malathion which prevents its conversion to an active inhibitor. Insects are deficient in such detoxification and therefore malathion is much more toxic to insects than to mammals. Isomalathion, trimethyl phosphorothioates (other impurities identified in stored malathion) and other organophosphorus compounds are direct inhibitors of the detoxifying carboxylesterases; thus, in their presence the toxicity of malathion to mammals increases and becomes closer to that for insects (Figure 9.2).

Dose–response is a vital component used for the identification of aetiological agents in poisoning of humans and animals. The essential steps are illustrated in Figure 9.3. Initial epidemiology may provide evidence of the vehicle for the poison and if the clinical signs and symptoms are recognised the identity of the poison may be suspected. If the signs and symptoms are not recognised but the vehicle for the poison is known then administration to experimental animals may cause toxicity similar to that seen in

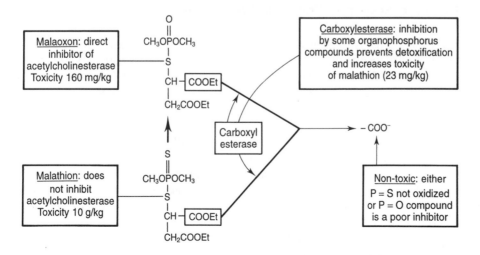

Figure 9.2 Mechanism of toxicity of malathion and its potentiation by other organophosphorus compounds (see Aldridge *et al.*, 1987)

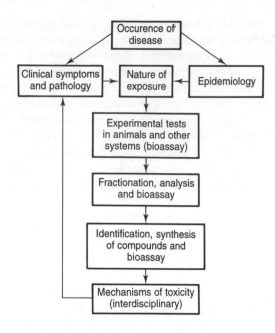

Figure 9.3 Pathways for the acquisition of information to establish the aetiology of chemical poisoning

humans. Extraction, purification and bioassay (using experimental animals if the symptoms are unusual) lead to the identification and synthesis of the intoxicant and to the initiation of research on mechanisms of toxicity. If at least some of the signs of poisoning cannot be produced in an experimental animal then bioassay is not possible and identification of the cause of poisoning becomes extremely difficult (see Chapter 10).

9.4 Exposure–Response: Chemical Carcinogens

Carcinogenesis is a multi-stage process extending over many months or years from initiation to the clinical recognition of the presence of a tumour. Some carcinogens produce tumours in most of the animals after a single exposure even when it is known that all the compound has been metabolised within a day or so, e.g. a single dose of dimethylnitrosamine to rats on a low protein diet causes kidney tumours in all of the rats (see sections 4.7 and 8.9).

The form of the exposure–response curve is essential information for taking decisions about 'safe' exposure and/or exposure leading to what has been decided as an acceptable risk. There is much loose talk about carcinogenic risk. Even if it were assumed that only one modification to the genome causes a cell to develop into a tumour it could be maintained that all that is necessary is the reaction of one molecule of carcinogen with one base of the DNA in one cell. This is a useless statement since many molecules will be required at the target (dose), as the laws of chemistry dictate, to ensure that reaction at a specific base takes place. A large amount of the carcinogen is needed (exposure) to overcome detoxification pathways and achieve this dose at the cell level (see Chapters 5 and 6).

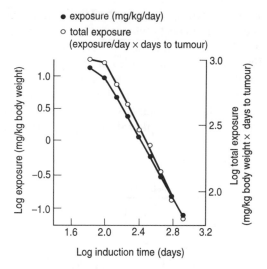

Figure 9.4   The relation between the exposure/day and total exposure of *N*-nitrosodiethylamine on the time of induction of liver tumours in rats. (*Source*: Data from Schmahl, 1979)

On general grounds it seems probable that some as yet incompletely defined modification(s) by chemicals of the DNA template in a cell, leading to a non-lethal mutation, is a process with no threshold, i.e. the relation between dose and effect will be linear. For tumour incidence, the time when the tumour appears is another variable (Figure 9.4).

Diethylnitrosamine in the drinking water of rats in concentrations ranging 256-fold from 20 down to 0.075 mg/kg/day and total doses ranging over a 10-fold range from 1,000 to 95 mg/kg causes tumours in almost all the rats (Schmahl, 1979). These results show that diethylnitrosamine is a powerful carcinogen capable of causing liver tumours in most of the rats after a life-time of exposure to 75 μg/kg/day (735 nmol/kg/day = 4.4×10^{17} molecules/kg/day). The total dose needed to produce tumours decreased the lower the concentration of nitrosamine in the drinking water. Whether this relationship would still hold if the delivered dose were known remains unanswered.

A huge experiment has been reported using 4,080 rats and *N*-nitroso derivatives of dimethylamine and diethylamine with exposures lower than in Schmahl's experiment and for the life-time of the animals which was, at the lower exposures, nearly normal (median survival 2.5 years; Peto *et al.*, 1991a,b). No threshold was found for liver cell, bile cell or oesophageal tumours.

Reviews on the exposure–response relationships for carcinogens are Crump *et al.* (1976); Doll & Peto (1978) and Christian (1985).

9.5   Structure– and Dose–Response Relationships: γ-Diketones and Acrylamide.

Exposure to *n*-hexane was first shown to cause neuropathy in 1967 during household sandal operations in Japan. Other episodes have occurred at work and solvent abuse such as glue sniffing has caused many cases. A large outbreak of a similar neuropathy occurred in 1974 in a textile printing plant in the USA when exposure to methyl iso-butylketone was changed to methyl *n*-butylketone. Typical symptoms following exposure included body weight loss, fatigue and distal sensory paresthesia followed by muscular weakness. Early experimental studies in several species have shown that the most characteristic morphological change is focal swellings in distal regions of peripheral nerves. The swellings consist of an accumulation of neurofilaments at the axonal constrictions at the nodes of Ranvier. Changes of the same type also occur in the brain which has lead to the term 'central/peripheral axonopathy' (Spencer & Schaumburg, 1976; Jones & Cavanagh, 1983a,b).

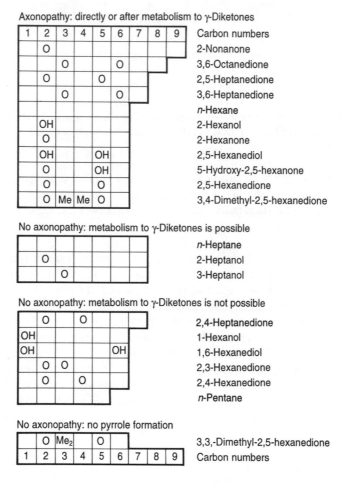

Figure 9.5   Structure–response relationships for production of central/peripheral neuropathy by hydrocarbons and metabolites. See text for clinical signs. From top to bottom: (1) all compounds are either γ-diketones or can be metabolised to them in sufficient amounts; (2) since the corresponding γ-diketones 2,5- and 3,6-heptanedione are active, these compounds do not cause neuropathy because they are not metabolised in sufficients amounts; (3) in these compounds the keto groups are neither in nor can they be metabolised to the γ-diketone configuration; (4) although it is capable of reacting with lysine, the 3,3-dimethyl compound cannot irreversibly form a pyrrole (see Couri & Milks, 1982)

2,5-Hexanedione causes central peripheral neuropathy in rats (Spencer & Schaumburg, 1975) and chemical evidence has been provided that this compound is the common active agent produced by metabolism after administration of a variety of 6-carbon compounds (DiVincenzo *et al.*, 1976; see Table 9.2 and Figure 9.5).

Structure–response relationships of a range of compounds indicate that a γ-diketone structure is essential, e.g. 2,3- and 2,4-hexanediones are inert (Figure 9.5). Compounds which are metabolised to γ-diketones in sufficient amount cause the same neuropathy (clinical and morphological changes). Some compounds which are metabolised are not active because sufficient γ-diketone is not produced. All those compounds whose structure will not allow metabolism to a γ-diketone do not cause neuropathy. 3,3-Dimethyl-2,5-hexanedione is inactive; this is probably because after reacting with lysine in proteins it cannot cyclise to form a pyrrole (see section 7.9).

Exposure–response studies of several hexacarbon compounds which are all oxidised *in vivo* to 2,5-hexanedione indicate that the rate of metabolism is inversely related to the time before clinical signs appear (Krasavage *et al.*, 1980; see Table 9.1); the clinical signs used in these experiments were severe hindlimb weakness or paralysis shown by dragging of at least one foot. Two measures of dose of 2,5-hexanedione are available: the peak concentration in the plasma and the area under the curve (AUC) which indicates the integrated dose. The total dose should be proportional to both parameters multiplied by the number of doses. The results in Table 9.1 show that over a 6-fold range of time to clinical effect the total dose is remarkably constant.

Acrylamide also causes an axonopathy lesion in the long nerves and different schedules of exposure indicate that, like 2,5-hexanedione, a constant exposure is required to produce the clinical condition over the first 50–70 days. Acrylamide, being unionised and very soluble in water, distributes uniformly throughout the body water and therefore exposure is directly proportional to the internal dose (see sections 5.3.1 and 7.7).

Table 9.1 Dose–response relationships for 2,5-hexanedione and central/peripheral axonopathy

Compound	Number of doses (mean) (A)	Peak 2,5-hexanedione (μmol/ml serum) (B)	Area under curve (C)	(A × B)	(A × C)
2,5-Hexanedione	11	5.0	4.2	55	46
5-Hydroxy-2-hexanone	15	2.8	2.9	42	43
2,5-Hexanediol	20	2.1	2.0	42	42
Methyl *n*-butyl ketone	40	1.0	1.0	40	40
2-Hexanol	59	0.66	0.2	39	12
n-Hexane	71	0.46	0.9	33	64

The axonopathy was produced either by the direct administration of or by metabolism of other compounds to 2,5-hexanedione. The compounds were administered to rats by gavage in equimolar doses of 6.6 mmol/kg once daily for 5 days a week except for *n*-hexane which was 46.2 mmol/kg. Separate groups of rats were used to determine the time course of 2,5-hexanedione in serum after a single dose of the various compound. The comparative area under the curve (AUC) was determined relative to methyl *n*-butylketone = 1.
Source: Data from Krasavage *et al.*, 1980.

Table 9.2 Amount and time of exposure of rats to acrylamide to cause clinical neuropathy

Period of exposure (days)	Type of exposure[a]	Mean rate of exposure (mg/kg/day)	Total exposure (mg/kg)
No clinical signs			
77	A	7.1	550
164	A	7.0	1160
Slight clinical signs			
21	C	25.0	525
28	C	15.1	422
28	A	7.8	500
42	B	14.3	600
70	B	10.0	700
84	C	12.0	1008
210	B	7.1	1500
280	C	7.5	2100
336	C	7.5	2520
Severe clinical signs			
15	A	40.0	600
21	B	28.5	600
56	B	14.2	800
56	C	25.0	1400
70	C	15.0	1055
112	C	12.0	1344
240	B	10.0	2400
392	B	7.1	2800

[a] A = daily oral 5 days/week; B = oral 100 mg/kg repeated at different time intervals; C = in the food.
Source: Data from Fullerton & Barnes, 1966; Barnes, 1970; Edwards, 1975; Aldridge, 1995b. The results have been arranged in the order of the period of exposure, i.e. time to clinical signs.

The results in Table 9.3 are a collation of data obtained by several exposure protocols. After the initial period of 50–70 days the exposure required to induce clinical signs increases. Acrylamide is excreted unchanged but most is detoxified by reaction with glutathione to yield a mercapturic acid which is excreted. The loss of acrylamide from the circulation is exponential with a half-life of less than 2 hours (Edwards, 1975; see section 5.3.1). The cumulative nature of the poisoning, therefore, cannot be due to the persistence of acrylamide.

It is tempting to suggest that the similarities in dose–response behaviour of acrylamide and 2,5-hexanedione are due to the time taken for neurofilaments to proceed down long axons; this may take as much as 50 days. This potential target (see sections 7.7 and 7.8) would then be available for chemical attack over this period. For high doses the necessary degree of chemical modification of the neurofilaments would be attained quickly, but for lower doses sufficient accumulation on the neurofilaments would take longer. This is a speculative hypothesis but the similar exposure– or dose–response

Table 9.3 Structure–response relationships for compounds causing neuronal necrosis or intramyelinic vacuoles

		Neuronal necrosis	Intramyelinic vacuoles	Mitochondria (B/A[a])
	TIN AND LEAD COMPOUNDS			
	4-Coordinate			
(1)	Trimethyltin	+	−	290
	Trimethyllead	+	−	850
	Triethyllead	+	−	640
(2)	Dimethylethyltin	+	+	32
	Methyldiethyltin	+	+	33
	Methylethyln-propyltin	+	+	11
	Trimethyltin/triethyltin	+	+	−
(3)	Triethyltin	−	+	15
	Tri *n*-propyltin	−	+	3.6
	Diethylphenyltin	−	+	1.6
	Ethyldiphenyltin	−	+	0.4
	5-Coordinate			
(4)	(2-[(Dimethylamino)methyl] phenyl)diethyltin	ND	−	0.01
	(2-[(Dimethylamino)methyl] phenyl)methylphenyltin	ND	−	0.05

ACIDIC PHENOLS AND PHENYLIMINO COMPOUNDS

		Neuronal necrosis	Intramyelinic vacuoles	Mitochondrial uncoupling
(5)	2,4-Dinitrophenol	ND	−	+
	Pentachlorophenol	ND	−	+
(6)	2,2'-Methylenebis[3,4,6-trichlorophenol] (hexachlorophene)	ND	+	+
	3,5-Diiodochloro salicylamide	ND	+	+
	2'-Chloro-2,4-dinitro-5',6-di(trifluoromethyl) diphenylamine	ND	+	+
	2,4-Dinitro-*N*-(2,4,6-tribromophenyl)-6-(trifluoromethyl)benzenamine	ND	+	+

[a] B/A is the ratio of the concentrations of the compound causing 50% of the maximum effect on ATP synthesis (B) and the Cl^-/OH^- exchange (A).
ND = no data.
Source: Data from Aldridge, 1995a.

relationship of these two neuropathic agents is not the same as that for delayed neuropathy caused by organophosphorus compounds; for the latter it seems as though sufficient intoxicant to cause 50% inhibition of NTE may be tolerated indefinitely (see section 9.7 and Figures 9.6 and 9.7).

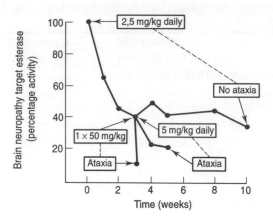

Figure 9.6 The effects of daily dosing of mono *o*-tolyl diphenyl phosphate to adult chickens on brain neuropathy target esterase and clinical signs of delayed neuropathy. (*Source*: Data from Lotti & Johnson (1980)

9.6 Structure–Response: Triorganotins, Phenols and Phenylimino Compounds

The neuronal necrosis caused by trimethyltin or triethyllead and the intramyelinic vacuoles caused by triethyltin have both occurred in humans as well as in several species of experimental animals (see section 7.12). The systems affected are therefore common to at least many mammalian species.

Although the uniqueness and location of the lesions are clear no explanation is available for the mechanism in molecular terms. The structure–response relationships are puzzling and show discontinuities (Table 9.3). The unexpected difference in the biological response of the mammalian nervous system to triethyltin and trimethyltin has been extended and, with successive substitution in trimethyltin of methyl by ethyl, both types of lesion are produced. Triorganotin and -lead compounds can be divided into several classes causing: (1) only neuronal necrosis, (2) neuronal necrosis and intramyelinic vacuoles, (3) only intramyelinic vacuoles, and (4) neither lesion. If both trimethyltin and triethyltin are administered simultaneously both lesions can be seen, and so far no triorganolead has caused intramyelinic vacuoles. These results reinforce the view that these two lesions are produced by independent mechanisms.

Following the human poisoning episodes with the phenolic hexachlorophene (Kimbrough & Gaines, 1971) other acidic substances have been shown to cause intramyelinic vacuoles in rats (Table 9.3). The acidic group may be phenolic or in others phenylimino. Not all acidic phenols are active.

All of the above chemicals affect energy conservation system in mitochondria. The acidic compounds cause classical uncoupling defined as an ability to reduce the phosphorylation of ADP to ATP while maintaining the consumption of oxygen. This activity is achieved by the carriage of protons across membranes and the consequent discharge of the H^+/OH^+ gradient essential for the synthesis of ATP. The trialkyltin and -lead compounds induce a Cl^-/OH^- exchange across mitochondrial membranes and also inhibit the ATP synthase reaction by binding to one of the components of the system.

146

Relative activity in bringing about these two effects varies from compound to compound (Selwyn, 1976; Aldridge *et al.*, 1977; Aldridge & Brown, 1988).

Triorganotin and -lead compounds and uncoupling agents are fairly specific and do not interact with many proteins. Their lipophilic properties and solubility in water also ensure that they are widely distributed; current information suggests that the cellular specificity in the central nervous system is not due to different cellular distribution (but see Toggas *et al.*, 1992). At present, any generally applicable hypothesis about mechanisms must be speculative. The production of intramyelinic vacuoles could be the disruption of an energy-requiring physiological system necessary to keep myelin sheaths together but with at least a film of extracellular fluid between them. The discontinuities in the structure–response relationships may be explained if more than one interaction is required. Perhaps a cell has to be affected by two actions at the same concentration of agent, i.e. the ability to transport chloride across membranes together with a reduction of energy requirements of the cell. Properties specific to the cell affected cannot be excluded, e.g. the presence of chloride in the myelin-forming cells, the oligodendroglia and Schwann cells. If this were a reasonable hypothesis for the trialkyltins, then their chloride-carrying property would have to be matched by the phenols and amino compound acting as carriers of sodium across membranes. Neuronal necrosis is caused by trialkyltins and trialkylleads with a relatively high activity in facilitating the Cl^-/OH^- exchange and could be associated with effects on systems in which chloride movement is linked to other transport, e.g. γ-aminobutyrate. Such primary effects need not necessarily be in the cells showing the lesions; influence from other cells removing inhibition could reduce their energy stores and compromise their viability.

9.7 Thresholds

A threshold exposure is that following acute or chronic administration of an intoxicant below which no toxicity occurs. The threshold is the point in the exposure–response curve at which if the exposure were increased toxicity would be seen and if decreased toxicity would not occur. A threshold is therefore always an extrapolation to zero biological effect. Exposure of experimental animals may yield a threshold exposure (a no-effect level for a defined form of toxicity; not the general no-effect level used in regulatory toxicology); such a threshold exposure is an operational value specific for the animal used and many other experimental conditions; it cannot be interpreted if the relationship between exposure and delivered dose is not known. Two questions will be addressed: (1) is there a single or few exposures below which no toxicity occurs, and (2) if the exposure is continuous or in divided amount, is the amount required to cause toxicity more, the same or less than for a single exposure?

Except for carcinogenesis, most intoxicants show a threshold exposure for acute administration, i.e. low doses cause no deleterious effect. The fundamental utility of a measured threshold is inversely proportional to the complexity of the biological system. In view of the expense of experiments giving data down to a low incidence (i.e. the large number of animals required) other parameters should be measured, e.g. delivered dose and effect showing a graded response, e.g. inhibition of a target enzyme. Many reactions affecting the delivery of the intoxicant can be eliminated by measurements of the relationship of dose in the cell or at the target to the relevant aspect of toxicity.

Thresholds demonstrated by such an approach are threshold doses rather than threshold exposures and can with greater confidence be used for cross-species comparisons.

In section 9.4 dose–response for carcinogenic nitrosamines have been discussed. Alterations to the DNA template leading to a mutation are probably processes without a threshold and large-scale experiments support this view (Schmahl,1979; Peto *et al.*, 1991a,b) although in the spirit of absolute correctness we do not and maybe never will have the data to answer the question. From a life-time study of exposure of rats to the powerful carcinogens *N*-nitroso-diethylamine and *N*-nitroso-dimethylamine the relationship follows the equation

$$\text{Exposure rate} \times (\text{Median time to tumours})^n = \text{Constant}$$

in which $n = 2.3$ for *N*-nitroso-diethylamine-induced liver cell and oesophogeal tumours, and $n = 1$ for *N*-nitroso-dimethylamine-induced liver cell tumours and $n = 2.3$ for bile cell tumours. The results from Schmahl's 1979 study (see Figure 9.4) show the same relationship for *N*-nitroso-diethylamine and liver cell tumours. No explanation is available for the different results from the *N*-nitroso-dimethylamine/liver cell study or for the fact that the total exposure decreases as the time to development of tumours increases (i.e. if $n > 1$). Measurement of delivered dose may help to clarify the position (Swenberg *et al.*, 1991).

In section 9.5 and Table 9.3 the relation between daily circulating doses of 2,5-hexanedione and clinical effect indicates that the total dose required is relatively constant for exposure times of 16–100 days. This is not due to the persistence of 2,5-hexanedione; its half-life in plasma is approximately 6 hours (Krasavage *et al.*, 1980) so that by the time each gastric intubation is given, four half-lives have elapsed. Some initiating reaction product must accumulate until it is sufficient to cause malfunction of the nerve axon. This does not imply that a threshold dose does not exist because in this same study no clinical evidence of hindlimb weakness was detected with total doses (peak concentration in serum × 64 daily exposures) of 13 and 25 whereas 33 was effective. A similar accumulation seems to occur with repeated administration of acrylamide (see section 7.7 and Table 9.2).

Cadmium accumulates in liver and kidney during exposure to low concentrations for a long time. The high affinity sites for cadmium in the kidney cortex and in other places ensure that the excretion rate is very low (half-life of 16–30 years; see Webb, 1979). Thus even with very low human exposures (30–60 μg/day) cadmium will continue to accumulate in the kidney until a steady state of 25–30 μg/g is reached. With higher exposure the concentration reached may be sufficient to impair tubular function. The delivered threshold dose for tubular dysfunction is usually taken to be 200 μg/g (i.e. 300–400 μg/g in the cortex); however, see section 12.6 for details of a study indicating subtle changes, not accompanied by renal insufficiency, occurring at much lower concentrations of cadmium in the kidney.

Some organophosphorus compounds cause delayed neuropathy after 70–80% inhibition of neuropathy target esterase, NTE (see section 7.6). If 2.5 mg/kg mono 2-tolyl diphenyl phosphate is administered to hens daily for 10 weeks no ataxia is seen even with the constant 50–55% inhibition of NTE (Figure 9.6). The hens do not become tolerant since one further exposure of 50 mg/kg caused ataxia and after 5 mg/kg daily from day 22 to day 35 the hens become ataxic by day 49 with 71–85% inhibition. The non-effective 2.5 mg/kg daily for 10 weeks is a total exposure to 2.5 × 70 = 175 mg/kg and this could probably be extended indefinitely. This experiment indicates that: (1)

the percentage inhibition of NTE required to produce ataxia is the same for a single and divided administration; (2) 14–21 days of 2.5 mg/kg were required to decrease NTE activity to 40–45% and that with daily treatment up to 70 days caused no further loss. Thus it appears that hens would remain healthy as long as inhibition does not increase above 50%, i.e. a low exposure for a long time leading to a large total exposure would not be neuropathic.

The same principles apply to acute toxicity to organophosphorus compounds due to inhibition of acetylcholinesterase (see sections 7.6, 11.7 and 11.8). Divided exposure which causes inhibition of the enzyme can be given for many weeks with no apparent toxicity. Metrifonate, which slowly changes in *in vivo* conditions into the acetyl-cholinesterase inhibitor dichlorvos, has been used for the treatment of Schistosoma haemotobium infections in large numbers of humans with no untoward effect following repeated administration (section 6.3.6; Holmstedt *et al.*, 1978; Plestina *et al.*, 1972).

Biological principles involved in these different responses to small and repeated exposures to intoxicants are illustrated (Figure 9.7). In a cell, the genome is one molecule of DNA which if modified can be repaired, but if mitosis occurs before repair then a mutated cell results (Figure 9.7a).

In contrast, for other macromolecules involved in toxicity (T_1) many molecules are present; sometimes they are present in excess of requirements and a substantial proportion must be modified to bring about dysfunction or death of the organism. Such macromolecules are continually being broken down and resynthesised (turnover). Such turnover may be slow and is of little significance in rapid toxicity due to a single exposure. However, as the exposure concentration is reduced and the time prolonged the turnover rate may be significant for covalent interactions. The turnover of phosphylated NTE is at the same rate as normal NTE (Meredith & Johnson, 1988) with a half-life of 4.5 to 5 days in hens (Figure 9.7b). If another esterase T_2 (say in the liver) competes for the organophosphorus compound then the faster it is resynthesised the better it is as a competitor.

For intoxicants which react reversibly with initiating targets T_1 (Figure 9.7c) resynthesis will have little influence on the concentration of modified targets since this is in equilibrium with the concentration of intoxicant and with other binding sites (T_2).

If it is accepted that the initiating event in the development of 2,5-hexanedione axonopathy is reaction with neurofilaments (see sections 7.9 and 9.5) then their length and rate of production may be significant factors (Figure 9.7d). Passage of neurofilaments is part of the slow component of axonal flow that moves down the nerve at 1–2 mm/day: passage down some long axons may take up to 50 days. During this time 2,5-hexanedione would, with repeated exposures, have the opportunity to react with the neurofilaments for a long time. This could explain its cumulative behaviour with a low dose threshold of certainly less than 0.6 μmol/ml equivalent to an exposure to approximately 0.4–0.5 mmol/kg/day. This biological property of long axons is entirely analogous to the accumulation of adducts on haemoglobin (compare Figures 9.7d and 11.4).

The foregoing discussion has concentrated on producing a framework for the dose–response relationships at or near to the threshold dose. Three different scenarios have been explored and the influence of normal turnover of macromolecules has been discussed. No account has been taken of repair mechanisms which can be beneficial or deleterious (see Chapter 8).

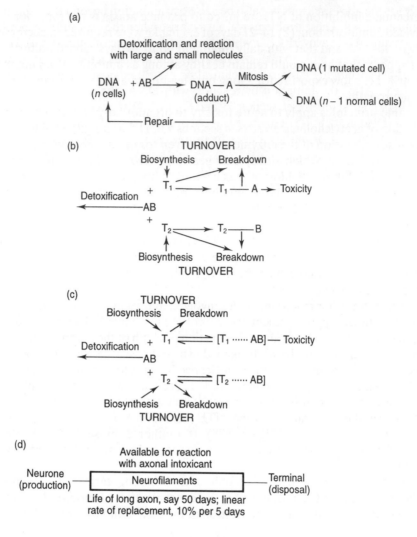

Figure 9.7 The influence of macromolecular turnover and detoxification on thresholds. (a) Carcinogenesis. (b) Covalent interactions. (c) Reversible interactions. (d) Covalent interaction with neurofilaments in long axons. T_1 = the initiating target; T_2 = other targets not causing toxicity; AB = the intoxicant

9.8 Discussion

The use of exposure–response as a bioassay (for the identification of the aetiological agent in poisoning in Pakistan) has been described. Such a bioassay consisting of oral administration to animals and the estimation of the exposure causing 50% of the animals to die is, for the purpose it was intended, an adequate procedure.

The determination of the exposure–response relationship for carcinogens produces a result which cannot be interpreted mechanistically (section 9.4). It is also difficult to use it to predict what will occur in other species or even in the same species with different dietary regimes. The use of the data for risk evaluation contains many pitfalls not only for the above reasons but also because extrapolation beyond the experimental range must be used. These problems will always arise when the exposure–response relationship required is at a low risk (i.e. when there is no evidence of a threshold). However, methods are now available to measure in experimental studies the dose at or near the target; effects occurring earlier than clinical or morphological diagnosis of tumours should help. After the initiation by reaction with DNA, the subsequent cascade is defined in biological terms (see section 8.9 and Figure 8.4). Current developments which may allow the identification of the relevant oncogenes may well help to provide a more molecular definition of earlier stages in tumorogenesis. These two developments (adducts for dose and oncogenes for effects) should help to bridge the gap between data from experimental animals and expectations in humans.

Structure–response and –activity relationships often lead to new hypotheses about the mechanisms involved. As with the γ-diketones, a particular molecular configuration is obligatory for the development of neuropathy (Figure 9.5 and section 7.8). Sometimes discontinuities are found in the structure–response and closely related compounds produce entirely different lesions. This certainly indicates that the targets will be different but it cannot be assumed that modification of only one target is required to cause one type of lesion. Naturally the usual approach is to try to establish the nature of a single target which, if modified, initiates a disease process. However, such a simplistic view has proved inadequate in chemical carcinogenesis and it is now accepted that several steps, perhaps taking place over an extended time period, are required. Discontinuities in structure–response appear in the toxicity of several chemicals previously discussed (see section 7.16), e.g. organophosphorus-induced delayed axonopathy (section 7.7), pyrethroid neurotoxicity (section 7.3) and the action of triorganotins producing neuronal necrosis and intramyelinic vacuoles (section 7.12).

Studies on the action of intoxicants on *in vitro* systems can provide valuable information about their biological properties. Whether these are relevant to effects (toxicity) seen *in vivo* must be checked. The first step is a comparison if the concentration of the intoxicant is similar *in vitro* and *in vivo* (dose–response); other intoxicants causing the same toxicity should also be checked in the same way (structure–activity).

9.9 Summary

1 Exposure–response relationships are operational constants which must be qualified by many factors which influence the amount of intoxicant delivered to the affected cell.

2 Dose (at the target)–response relationships are unaffected by these factors and define the intrinsic activity of the intoxicant.

3 Structure–response relationships provide qualitative information about what chemical structures cause the same biological effect.

4 Structure–activity relationships suffer from the same problems of interpretation as when only the exposure relationships are known; if dose at the target or a realistic estimate of it is available, then the influence of chemical structure on activity of the intoxicants may be compared.

5 The beneficial effects of many exogenous (drugs, vitamins, metals) or endogenous (hormones) substances are limited by exposure and dose; higher exposures or doses may be toxic.

6 Exposure–response relationships are used as bioassay systems for the identification of aetiological agents causing poisoning.

7 A threshold is the exposure or dose (defined by amount, frequency, time) below which no biological effect will occur. Most intoxicants have thresholds.

8 Chemical-induced mutations can have no threshold but many are without biological effect.

9 Genotoxic chemical carcinogenesis may have no threshold. There is much debate about non-genotoxic carcinogenesis.

10

Selective Toxicity, Animal Experimentation and *In Vitro* Methods

10.1 Introduction

Selective toxicity has been used in Chapter 7 in a rather restricted sense but historically it has had other meanings. An all embracing definition is 'selective toxicity means the injury of one kind of living matter without harming some other kind with which the first is in intimate contact' (Albert, 1985). This definition fits well with the previous definition that selectivity should be used down to the cell level and specificity for subcellular components; Table 10.1 lists many examples of selectivity. The last few items in the table, selectivity occurring within a species such as effects confined to one tissue or one cell type (class 5), has been considered in Chapters 7 and 8. Class 1 contains substances which are highly toxic to most organisms and are often volatile such as methyl bromide and phosphine; their selectivity is not biological but brought about by their pattern of use. Classes 2 and 3 have been designed to attack an unwanted organism and to be relatively non-toxic by virtue of their biological properties and/or their pattern of use, e.g. rodenticides (Meehan, 1984). Class 4 is the modification of physiology for the benefit of humans or animals. Many of the current drugs are designed to rectify derangements in normal physiology, to modify normal physiology, to remove cells with uncontrolled growth or to substitute deficient (or mutated) genes. Class 5 is relevant to all chemicals in classes 1–4 which may cause unwanted effects during medical treatment and occupational and environmental exposure. Definition of the selectivity of such exposure in terms of organs, cells and subcellular constituents is important in the assessment of risk of exposure. Inherent in these procedures are problems of predicting from animal data what will be the risk of exposure of humans.

Unfortunately there are many differences in the toxicity of a particular chemical in different species. As has been shown in previous chapters most of these are quantitative with the same signs of poisoning being produced in a wide range of different animal species even though very different doses are required to produce them. The assumption behind most toxicological studies using animals is that the system which is attacked is basic to many species, e.g. most of the transmitter systems are present not only in most vertebrates but also in many invertebrates. Thus although the basic building blocks for the nervous system may be similar the organisation (the structure and complexity

Table 10.1 Biological selectivity of chemicals

Purpose of agent		Selectivity required or found
1	Fumigants	Usually toxic to many organisms
	Sterilants	Selective by use pattern
2	Insecticides	Improvement of crop yields and animal
	Moluscicides	husbandry
	Fungicides	Removal of organisms acting as vectors
	Acaricides	of human and animal diseases
	Herbicides	
	Rodenticides	
3	Bacterial pathogens	Selectivity between organism and
	Viruses	human and animal hosts
	Parasites	
4	Diseases of abnormal	Selectivity for a given physiological
	physiology (e.g. diabetes,	system or cell within human or animal
	neurological)	
	Modification of normal	
	physiology (e.g. contraceptive	
	agents)	
	Removal of unwanted cells	
	(cancer chemotherapy)	
5	Unwanted effects of	Selective effects on an organ,
	chemicals	type of cell, subcellular system,
		macromolecule leading to toxicity

of connections) is very different across species. Similarly, the mitochondrial system of enzymes used to produce ATP for a variety of energy-requiring reactions, e.g. muscular effort, osmotic differences, synthesis of essential metabolites required for the maintenance of structure (macromolecules including protein, carbohydrate and lipid) etc., is present in many species. Even in plants, although there are unique features required to trap the energy from sunlight, many of the components of the energy conservation system are similar to those present in mitochondria and are sometimes inhibited by the same chemicals. Nevertheless the wider the range of species being considered the more likely it is that systems will be found which are not common. This has beneficial results since herbicides and bactericides may be designed to attack unique systems not found in humans or other mammals. However, even when the same basic physiological system is involved, the range of toxicity across species can span many orders of magnitude (Figure 10.1). An exact comparison across such a large range of species is difficult but in the case of Figure 10.1, the toxicity range approximates to 10^7 and overwhelms problems of comparison of exposure of fish to X ppm in water with oral administration to rats in X μg per g. Table 10.2 illustrates that for 2,3,7,8-tetrachlorodibenzo-*p*-dioxin (dioxin, TCDD), amongst the more usual experimental animals and strains within them, differences of over 1,000 in the range of lethality (1–6 weeks) occur after a single administration (Pohjanvirta & Tuomisto, 1994). If the same disease syndrome is caused by a chemical in several species but the exposure needed varies, this suggests that the differences are in delivery of intoxicant following exposure. Such differences may be much reduced if the dose delivered to the affected cells is known (see Chapter 9), i.e. dose–response indicates intrinsic toxicity.

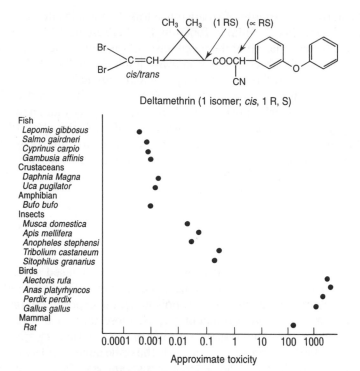

Deltamethrin (1 isomer; *cis*, 1 R, S)

Figure 10.1 The toxicity of deltamethrin to different species. Approximate LC_{50}s are expressed for fish, aquatic invertebrates and grain storage pests in ppm; LD_{50}s for house flies and honey-bees toxicity in μg per insect; for rats in μg per g; for birds the actual LD_{50}s are more than the values (μg per g) in the graph. (*Source*: Grieg-Smith, 1993)

Table 10.2 Acute lethality of TCDD to various species and (sub)strains

Animal	Route of administration[a]	Toxicity LD_{50} (μg/kg)	Time of death (days)
Guinea pig (Hartley)	po	2	5–42
Chicken	po	<25	12–21
Rhesus monkey	po	ca. 70	14–34
Rabbit (New Zealand White)	po	115	6–39
Hamster (Golden Syrian)	po	1,157	2–47
Rat (Long Evans; Turku AB)	po	10–18	13–35
	ip	10	15–23
Rat (Sherman–Spartan)	po	22	9–27
Rat (Sprague–Dawley)	ip	25–60	–
Rat (Fischer)	po	340	28
Rat (Han–Wistar, Kuopio)	po	>7,200	17–42
	ip	>3,000	23–34
Mouse (C57BL/6)	po	182	Mean 24
	ip	132	–
Mouse (DBA/2)	po	2,570	Mean 21
	ip	620	–
Mouse (B6D2F$_1$)	po	296	Mean 25
	ip	300	–

[a] po = by oral route; ip = intraperitoneal.
Source: Data from Pohjanvirta & Tuomisto, 1994.

:ication is the response of an organism to a chemical insult and is always defined
of changes in behaviour or function. Further research, often by *in vitro* studies,
may result in the elucidation of the mechanism of toxicity including the initiating reaction of chemical with target. If this is known then it is usually possible to devise an *in vitro* technique which will predict that a particular chemical has the potential to cause a particular type of toxicity; it is rarely possible to predict the exposure which will cause it in whole organisms including humans. New types of toxicity and new biological pathways (i.e. physiological control mechanisms) are often found after administration of or exposure to a chemical of a whole organism. It is by the interplay between *in vitro* experiments and research involving whole animals that new tests can often be devised for particular types of toxicity; understanding the reasons for species differences in the exposure required often follows.

10.2   Differences in Metabolism: Methanol

Methanol as a constituent of illicit distilled liquor has caused several outbreaks of poisoning (Wood & Buller, 1904). It is used industrially as a solvent and could be used as a constituent of fuel. In epidemics of poisoning, the exposed fall into three groups: those that recover with no permanent effects, those that have severe visual loss or blindness, and those who die. When symptoms of visual deficiency are reported, hyperaemia of the optic disc is present. Ultimately the optic nerve head will be swollen along with the retinal vasculature. If the oedema persists and is sufficiently severe, optic nerve atrophy will follow accompanied by lesions in the basal ganglia (Potts *et al.*, 1955). The progression of the disease in human and primates is identical and proceeds through three stages: (1) organic solvent central nervous depression (also seen in rodents), (2) systemic acidosis, and (3) specific central nervous effects including changes in the eye and the basal ganglia.

   Methanol, like ethanol, is readily metabolised in mammals; the products are formaldehyde, formic acid and carbon dioxide. For many years it was accepted that formaldehyde was the proximal intoxicant but the fact that ocular toxicity is seen in humans and monkeys but not in rodents, dogs and cats was difficult to reconcile with similar metabolites in these species (Gilger & Potts, 1955; Tephly, 1977). The primary step in metabolism is to formaldehyde but the pathways can be different; in rodents oxidation is via a catalase-dependent pathway whereas in humans and primates alcohol dehydrogenase is the main oxidant (Tephly *et al.*, 1964). Formaldehyde is the product for all species but even after ingestion of large amounts of methanol by humans, primates and other species no formaldehyde can be detected. Formaldehyde is oxidised rapidly to formic acid mainly by formaldehyde dehydrogenase but with contributions from other enzymes; the subsequent oxidation of formic acid is to carbon dioxide by a folic acid-dependent pathway (Figure 10.2; Kavet & Nauss, 1990). Severe acidosis in humans and primates follows large amounts of methanol whereas this does not occur in rodents (Tephly, 1991) because of differences in the balance of rates of production and removal. In humans and primates formic acid is produced rapidly but removed slowly; it thus accumulates causing the acidosis (Röe, 1982). Although there is this association between the accumulation of formic acid and acidosis, experience with poisoned patients has shown that treatment of the acidosis by infusion of base does not prevent ocular toxicity. A more direct effect of formate seems likely since intravenous infusion of formate into monkeys while maintaining the blood pH within normal limits causes

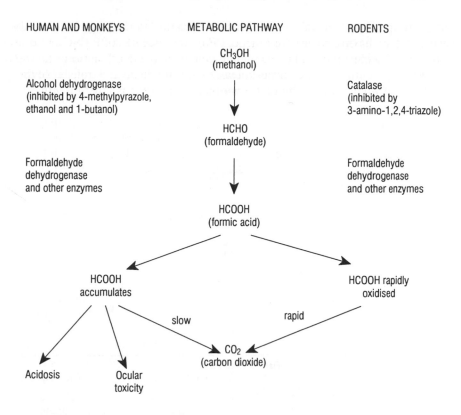

Figure 10.2 Current hypotheses on the species differences in the toxicity and metabolism of methanol. (*Sources*: Kavet & Nauss, 1990; Tephly, 1991)

ocular toxicity (Martin-Amat *et al.*, 1978; Tephly, 1991). The mechanism of action of formate has not yet been established nor is it clear if formate will cause ocular toxicity in other mammals such as the minipig (Makar *et al.*, 1990) which has a low rate of formate oxidation but no formate accumulation or acidosis (Dorman *et al.*, 1993) or in rodents made tetrahydrofolate deficient. In experimentation there are several possibilities of manipulation of the rate of delivery of formaldehyde to the formate oxidation step (see Figure 10.2) and in humans ethanol can prevent methanol toxicity by competing in the primary oxidative step, alcohol dehydrogenase. Therapeutic measures, therefore, are based on methods to reduce the rate of oxidation of methanol and thus prevent the accumulation of formate.

10.3 Differences in Detoxification and Reaction with Target: Chlorfenvinphos

Chlorfenvinphos is a direct-acting organophosphorus compound used in crop protection particularly against soil organisms. Its LD_{50} varies widely between species of mammal (Figure 10.3b). Toxicity is highest in the rat decreasing with mouse and rabbit and least in the dog with an estimate of >5,000–12,000 mg/kg. The ratio of the LD_{50}s dog : rat is >500. The main route of metabolism of chlorfenvinphos is via removal of an ethyl group (Figure 10.3a) and the main metabolite in the dog is the monoethyl derivative which having a negative charge, P-O$^-$, in place of the P-O-C$_2$H$_5$, does not inhibit acetylcholinesterase. The two main mechanisms of deethylation are oxidative attack by the cytochrome P$_{450}$ enzymes releasing acetaldehyde and transfer of the alkyl group to glutathione by glutathione transferase. The latter is most effective for the

(a)

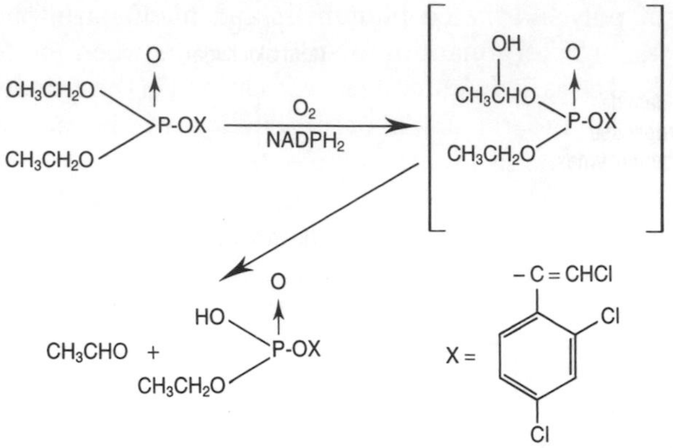

(b)

Species	Rate of deethylation		LD$_{50}$ (oral, mg/kg)
	(nmol/min/mg microsomal protien)*	(nmol/min/nmol cytochrome P$_{450}$)**	
Rat (Wistar)	0.02	0.13	20–30
Rat (Aroclor induced)	–	2.27	–
Mouse (CF1)	0.65	–	100–200
Human	–	1.0	–
Monkey	1.0	–	–
Rabbit	–	1.3	500–1000
Dog	2.0	–	>12000

Sources:
Data taken from Donninger (1971)* and from Hutson and Milburn (1991)**.

(c)

Species	pI$_{50}$ (–log pI$_{50}$)	Bimolecular rate constant* (M^{-1}, min^{-1})	Ratio of rate constants (rat : dog)
Rat	5.9	1.8 × 10^4	
Dog	5.1	2.9 × 10^3	6.2

Note:
The conditions of incubation before adding the substrate acetylcholine were for 30 min at pH 7.15 at 30 °C. *Rate constants are calculated from the pI$_{50}$ values. *Source:* Hutson and Hathway,1967.

Figure 10.3 Factors involved in the species differences in the toxicity of chlorfenvinphos. (a) Enzymic dealkylation of organophosphates. (b) Rate of deethylation of chlorfenvinphos in relation to its acute toxicity in several species of mammal. (c) Inhibition by chlorfenvinphos of acetylcholinesterase from dog and rat

transfer of methyl groups and less active with alkyl groups with more carbon atoms whereas the oxidative route is more generally active. Liver slices convert the triester to the diester in the increasing order rat, mouse, rabbit and dog, and microsomes from liver supplemented with a NADPH generating system are active in the same order (Figure 10.3b); this order is in inverse relation to the LD_{50}s. The low activity in the rat can be increased by as much as 40–600-fold by pretreatment with dieldrin, Aroclor (a mixture of polychlorinated biphenyls) and phenobarbitone (Hutson & Wright, 1980). The major determinant of the difference between the toxicity of chlorfenvinphos to rats and dogs is the rate of detoxification via the oxidative deethylation route and therefore in the rat a bigger proportion of the active inhibitor of acetylcholinesterase (the target) reaches the nervous system. Another contributing factor is the sensitivity of the target to inhibition: rat acetylcholinesterase is approximately six times more sensitive than that from the dog (Figure 10.3c; Hutson & Hathway, 1967). Thus two factors, both acting in the same direction, influence the higher toxicity of chlorfenvinphos to the rat. Both can be evaluated using human liver microsomes and acetylcholinesterase from erythrocytes; the results suggest that toxicity to humans will be lower than to the rat and be in the region of 500–1,000 mg/kg. This compound therefore, has a toxicity which the World Health Organization normally accepts for routine use in vector control programmes.

10.4 Species Difference in Induction of Peroxisomes in Liver

In research to understand the mechanisms of species differences, much use is made of *in vitro* techniques devised to answer precise questions under controlled conditions. Such techniques play a vital role in research into mechanisms but to establish their relevance to toxicity requires a continual to and fro between *in vitro* and *in vivo*. An example is the extensive research to understand the mechanisms of peroxisome proliferation (section 7.9) and to examine whether it is associated from a mechanistic viewpoint with carcinogenesis in rodents. Hypolipidaemic drugs seemed to be species-specific and cause an increase in peroxisomes in rats and mice but not in guinea pigs, rabbits, chickens and squirrels (Reddy & Lalwani, 1983). A more active compound, ciprofibrate, causes peroxisome proliferation as judged by morphological changes and enzymes induced, in cats, chickens, pigeons, rhesus and cynomologous monkeys as well as rodents (Reddy *et al.*, 1984a). Liver biopsies from patients taking hypolipidaemic drugs have shown a marginal or nil excess of peroxisomes (Lock *et al.*, 1989); however, the amounts of drugs taken were relatively small compared with experimental research. Cultured hepatocytes also show a marked species difference in response: mouse and rat are positive whereas guinea pig and human hepatocytes showed no induction of either peroxisomes or associated enzyme activities (see section 7.9). After exposure to trichlorethylene the mouse produces more trichloracetic acid than the rat and, using cultured hepatocytes, the decreasing order of production is mouse, rat and human. Peroxisome proliferation by trichloracetic acid in mouse and rat hepatocytes is similar and few, if any, are produced by human tissue (Elcombe, 1985). Cross-species transplantation techniques have also been developed (Reddy *et al.*, 1984a,b,c; Rao *et al.*, 1986). Recent research implicating a nuclear receptor mechanism (Green *et al.*, 1992; see section 7.9) may allow experiments to decide if peroxisome proliferation across species is a dose-dependent or a species-specific phenomenon.

10.5 Human Chemical-induced Diseases with No Animal Model

In Table 10.3 are a few examples of human diseases for which there is no experimental animal model. Although the vehicle carrying the aetiological agent via the oral route is known from epidemiological evidence for all five episodes its chemical identity is still unknown for toxic oil syndrome, eosinophilic myalgia syndrome and margarine disease. The proximal intoxicant in aminorex pulmonary hypertension and for the practolol syndrome may not be the parent compound and could be a metabolite produced by a small number of the population. The incidence among those consuming the products is low for the late and chronic phase of toxic oil syndrome and the other diseases. The incidence for the primary respiratory insufficiency in toxic oil syndrome is not known but may be high. Should the aetiological agents for these severe human diseases occur and be consumed again there is no biological testing system available to detect them. Without an animal model for at least part of these syndromes, progress is difficult and the relevance of any *in vitro* study is difficult to decide.

10.6 The Ames Test

Based on the results of much research the view was formed that exposure to electrophilic reagents or to compounds bioactivated to electrophilic reagents was followed by reaction with nucleophilic centres in DNA, and that if cell mitosis occurred before repair a mutated cell resulted. Although this alone was not sufficient to cause cancer much later, a mutation came to be regarded as an obligatory step. Bacteria, with their rapid cell turnover, are suitable test systems for induced mutations. Ames and his colleagues introduced the use of *Salmonella* bacteria for such a test. These organisms are histidine-dependent but may be induced to back-mutate by DNA-reacting chemicals to become histidine-independent and thus grow rapidly in a histidine-deficient medium (Ames *et al.*, 1975a). Thus it became possible to detect chemicals which react with DNA and cause such a mutation. Unlike experiments exposing animals to potential carcinogens and then waiting until tumours appeared, the test was rapid. Many variants of this test have been devised (Maron & Ames, 1983), some using different cells, e.g. with different capacity to repair damaged DNA and different measured responses. Also, because most of the organisms do not, unlike many mammalian tissues, possess the enzyme systems capable of bioactivating stable compounds to electrophilic reactants, enzymes (usually a supernatant from homogenised rat liver) have been incorporated into the test. All of these tests detect the ability of chemicals to interact with DNA and induce mutations and also give a semi-quantitative indication of their capacity to do so.

The Ames type test systems have been incorporated into the battery of tests required by the regulatory bodies and for tests for potential carcinogenic activity. Thus they are an essential component for screening of compounds to which the public may be exposed during medical treatment, and in their occupations and the environment generally, e.g. drugs, pesticides, herbicides, food additives, and 'normal' contaminants such as those caused by contamination of food by micro-organisms, water treatment procedures to remove organisms (see section 13.5), in motor vehicle exhaust gases, in urban air, following high temperature cooking, etc.

The significance of these tests for human risk is a continuing debate. Many but not all positives are either mutagenic or carcinogenic *in vivo* in rodents. There are a signif-

Table 10.3 Chemically-induced diseases in humans with no experimental animal model

TOXIC OIL SYNDROME

Disease characteristics	Pulmonary disease (endothelial damage) and a chronic non-necrotising vasculitis (section 8.10)
Cases	>20,000 with lung damage; an unknown proportion became chronically ill
Number exposed	Not known
Intoxicant carrier	Rape seed oil refined after denaturation with 2% aniline (Chapter 12)
Intoxicant	Not known
References	WHO, 1983, 1992; Aldridge, 1992c

EOSINOPHILIA MYALGIA SYNDROME

Disease characteristics	Incapacitating myalgia and peripheral eosinophilia (section 8.10)
Cases	1,500
Number exposed	Not known
Intoxicant carrier	1-Tryptophan
Intoxicant	Not known
References	WHO, 1991, 1993; Swygert *et al.*, 1990; Slutsker *et al.*, 1990

MARGARINE DISEASE

Disease characteristics	Extensive and often whole body rash including mucosae, fever and itching
Cases	Estimated 50,000
Number exposed	Estimated 600,000
Carrier of intoxicant	Margarine with new emulgator
Intoxicant	? emulgator; ? impurity
References	Grimmer & Joseph, 1959; Doeglas *et al.*, 1961; Mali & Malten, 1966

AMINOREX PULMONARY HYPERTENSION

Disease characteristics	Chronic pulmonary hypertension of vascular origin
Cases	582
Number exposed	Not known
Carrier of intoxicant	Aminorex (appetite suppressor)
Intoxicant	Not known
References	Gurtner, 1979

PRACTOLOL SYNDROME

Disease characteristics	Oculmucocutaneous syndrome: psoriasis rash with hyperkeratosis, keratoconjunctivitis, otitis media, sclerosing peritonitis
Cases	>1,300
Number exposed	Approx. 1 million patient years
Carrier of intoxicant	Practolol
Intoxicant	Not known
References	Amos *et al.*, 1975; Felix *et al.*, 1974; Wright, 1975; Reeves *et al.*, 1978; Cruikshank & Prichard, 1988

icant number of chemicals which are not mutagenic in the Ames test or in other short-term tests which, nevertheless, are carcinogenic in rodents. In addition to this uncertainty, the significance of carcinogenic potential in rodents for human risk is problematical. Thus while 'complete' and active electrophilic carcinogens are relatively easy to detect and are almost certainly a hazard to humans, such decisions about non-genotoxic chemicals carcinogenic to rodents, are difficult to make: the chemicals may have quite different dose–response relationships and also be species specific (Purchase, 1994). For a discussion and survey of known human carcinogens and their performance in short-term tests and their chemical structure see section 7.14.

Thus this *in vitro* test has been and is extremely valuable in research, but in detecting carcinogenic potential its accuracy for prediction of human risk is not absolute. Positive results, however, are a good indication that the compound or its metabolites react with DNA and cause mutation.

10.7 *In vitro* Techniques and the Use of Animals

There is much current discussion, even agitation, about the use of animals for experimental purposes. On the one hand there are those who claim that it is wholly immoral to use animals to try to establish if there is a likely hazard from exposure of humans or animals to various chemicals. On the other side are those who consider that, under defined conditions, it is justifiable to obtain the best information possible, using animals if necessary, for the risk–benefit debate. The regulatory process as we now know it has existed only for the past half-century. Previously humans were exposed in many ways and if ill-health resulted conditions were improved. The whole of this book is based on the view that the controlled use of experimental animals is justified. If the former view is held, which takes no account of past and future benefits, including the advance of biological knowledge, and rests on perceptions and beliefs which apply the sanctity of human life ethic to animals, there is little chance for consensus.

There can be no doubt that the use of animals for biological (usually medically driven) research in the past has proved worthwhile with consequent benefit to human and animal health. For the foreseeable future it seems likely that the discovery of new biological knowledge will depend to some extent of the use of experimental animals. The design of the experimental procedure, the choice of animals for the experiment, the conduct of the experiments, animal husbandry, the use of inbred strains or transgenic animals are all open to discussion in relation to the purpose of the experiment and whether the design will allow conclusions to be drawn. In basic biological and medical research it is often difficult to predict the benefit which will result from potential new findings. For the testing of chemicals which governments now demand to fulfil their duty of protection of the public, there is and must be much debate about the updating of procedures so that fewer animals are used and more information is acquired from each animal. This comes under the aims of the three Rs: reduction of the number of animals used, refinement of the end-points of the experiment, and replacement of the animal by other techniques not involving the use of animals – aims which are slowly being achieved in toxicity testing. In biological research, particularly that which aims to understand processes at the molecular level, many *in vitro* controllable techniques are used; hypotheses developed from results using such techniques always require verification in experimental animals. Those wishing to pursue the arguments used in the debate about the use of animals should consult for the philosophical discussion Singer

(1983) and Regan (1983), for the practical issues involved in the need for biomedical research, Paton, (1984), and for the ethical issues, Institute of Medical Ethics (1991).

10.8　Discussion

In research on species differences the first question to ask is can a particular clinical pattern or a substantial part of it be produced in several animal species and then what is the effective exposure? This question may not be simple to answer when the range of effective exposure is large; in mechanistic terms we are asking whether the same target is involved across species. This is a fundamental question not directly connected to risk assessment and essential for understanding of structure–activity relationships. If the same target is involved and a range of exposures is required to bring about the clinical effect in different species, then three further questions may be asked about the quantitative contribution of various systems in the stages of developing toxicity: i.e. in stage 2, in the delivery of intoxicant to its target, in stage 3, in different susceptibility of the target to intoxicant attack, and in stage 4, in the various parts of the biological cascade leading to signs and symptoms of toxicity.

Biological research has established that the major components of metabolism and control mechanisms are similar across a wide range of species although there may be quantitative differences in their affinity for or rate of reactions with intoxicants. Examples discussed in preceding chapters have illustrated this point and underline the view that experimental models of chemically induced disease are usually available in several species. However, the exposure required often varies markedly; in many cases factors in stage 2 are the major cause. Such differences in stage 2 are expected since they have evolved due to the fact that different species are exposed to different chemicals in their respective environments of food, air and water (see Chapter 6). If a species difference in the effective exposure is found then the first hypothesis should be that it is due to delivery of intoxicant. New techniques are available to determine the dose reaching the target and to compare the dose–clinical response across species. If these doses are different then other explanations must be sought such as intoxicant affinity for or reactivity with the target (stage 3; see methanol, section 10.2; chlorfenvinphos, section 10.3) or in the consequent biological responses (stage 4; e.g. fibrosis after injury, section 8.3.1). The major differences found between strains within the same species (e.g. rat and mouse strains and TCDD; Table 10.2) reinforces the possibilities and problems of differing susceptibilities within the human population (section 11.2). Other factors such as age may play a role in susceptibility. The adult hen is a good experimental model for organophosphorus compound delayed neuropathy but the chick is not (section 7.9), nor could clinical signs be produced in the rat. This difference has now been explained, and provided older (than normally used) rats are used they are as susceptible as hens; the period of insensitivity of young chicks (to 30% of its adult weight at 60 days) is much extended in the rat (to 70–80% of adult weight at 105 days; Moretto *et al.*, 1992).

The extent to which genetic differences can influence susceptibility to intoxicants is illustrated by the development of resistance of insects to insecticides. Minority mutants survive and reproduce rapidly under the selection pressure of insecticides. Resistance may be caused by increases in detoxifying systems but also by changes in the target. Two are well known: a single recessive *kdr* gene (knock down resistance gene) after prolonged exposure to DDT and pyrethroids considered to be due to a change in the molecular configuration of the voltage-dependent sodium channels (see Hassall, 1990, for discussion) and a change in the acetylcholinesterase so that it requires higher concentrations of organophosphorus compounds to cause inhibition (Tripathi & O'Brien, 1973; Tripathi, 1976; O'Brien *et al.*, 1978; Devonshire and Moore, 1984). It is remarkable that sensitivity to organophosphorus compounds is reduced by 2–3 orders and yet the enzyme is still able to serve its physiological function of hydrolysing acetylcholine. The mechanism of reaction for acetylcholine and inhibitor is identical and illustrates the influence of probably quite minor changes in the tertiary structure on the catalytic activity of enzymes (Hassall, 1990). This change gives a glimpse of the many possibilities of silent mutations which may influence susceptibility to intoxicants. Controlled genetic manipulation is now possible in most organisms; those in plants and animals for food purposes, in micro-organisms to increase production of defined biological material and in experimental animals for particular testing or research purposes.

The preceding discussion has illustrated that the mechanisms involved in species differences in response to chemicals are many and sometimes complex. There are many problems in establishing alternatives to animal models. These include the complex physiology of tissues, the variations in biochemistry and physiology in the many differentiated cells, the compartmentalisation into organs and the relationships between cell types within them and the huge losses and gains in intoxicant between exposure and dose at the target. It is the variation in these factors which creates the problems in the extrapolation of *in vivo* effects between mammalian species and imposes stumbling blocks to developing *in vitro* procedures of direct value in risk assessment. *In vitro* techniques play an important role in research but at present are less useful in testing procedures for regulatory purposes. There is no immediate likelihood that *in vitro* alternatives will replace experimental animals in the assessment of the acute or chronic effects of chemicals. Use of *in vitro* methods in research in conjunction with experimental animals will increase understanding so that reliable non-animal procedures may be developed for the detection of the ability of chemicals to cause a defined type of toxicity. The mutagenicity testing using Ames type systems have proved useful for screening for chemicals (or their metabolites) able to react with DNA and cause mutations. The gap between these tests and the risks of cancer due to exposure of humans is still large (for a historical review of information relevant to risk assessment of vinyl chloride see Purchase *et al.*, 1987). It may be that, following a positive result in an *in vitro* test, the cost of unnecessarily discarding a potentially useful drug is worth bearing but there are also problems of false negatives. For a discussion of the issues in testing for potential cancer-producing chemicals and the future possibilities of *in vitro* tests see Grasso *et al.*, 1991, and Purchase, 1994.

Understanding of the mechanisms of chemical-induced toxicity may lead to reliable *in vitro* tests. Information flow usually follows animal experimentation to identification of the cell and/or target to *in vitro* tests for a particular biological activity to validation against animal tests to acceptance by regulatory bodies and experience in use. Sound *in vitro* tests are in principle better than tests on animals because the conditions of their use are more rigidly under the experimenter's control but they will often only answer a specific question. Developments in the isolation of specific cell types or parts of organs in a functioning state are providing opportunities for research and for new test systems. Once the mechanism of a toxicological response or the initiating reaction has been identified then more readily available or convenient indicator cells other than those affected *in vivo* can potentially be developed for testing purposes. This increasing knowledge will certainly play a significant part in the reduction and refinement of animal experimentation; replacement is some way off. The same research-derived knowledge may allow measurements of early change in humans (i.e. biological effect monitoring) before meaningful changes in function can be detected.

10.9 Summary

1 Selective toxicity can occur between widely differing organisms, mammalian species, different organs within a species and between cells within an organ.

2 A major cause of selective toxicity between mammalian species is differences in the delivery of the intoxicant to its site of action (detoxification, bioactivation). Differences in the properties of the target contribute less frequently and to a lesser extent.

3 For some chemical-induced diseases in humans no animal model has been found.

4 *In vitro* techniques are used extensively to elucidate mechanisms.

5 *In vitro* techniques answer specific questions and therefore their application for prediction of human and animal toxicity and risks of exposure often presents difficulties.

6 Genetic differences can influence susceptibility to intoxicants while being compatible with normal life.

11

Biomonitoring

11.1 Introduction

Biomonitoring is measurement which indicates conditions *in vivo*. The aim is to obtain dose–response relationships of internal dose (as near to the target as possible) related to biological changes occurring before clinical signs of poisoning appear. For humans the material available for examination is limited and only accessible samples such as blood, urine or excretions, e.g. exhalation or saliva, can be used. For experimental animals such restrictions do not apply and measurements in individual tissues may be made after death.

In the context of biomonitoring, dose is defined as the internal concentration of intoxicant and does not have the wider connotation used in medicine where it includes what we have called exposure. The emphasis is to measure the concentrations of the intoxicant available to tissues; because of bioactivation, this may not be the chemical to which humans or animals have been exposed.

Biomonitoring serves the three different purposes of identifying and using:

1 biomarkers for susceptibility of an individual within a population of one species to exposure to an intoxicant – genetically determined susceptibility;
2 biomarkers for internal dose of the intoxicant – dose monitoring;
3 biomarkers for early biological changes following exposure – effect monitoring

Drug or chemical idiosyncrasy is a genetically determined reactivity to a drug or chemical. The observation that an individual is more or less sensitive to administration of a chemical is not sufficient to qualify as an idiosyncrasy in the sense defined above. Many dose–response curves show a wide variation between the most and least sensitive. Other evidence is required to establish that the difference has a genetic basis; this is often based on familial patterns of the differences. In animals the variation is less in inbred than in outbred strains. The characteristic feature in idiosyncratic low exposure–dose sensitivity or high exposure–dose resistance to chemicals is a discontinuity from the ordinary pattern of dose–response. Biomarkers of genetically inherited characteristics are often single proteins, e.g. an enzyme. Mutational changes, presumably leading to altered protein, are sometimes lethal and sometimes cause disease. In the context of biomonitoring we are concerned with changes leading to susceptibilities in apparently healthy individuals. A large number of factors contribute to the eventual toxicity and therefore there are many opportunities for silent mutations, e.g. in detoxification systems (LaDu, 1972). These include a wide range of possibilities and may involve, for example, the rate of metabolism of a test substance by a particular isozyme of cytochrome P_{450}. As generally understood, biomonitoring is not used to indicate the sensitivity of individuals to exposure to chemicals owing to intercurrent disease and differences between species. However, these and differing sensitivity due to age (early development and later life) may be detected by biomonitoring. The boundaries of research in this area are difficult to define and are changing, e.g. different strains within a given species of experimental animal and transgenic animals now available provide opportunities for research.

Dose and effect monitoring overlap although the measurements made are different. The overlap occurs in stage 3 (Figure 11.1) when the intoxicant interacts with a particular macromolecule (target):

$$M + AB \xrightleftharpoons{K_{aff}} [M\cdots AB]$$

$$M + AB \xrightarrow{k} MA + B$$

At stage 3 the concentration of intoxicant ([AB]) defines the dose and the modified M ([M$\cdots$AB] or MA) defines the beginning of the biological effect. The concentration

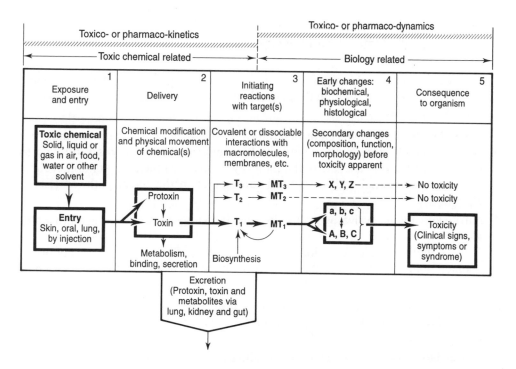

Figure 11.1 Scheme for developing toxicity due to chemicals. The stages covered by the terms toxico- or pharmacokinetics and toxico- and pharmacodynamics are marked on the figure. (*Source:* Adapted from Aldridge, 1981, 1986; see also legend to Figure 2.1)

of the intoxicant and the degree of reaction are related to each other and are defined by affinity constants (K_{Aff}) or rate constants (k). This overlap between chemical related and biology related events is the same overlap that there is between the terms toxico- or pharmacokinetics on the one hand and toxico- or pharmacodynamics on the other (Figure 11.1). In dose and effect monitoring the aim is to find the clues that the chemical/intoxicant is or has been there and has caused effects while there.

It is ideal if the concentration of intoxicant at the target T_1 (see Figure 11.1) and its degree of reaction can be directly related to a biological event on the way to clinical manifestation of disease. Often this is not possible and surrogates for dose at the target have to be used and the internal or circulating dose may be derived from the degree of reaction of the intoxicant with targets T_2, T_3, unrelated to subsequent toxicity. Measured biological effects are various, e.g. repair, mitosis, enzyme induction. The evidence for a relationship between target dose and disease is not yet extensive. For example, for carcinogens the target may be a single base in a particular gene, and the most sensitive human monitoring technique cannot quantify such modifications satisfactorily, i.e. surrogates are measured and 'target' doses are not directly measured. Beland & Poirier (1993) have summarised current DNA adduct–tumour relationships in animal models.

The three different kinds of biomonitoring listed above may be linked. Dose–response relationships resulting from dose and effect monitoring may indicate that there is more than one population within the group examined. Further research would aim to establish a difference between these populations which may become diagnostic for their subsequent susceptibility to exposure to a particular chemical.

11.2 Genetically Determined Susceptibility

The essential feature of abnormal susceptibility is that it is genetically determined and it is a difference of a group within the general population which does not directly cause illness. Examples are:

1 The induction of porphyria cutanea tarda syndrome by hexachlorobenzene and other chloro-aromatic compounds where the biochemical abnormality is sensitivity to induction of the first enzyme in the pathway of haem synthesis, 5-aminolaevulinic synthetase associated with a reduced throughput in the haem pathway (Elder, 1978).

2 Nitrite and aniline derivatives cause in some individuals a long-lasting methaemoglobinaemia which is due to a reduced capacity to regenerate haemoglobin via NADH methaemoglobin reductase (Smith, 1986). Some genetically abnormal haemoglobins may show an abnormal propensity for oxidation by agents such as nitrite.

3 A reduced capacity in *N*-acetylation of chemicals may decrease rates of detoxification and lead to increased toxicity of isoniazid (Evans *et al.*, 1960) and also of bladder cancer in smokers (Vineis *et al.*, 1990).

4 *O*-acetylation is important in the bioactivation of certain arylamines; low activity may have significance in susceptibility to cancer (Hein *et al.*, 1992).

5 Individuals with a high debrisoquine activity appear to run an increased risk of lung cancer (Caporaso *et al.*, 1990).

11.3 Succinyldicholine

Succinyldicholine is a depolarising neuromuscular blocking agent which is used to induce muscular relaxation during surgery. Its infusion causes muscular relaxation of short duration and recovery is rapid when infusion is stopped. While infusion is taking place and the concentration of succinyldicholine is maintained, muscular relaxation persists, but as soon as the infusion is stopped the concentration of drug falls rapidly due the drug's hydrolysis, mainly by plasma cholinesterase, to the inactive succinyl-monocholine. However, in some patients infusion of succinyldicholine results in a very prolonged muscular relaxation and apnea lasting sometimes several hours. These patients have an atypical plasma cholinesterase which hydrolyses the drug at greatly reduced rates. The capacity of the atypical cholinesterase to hydrolyse succinyldicholine is not much reduced, i.e. the V_{max} is the same but the relation of activity to concentration of substrate is different, i.e. the K_m is raised by about two orders so that at the concentration of circulating drug the rate of its hydrolysis is much reduced and its half-life is prolonged.

The presence of the atypical cholinesterase can be detected by the high K_m for both succinyldicholine and for benzoylcholine and by the low affinity for the inhibitor dibucaine. A 'dibucaine number', defined as the degree of inhibition of benzoylcholine hydrolysis under standardised conditions (Kalow, 1962), is used as a predictive test for patients who would have a high sensitivity to succinyldicholine. Normal populations have dibucaine numbers of around 80 whereas those of high and intermediate sensitivity are 15 and 60 respectively.

Studies of families indicate that the presence of atypical cholinesterase is a genetically determined characteristic. The gene is widespread throughout the world with a frequency of around 20% in many groups but in others the gene is absent or of very low frequency. As often happens when new methods of measurement are devised, further research reveals that there are other variants of cholinesterase distinguished by their dibucaine number and by resistance to inhibition by fluoride; a variant is also known which has an abnormally high enzyme activity.

This genetically determined abnormality first detected by the abnormal sensitivity of patients to challenge with succinyldicholine is an excellent example of an abnormality which under normal circumstances causes no illness. No function is known for the cholinesterase present in human and animal plasma or in their tissues. Inhibition of this enzyme by exposure to organophosphorus compounds produces no evidence of toxicity.

11.4 Exposure, Dose and Effect Monitoring in Humans

Measurements of exposure are often difficult to interpret. Concentrations in factories or in the outside environment as in spraying programmes are always extremely variable and depend on the sampling points and working practices and at best are average values. Personal air samplers and concentrations found on skin (or on clothing worn for sampling purposes) are in theory more indicative of individual exposure but do not give any information about the amount which has penetrated (dose). In some cases, as for inhalation of reactive gases such as phosgene or methylisocyanate which cause direct toxicity to the lung, only measurements of their concentration in the inhaled air is possible. Acrylamide is particulate, uncharged and very soluble in water; it can be inhaled and significant entry can occur via the skin and mouth. The amount gaining entry can be measured by the determination of haemoglobin adducts in which the acrylamide has reacted with a cysteine (Bailey *et al.*, 1986) or valine residue (Bergmark *et al.*, 1993). Such measurements yield values for individuals. This kind of data improves epidemiological surveys and reduces the variation due to the use of average exposures (see Chapter 12). In research using experimental animals more and more emphasis should be placed on dose rather than exposure (concentration in the inhaled air, applied to the skin or administered by mouth) so that dose–response relationships may be obtained in which the dose approximates to that dose reaching the affected tissue, cell or target.

It is important to distinguish three questions:

1 Has the person or animal been exposed?
2 What has been absorbed?
3 What is the relation between dose and effect?

Detoxification products in blood and/or urine give a reliable indication that the chemical has been present *in vivo*. As discussed previously, there are many pathways of metabolism and which is the best metabolite to measure will depend on previous research.

If the chemical/intoxicant is sufficiently stable then previous exposure can be deduced from analysis of urine but quantitative evaluation of dose requires blood or tissue. The time factor can be evaluated by clearance curves; the peak concentration and the total concentration × time can be calculated. For many stable compounds reactions with components of the affected cell are reversible. Concentrations in circulating blood are assumed to be in equilibrium with other compartments, e.g. concentration of an intoxicant in erythrocytes should be a function of that in the affected cell.

Concentrations of reactive chemicals/intoxicants are often difficult to measure directly in biological material. Electrophilic species react with the many nucleophiles *in vivo*; mainly inactive products result but some react with initiating targets to cause toxicity. Some nucleophiles such as glutathione are small molecules but many are macromolecules such as proteins or nucleic acids each possessing a variety of nucleophilic centres. If the modified macromolecule does not have a rapid turnover then adducts accumulate. The following two examples illustrate the principles involved in biomonitoring intoxicants which interact reversibly or covalently with macromolecules.

11.5 Dose Monitoring in Humans: Methylmercury (Epidemic in Iraq)

From 1953–1971 there have been eight episodes of poisoning by alkylmercury compounds (mainly methylmercury) with over eight thousand reported cases. The first from Japan (see section 13.4) was due to the consumption of fish contaminated by methylmercury discharged in the effluent from a chemical plant engaged in the manufacture of acetaldehyde (Tsubaki & Irukayama, 1977). Other major outbreaks occurred in Iraq and were caused by seed grain pretreated with methylmercury fungicide being used for the preparation of bread (Bakir *et al.*, 1973; Clarkson *et al.*, 1976; WHO, 1976).

After a latent period, usually of several weeks, the symptoms were sensory (paresthesia and numbness of hands, feet, lips and tongue), motor (ataxia, gait and speech) and visual (particularly restriction of the visual fields). Methylmercury is therefore highly neurotoxic often causing physical and mental incapacitation.

Alkylmercury compounds form chlorides and hydroxides and, being uncharged and lipophilic, they are rapidly absorbed and distributed throughout the body. They also have a high affinity for thiols and become attached to many small and large molecules *in vivo* (e.g. thiol groups of glutathione and haemoglobin). Although the affinity constants of methylmercury for protein thiols are very high it is a reversible attachment and is presumably in equilibrium with all other binding sites throughout the body. Blood mercury concentrations (methylmercury bound to haemoglobin) may be correlated with symptoms. In the first few months after the outbreak in Iraq paresthesia was present in only a few cases where blood concentration was <250 ng/ml; the incidence became much higher and increased with concentrations from 300 up to 3,000–4,000 ng/ml (Table 11.1). The exposure took place in November and December 1971 and the first blood samples were collected in February 1972, 60–70 days later. The rate of fall in the concentration of methylmercury in the blood was exponential over the five months from the end of February to the end of July and the first-order rate constant was 0.0106/day indicating a half-life of 65 days. If this rate can be used to extrapolate back to November/December 1971 the initial concentrations will then have been much higher.

Another approach was to analyse samples of hair. The concentration in blood is in equilibrium with the concentration in hair at the time it is biosynthesised and as the hair grows out from the scalp the methylmercury retains its position. By sampling the hair and cutting into 1 cm lengths and linking analyses with those of blood the rate of decrease of concentration of methylmercury in the growing hair is the same as the exponential decay of concentrations in blood (Figure 11.2). The ratio of the concentration of mercury in hair (per gram) to that in blood (per millilitre) is approximately 300. Since the growth of hair is about 1 cm/month the sampling of the long hair of females and cutting into 1 cm portions would allow a recapitulation over periods of several years. Sampling of hair at different dates also yields an approximate date when the exposure to methylmercury took place. Figure 11.2 illustrates this procedure for samples of long hair sampled from the same individual at different times; the date of her exposure appears to have been December 1971.

These studies have provided much information about the toxicokinetics of methylmercury in humans. The results show that blood mercury if measured early after

Table 11.1 The relationship between the concentration of methylmercury in blood and the incidence of paresthesia

Methylmercury in blood (ng/ml)	Mean period of ingestion (days)	Latent period (days)	Paresthesia %	(No./group)
0–100	43	–	9	(2/21)
101–500	43	–	5	(1/19)
501–1000	43	16	42	(8/19)
1001–2000	41	18	60	(10/17)
2001–3000	55	26	79	(20/25)
3001–4000	58	32	82	(14/17)
4001–5000	68	38	100	(4/4)

Note: Blood was analysed approximately 65 days after the end of exposure and the individuals were sorted into groups according to the concentration of mercury. A similar relationship was found for ataxia and visual effects with dysarthia and hearing defects being correlated with higher concentrations.
Source: Data from Bakir *et al.*, 1973.

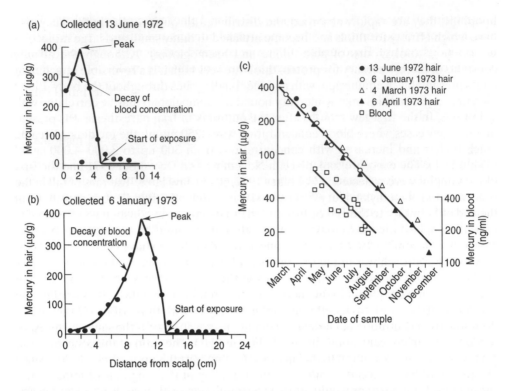

Figure 11.2 Measurement of the concentrations of methylmercury in human hair and blood after exposure has ceased. The exposure took place in Iraq and was due to the consumption of contaminated grain. Graph (c) shows the relationship between blood and hair for many exposed patients. The values in (a) and (b) for the 1 cm sections of hair sampled on two dates six months apart were from the same individual. (*Source*: Data from Clarkson *et al.*, 1976)

exposure can be used to predict the subsequent clinical outlook and thus allow intervention with therapeutic procedures. This is possible because the compound binds tightly to a macromolecule in an accessible tissue (haemoglobin in blood). The clearance rate is probably proportional to the free methylmercury concentration in equilibrium with methylmercury bound to high affinity sites in haemoglobin and other macromolecules. The use of hair illustrates the value of this long-lived protein as a collecting device to provide retrospective data. It is reasonable to assume that concentrations bound to both hair and haemoglobin would have been proportional to those in toxicologically relevant sites, e.g. in the nervous system. The use of hair for biomonitoring has been used for the detection of exposure to arsenic; potentially it should be applicable to any electrophilic compound which reacts, as hair protein is being formed, with the nucleophilic sulphydryl groups.

11.6 Dose Monitoring in Humans: Ethylene Oxide

Ethylene oxide is a widely used chemical both as an intermediate in large-scale synthetic processes (polyester fibres) and surface active agents (glycol ethers, polyethylene glycols, etc.) and as a sterilant (for health care products) and as a fumigant (for spices, book preservation in libraries, dairy packaging, animal and plant quarantine services). There are, therefore, opportunities for the exposures of humans and animals, particularly in its non-industrial use. Exposure to both exogenous and endogenous ethylene (ethene) which is oxidised *in vivo*, is also a potential source of ethylene oxide.

$$H_2C=CH_2 \qquad H_2C \overset{O}{\overset{/ \backslash}{-}} CH_2 \qquad HO-CH_2-CH_2-\begin{cases} \text{N terminal valine} \\ \text{or} \\ \text{N—1 histidine} \end{cases}$$

Ethylene oxide is a colourless gas (BP 10.7°C), is soluble in water, alcohol, ether and other lipophilic solvents and, when absorbed, mixes rapidly with the body water (see section 5.3.1). It is a reactive substance and is highly irritating to eyes and mucous membranes. For a chemical with such properties and uses, direct assessments of representative exposure levels in places of work are difficult and the relationship between exposure level and *in vivo* dose is uncertain. Current epidemiological evidence does not support the view that it is a major cause of cancer in those exposed at work. Animal studies indicate that ethylene oxide is a weak carcinogen to rodents although there is abundant evidence that it is a mutagen. It is presented here as an example of the principles of dose monitoring and how increasing finesse in analytical chemistry now allows dose monitoring down to an acceptable carcinogenic risk level. Instead of relying on the highly variable exposure in the workplace and individual variability of absorption via the respiratory system, skin and gut, measurement of adducts with proteins or DNA yield values proportional to absorbed dose.

Ethylene oxide will react with many macromolecules although not all are suitable for dose monitoring purposes. As discussed below (section 11.3.3) human red cells have a long life (120 days) so that the determination of the extent of reaction with amino acids in haemoglobin will provide a measure resulting from current and previous exposure. Haemoglobin is a surrogate for DNA, the real target in initiation of cancer. Lymphocytes are an available source of DNA but although many lymphocytes are long-lived there are doubts about variable DNA repair and cell renewal. Haemoglobin is a good monitor for circulating ethylene oxide (Ehrenberg *et al.*, 1974) and since it is distributed throughout the body water reaction with haemoglobin should be directly proportional to reaction with 'relevant DNA'. Reaction of several compounds including ethylene oxide (Osterman-Golkar *et al.*, 1983) with haemoglobin has been shown to be proportional to absorbed dose. Using a 10^5-fold dose range of trans-4-dimethylaminostilbene the haemoglobin : DNA adduct level ratio remained constant down to a dose of 0.5 nmol/kg b.w. and binding to globin of 0.3 pmol/g globin (Neumann, 1980).

Ethylene oxide, an electrophilic reagent, reacts with nucleophilic centres in several aminoacids in haemoglobin (SH in cysteine, N–1 in histidine, N terminal-N in valine) and with bases in DNA (N–7 and 0–6 in guanine and N-1, N–3 and N–7 in adenine (Farmer *et al.*, 1986). Analytical methods have been based on high pressure liquid chromatography (HPLC) with fluorescence detection and gas chromatography–mass spectrometry (GC–MS) with various work-up procedures to isolate the globin, hydrolyse the protein and separate and perhaps derivatise the adduct. A technique has been developed for the selective liberation of valine adducts from globin and has now achieved a detection limit of 1 pmol valine adduct per gram of globin. For a discussion of the methodology see Farmer *et al.* (1987) and Farmer (1994). In a comparison of haemoglobin for workers exposed to ethylene oxide measurement of the 2-hydroxyethyl histidine and valine adducts gave consistent results (Farmer *et al.*, 1986) and in an

Table 11.2   Haemoglobin adducts after exposure of humans to ethylene and ethylene oxide

N-2-HYDROXYETHYLVALINE ADDUCTS[a]

Exposure	Adducts (pmol/g globin)
Ethylene oxide (1 ppm, 40 h/week)	2,400
Ethylene (1 ppm, 40 h/week)	120
Background (controls)	20

N-(2-HYDROXYETHYL)- AND *N*-METHYLVALINE[b]

10 Monozygotic twins discordant for smoking habits were examined

Adducts	Smokers(10)	Non-smokers(10)	Due to smoking
	(Concentration pmol/g globin)		
N-2-Hydroxyethylvaline		146 ± 26	16 ± 2 132 ± 25
N-Methylvaline	271 ± 14	219 ± 11	52 ± 10

[a] Data from Ehrenberg & Tornqvist, 1992.

occupational exposure study it has been shown that haemoglobin adducts are quantitatively related to biological effects such as sister chromatid exchange (Tates *et al.*, 1991).

A comparison of the amount of valine adducts under different circumstances is shown in Table 11.2. Ethylene exposure leads to one-twentieth of that from the same exposure to ethylene oxide; in an unexposed individual a background level of 20 pmol/g globin was obtained. In a comparison of ten pairs of identical twins separated by their tobacco-smoking habits most of the 2-hydroxyethylvaline but only 19% of the methylvaline adduct was due to smoking. Ethylene is present in tobacco smoke and the low background probably arises from ethylene from intestinal flora, dietary factors and perhaps from passive smoking. The origin of the high non-smoking background of *N*-methylvaline is unknown.

The relationship between exposure (measured as adducts) and cancer incidence requires discriminating epidemiology (see Chapter 12). By the use of adducts two factors, inaccurate measures of individual exposure and variable absorption, are eliminated. The expected genetic damage by mono-functional alkylating agents has been compared with that observed in experimental systems using radiation as the standard mutagen (Ehrenberg *et al.*, 1974). The degree of risk is expressed in terms of rad equivalent dose, i.e. the number of rads of acute radiation that would give the same genotoxic effect as a unit dose of test chemical. This procedure is, therefore, a calibration of dose of genotoxic chemical (expressed in terms of haemoglobin adduct) against the much better defined effectiveness of radiation as a mutagenic and carcinogenic agent. This predictive procedure will have to checked against measured incidences in exposed populations.

11.7   Dose and Effect Monitoring in Humans: Anticholinesterases

Human blood and that of many but not all species contain different cholinesterases in the red cell membrane and in plasma. They may be distinguished by their different

Table 11.3 Hydrolysis of choline esters by acetylcholinesterase (AChE) and cholinesterase (ChE) in human blood

RELATIVE HYDROLYSIS OF CHOLINE ESTERS

Enzyme	Acetyl-	Choline ester Propionyl-	*n*-Butyryl-
Red cell and brain AChE	100	55	2
Plasma and serum ChE	100	165	205

RELATIVE HYDROLYSIS OF ACETYLTHIOCHOLINE BY ACHE AND CHE

	Activity (μmol/min) per ml fraction	per ml blood[a]
Whole blood	3.6–7.2	3.6–7.2
Plasma	0.3–2.4	0.17–1.37
Erythrocytes	7.4–13.4	3.4–5.8

[a] The activity per ml blood was calculated using an average haematocrit value of 43%

relative catalytic activity in the hydrolysis of choline ester substrates (Table 11.3). Both are serine or B-esterases and are thus inhibited by organophosphorus compounds and esters of substituted carbamic acids. No biological function is known for the cholinesterase (ChE) in the plasma or for the acetylcholinesterase (AChE) in the red cell membrane.

AChE in red cells is identical to that in the nervous system where its function is the removal of acetylcholine after its release at synapses, myoneural junctions, etc. Since most organophosphorus compounds and carbamates used as pesticides are uncharged and lipophilic they readily penetrate all cells, and therefore inhibition of AChE in erythrocytes and the nervous system is equal. AChE is the target for acute toxicity by organophosphorus compounds and carbamates (see section 7.6) and therefore measurement of inhibition of AChE is a biomarker for both dose and effect. There is little or no sign of poisoning up to 50% inhibition, signs and symptoms of increasing severity from 50–85%, and death at 90% inhibition and above. The degree of inhibition is proportional to the concentration of inhibitor [AB] and time (t) of contact of enzyme with inhibitor; if the rate constant for inhibition (k_a) is known then the dose (concentration × time = [AB] × t; see Figures 3.1 and 3.5) may be calculated. Since red cells have a long life the stable inhibited enzyme accumulates.

ChE, either in plasma or tissues, has no known function but is inhibited by organophosphorus compounds and carbamates and can be inhibited *in vivo* almost completely without any intoxication. Since AChE and ChE are different enzymes, i.e their structural environments around their catalytic centres containing serine are different, the rate constants for reaction with the above inhibitors are different; often ChE is inhibited more than AChE. Therefore inhibition of ChE is a biomarker for dose but not effect. Plasma ChE is synthesised by the liver and at a much faster rate than red cell turnover so that return of activity is faster in plasma than in red cells.

Nothing is absolutely simple and defined and other factors influence the inhibition of AChE, e.g. variation in the controls, rate of spontaneous reactivation (see Figure 3.7) and the rate of aging of the inhibited enzymes (see Figures 7.7 and 7.8). Monitoring of workers should preferably be done using control values determined before exposure.

If this is not possible then account must be taken of conditions which lower the red cell count (anaemia) and liver conditions which may affect the synthesis of ChE. These complicating factors in the interpretation of low values is important in developing countries where intercurrent disease and malnutrition occur.

11.8 Dose and Effect Monitoring in Humans: Dichlorvos

Spontaneous reactivation and aging are illustrated in Figure 11.3 for dimethylphosphorylated AChE produced, in this instance, by reaction with dichlorvos. The rather rapid spontaneous reactivation (half-life 0.85 h) can cause problems in obtaining an accurate measure of inhibition at the time of sampling. Special precautions must be taken to slow down reactivation in the blood after sampling by storing cold and perhaps by making the sample slightly acid and performing the analysis as soon as possible (Vandekar, 1980). The rate of spontaneous reactivation is 4.5 times faster than the rate of aging and the two reactions proceed at a comparative rate proportional to the ratio of their rate constants. Thus after exposure to dichlorvos sufficient to produce 60% inhibition then next day 49% will have reactivated and be fully active enzyme while 11% inhibition will remain as irreversible aged enzyme. Thus with repeated exposure the proportion of aged enzyme will increase and when further exposure does not occur will

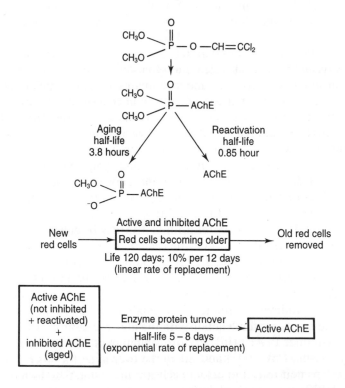

Figure 11.3 The return of acetylcholinesterase (AChE) in human red cells and brain after inhibition by dichlorvos. (*Sources:* The half-lives for aging and reactivation are calculated from the rate constants determined by Skrinjaric-Spoljar *et al.*, 1973). The rate of turnover of AChE in human brain is assumed from animal data)

disappear only as new red cells are made (average life span 120 days = 10% every 12 days). Since new cells are made in response to the removal of old cells, the rate of replacement is linear. From results in experimental animals the rate of synthesis (turnover) of AChE in the nervous system is exponential and is much faster than the turnover of red cells. The comparative data are for 10% and 90% resynthesis of red cells 12 and 108 days where for resynthesis of AChE in the brain approximately 1 and 22 days. Thus biomonitoring of erythrocyte AChE following repeated exposure of humans will probably overestimate the inhibition in brain, particularly during the recovery phase.

For dose and effect monitoring for organophosphorus-induced delayed neuropathy, inhibition of neuropathy target esterase (NTE) which is present in lymphocytes is possible. There seems little doubt that such a measurement will be a reliable monitor of dose. Its use as an effect monitor is still under review and must take into account the recent findings on mechanism (see section 7.7; Lotti, 1987).

The use of plasma ChE, erythrocyte AChE and lymphocyte NTE illustrates the general principles behind dose and effect monitoring for substances which react covalently with proteins. The ideal is if the initiating target in tissues is also present in blood as well as the affected tissue (e.g. T_1 in Figure 11.1; AChE and NTE). Inhibition of targets irrelevant to toxicity (e.g. T_2 and T_3 in Figure 11.1 and ChE) are not useful for effect monitoring but are valuable for ascertaining whether prior exposure has taken place and also what is the dose delivered *in vivo*.

11.9 Dose Monitoring in Experimental Animals

There are obviously fewer constraints on what can be measured in experimental animals. To interpret the toxicity testing procedures, more information is required about absorbed dose so that meaningful dose–response relationships may be available. The concentration of the parent intoxicant and, where applicable, the bioactivated species should be determined in the affected tissue. For reactive intoxicants, adducts may have to be determined.

11.10 Effect Monitoring

In humans effect monitoring is common in clinical biochemistry and physiological measurements of changes in function for the early detection of many diseases; standard textbooks should be consulted. This is a rapidly advancing field as, following the discoveries of cell-specific proteins, procedures are developed for their measurement in accessible tissue. For examples of measurements now available for the detection of early changes in the kidney see section 12.6. Two recent publications illustrate the potential: the measurement of intestinal-type alkaline phosphatase in urine as an indicator of mercury-induced effects in a particular segment of the proximal tubule in the human kidney (Nuyts *et al.*, 1992) and the measurement of a decrease in serum of a specific Clara cell protein as an indicator of cell-specific changes in the lungs of smokers (Bernard *et al.*, 1992).

In animals the scope is obviously much greater and increasing finesse is allowing many more measurements to be made on individual animals thus reducing the number of animals used. Chapters 7 and 8 should be consulted for the variety of measurements which have been used and will allow dose–response relationships to be established at early times and before clinical signs of dysfunction. For research which provides the basis for such monitoring, there are now many possibilities for the detection of changes in targets, isolated cells, tissue slices, perfused functional tissue units and whole animals. Studies *in vitro* of the effects of chemicals on isolated biological systems and the examination of tissues isolated from animals exposed to chemicals allow *in vitro/in vivo* comparisons necessary for the testing of mechanistic hypotheses and also the validation of biomonitoring procedures (Aldridge, 1992).

11.11 Discussion

The object of human biomonitoring is to obtain accurate indicators of the internal dose of the intoxicant and information about early biological effects as indicators of changes before toxicity appears. Sometimes the intoxicant is the chemical absorbed and sometimes it is another chemical species bioactivated *in vivo*. Sometimes the early effects are the beginning of a short or long silent period. Examples of the types of option are illustrated in Figure 12.1 but, in most cases, predictors of future disease suitable for use to detect chemical-induced human disease have not yet been identified.

Biomonitoring of the same parameters in experimental animals supplemented with tissue doses and/or sometimes target doses and by early biological responses allows the relationship between dose and response to be defined. The relationship between such animal data and what data are available for humans may allow an assessment of risk and whether a threshold exists. Prediction of toxicity in different species is very difficult if many of the species differences affecting the delivery of the intoxicant to its site of action are not eliminated.

Measurement of internal or circulating dose is useful not only for exposure at work and in the environment but also to control the dosage of drugs when continuous treatment is required, e.g. cancer chemotherapy.

There are limitations to human biomonitoring of intoxicants arising from bioactivation to highly reactive species. In some cases these species are so reactive that little intoxicant escapes into the circulating blood from the cells where the bioactivation occurs, e.g. the highly reactive carbonium ion resulting from oxidation of dimethylnitrosamine produces little methylation of haemoglobin. Comparison of results from human accessible tissue and from experiments with animals, including adducts of tissue protein and nucleic acid, is essential.

Besides exposure to known chemicals it is now recognised that we are exposed to a variety of chemicals arising from our diet or endogenous by-products of metabolism (Higginson & Muir, 1979). Most of the biomonitoring techniques are dedicated to specific chemicals and possibilities for the detection of adducts and their identification and quantitative determination are continually emerging (e.g. see Bergmark *et al.*, 1991). For screening virtually all exposure to carcinogens the [^{32}P]-postlabelling technique for DNA adducts is capable, with high specific activity [^{32}P]-ATP, of detecting very small amounts of adduct separated by chromatographic methods (Randerath *et al.*, 1981, 1985; Gupta, 1985). Valine adducts can be selectively released from haemoglobin and identified using GC–MS techniques (Farmer *et al.*, 1986). The latter instrumental techniques have been improved not only in their ability to separate and identify unknowns but also in their sensitivity.

Several adducts are formed by the reaction of a single intoxicant both with different residues in haemoglobin and with different bases in nucleic acids. The ratio of the extent of reaction with these different sites provides information about the type of reactant involved. Using dedicated methods, unexpected background levels have been found (see Table 11.2; Farmer *et al.*, 1993; Tornqvist & Kantiainen, 1993). The origin of all these unexpected adducts must be found.

The development of sensitive techniques for human biomonitoring has been driven by the need for risk assessment for exposure to carcinogens. In principle they can be used for any reactive intoxicant, e.g. acrylamide (Bailey *et al.*, 1986; Bergmark *et al.*, 1993). The major advantage of their use is that results are obtained on an individual basis thus eliminating extrinsic factors affecting the exposure and intrinsic factors influencing the delivery and stability of the intoxicant in the internal milieu.

Measurement is now possible of low concentrations of adducts in tissues from experimental animals where bioactivation activity is low (but maybe in specific cells only); such information may help to understand tissue selectivity of intoxicants.

11.12 Summary

1 Biomonitoring serves the three purposes of identifying and using biomarkers for genetic susceptibility, internal dose and biological effect.

2 When the target is known, the degree of reaction at the target can be measured; this indicates the dose at the target (dose biomonitoring) and the primary biological response (effect biomonitoring).

3 Often the macromolecular target is not known and surrogates for target dose must be used.

4 Accessible long-lived macromolecules often provide useful biomarkers for dose monitoring.

5 Intoxicants interacting reversibly with several macromolecules remain in equilibrium and provide an estimate of the internal dose at the time of measurement.

6 The degree of covalent reaction with a macromolecule depends on the time of contact and concentration of the intoxicant, and the reaction product persists for a time dependent upon the resynthesis of the macromolecule (not on the persistence of the intoxicant).

7 Biomarkers for effect monitoring can potentially arise from any stage of developing toxicity after the primary reaction with the target (biochemical, physiological and functional).

8 Effect biomonitoring in humans is restricted to accessible tissue or clinical examination. In animals more invasive techniques may be applied to obtain dose–early response relationships; these can be important for the assessment of the risk of human exposure.

12

Epidemiology

12.1 Introduction

Epidemiology is the study of factors determining and influencing the frequency and distribution of disease, injury and other health-related events and their cause in a defined population. Such studies have made and will continue to make a major contribution to the discovery of human diseases caused by exposure to exogenous materials, both natural and synthetic. The problems may be sudden with a sharp rise in poisoning or may involve a late increase in incidence of a disease over many years. The outbreak of poisoning in Pakistan of spraymen handling the malathion for mosquito control in a malaria eradication programme is an example of the former. Malathion is normally a particularly safe pesticide but in this instance contained an impurity which can increase its toxicity 100-fold (Baker *et al.*, 1978: Aldridge *et al.*, 1979). An example of a late development is the increased incidence of vaginal adenocarcinoma in the young daughters of women who had been treated with diethylstilboestrol during pregnancy prior to the eighteenth week (Poskanzer & Herbst, 1977; Herbst *et al.*, 1977; Marselos & Tomatis, 1992). Abnormalities in the reproductive systems of male offspring were also found (Bibbo *et al.*, 1977) which has recently been extended to testicular carcinoma.

Although human disease is the usual focus of epidemiology there is no reason that this should be so; outbreaks of disease in animals require similar techniques to establish the cause and may provide information about potential problems for human population, e.g. disease and deaths in turkeys following the inclusion of fungal contaminated groundnuts in feedstuff which led to the recognition of aflatoxins as potent liver-damaging as well as carcinogenic agents. However, studies on the epidemiology of chronic and rare diseases would require knowledge of the size and age structure of the population at risk; this is rarely available.

Techniques developed in epidemiology are used in diverse fields, e.g. the efficacy of control measures to eliminate the cause of disease, the relationship between various biomonitoring procedures and the incidence of disease, the proper design for studies to establish whether there are late consequences of an acute poisoning episode, etc. The following epidemiological aspects are important for those concerned with the

180

toxicity of chemicals:

1 The correct approach to the collection of data from humans.
2 The selection of the population to be studied.
3 The selection of the control population.
4 The measurements to be made and at what time.
5 The statistics applicable to the study.
6 The statistical power of the study.

The problems can be relatively simple if there is a low incidence of a particular condition in the general population, e.g. the increase of angiosarcoma of the liver in workers in chemical industry handling vinyl chloride (Purchase *et al.*, 1987; Creech & Johnson, 1974; Beaumont & Breslow, 1981). Others, such as in changes in the incidence of heart disease in populations with a high background incidence, may pose great problems in the size of the study necessary to obtain statistically significant results. Epidemiological studies are required to establish if the findings derived from experimental studies in relatively inbred strains of animals are relevant to humans with their wide genetic mix.

Figure 12.1 illustrates the range of potential information usable in epidemiological

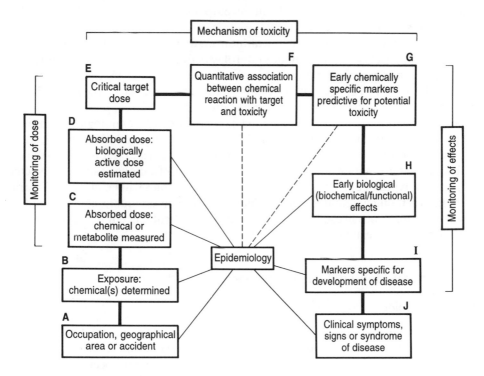

Figure 12.1 Epidemiology of chemical-induced toxicity related to measures of exposure, dose and biological effects. The various boxes linked by a heavy line indicate the route, by experimental studies, to establish mechanisms of toxicity (boxes E, F and G) and to establish the relationship between exposure (B) and disease (J). The thin lines indicate the routes that epidemiology may take to establish such a relationship in humans. The dashed lines indicate that in only a few cases can early specific markers (G) be measured in humans. There is no line between 'epidemiology' and critical target dose (E) because (E) can only rarely be measured in accessible tissues in humans.(*Source*: adapted from Aldridge, 1989b)

studies of exposure to chemicals and relationships between such studies to the advancing knowledge of mechanisms of toxicity and development of disease. A study may show an association between an occupation (A) and the clinical symptoms, signs and/or syndrome of disease (J). The occupation (A) may involve exposure to one or more chemicals (B). Such chemicals may be measured in the contact environment but more defined measurements of individual absorbed dose (C, D and E) of the chemical or in some cases of the metabolite which is the actual intoxicant are now possible. More finesse in the range of potential measurements follows from experimental studies which develop knowledge inherent in D–I; E, F and G are the essence of mechanisms of toxicity when the target has been identified and a quantitative relationship between reaction with the target and the toxicity is known (see Chapter 7). Other developments are measurements of chemically specific markers which are predictive (i.e. increased probability relative to control) for future chemical-induced disease (G), e.g. the inhibition of lymphocyte neuropathy target esterase (NTE) to indicate the future development of delayed neuropathy (see section 11.8). Measurements of the release of enzymes and or macromolecules from particular tissues/cells (H) indicate at an early stage developing changes in these tissues. Markers specific for diseases with a long latency are rarely attained, e.g. there is, as yet, no measurement which will enable predictions to be made that a particular individual will develop a tumour. Figure 12.1 is, therefore an idealised summary of potential aims, particularly with respect to markers to indicate progression towards future chemical-induced toxicity (e.g. G, H and I).

It is obvious the close and continuous interplay between the types of study illustrated in Figure 12.1 and experimental studies is needed (Lauwerys, 1986; Lauwerys & Lois-Ferdinand, 1984). The applicability of findings from experimental studies to the human population is a question which must be constantly addressed.

This book is not the place for a detailed exposition of epidemiological techniques and principles. For this other texts should be consulted (e.g. Alderson, 1983). In this short commentary the aim is to present enough information and references so that the route to more information and examples is clear. After definitions of some of the characteristics of types of epidemiological study, three examples will be given to illustrate the mode of thought required, the problems of finding adequate controls and the increase in confidence in establishing causality of a particular event if a dose–response relationship can be established.

12.2   General Methodological Approaches

The aims of epidemiological studies are:

1   To obtain clues about the causes of disease by examining the variation in its incidence in different populations, e.g. sex, country, region, time etc., (descriptive or ecological studies) or by enquiries about the past behaviour, occupation, etc., of people with and without the disease (case-control studies).
2   To test the relevance of clues obtained as above by seeing whether people with disease are characterised by more exposure to the suspected agent than comparable people without it (case-control or cohort studies).
3   To test the correctness of conclusions obtained by previous studies by testing whether the incidence of the disease is reduced when the agent is removed (by randomly allocated and controlled studies); this is seldom possible but sometimes it can be done, e.g. by changing procedures in industry.

There are five major modes of epidemiological study. The first is the collection of morbidity or mortality data for statistical analysis. These data are often derived from standard population statistics or from national registers for particular purposes. Results from such collation and analysis of data can be the first indication that a problem exists, e.g. by demonstrating an increase in incidence, and that further study is necessary. The second is the conduct of surveys, i.e. special enquiries for the collection of planned information from a sample of individuals by questions, clinical examinations and information from other sources. These are particularly valuable when the effects are chronic or non-fatal, e.g. dermatitis. Cross-sectional studies are undertaken with more intensive clinical and functional studies. They may indicate an increasing incidence of the disease. Such studies are usually only of value when the prevalence of the disease is relatively high and fatality is low, when there are sensitive measures of changes in function and when there is an identifiable precursor indicative of future disease.

The third and more common is case-control study. Case-control studies are retrospective and may be carried out to look for unexpected causes or, preferably, to test a hypothesis about a possible cause. Populations are identified with a particular disease and they are then interviewed to obtain information about employment history as well as other confounding factors such as alcohol consumption and smoking habits. Such studies can be very useful but there are often problems in obtaining accurate histories and there may be difficulties in securing a representative control group for comparison. In many instances of toxicity caused by a particular chemical the aetiology becomes clear for a variety of reasons. These reasons include information about the nature of the exposure (route, solvent, etc.), what the chemical was, the clinical signs and symptoms of the poisoning, suitable analytical methods for the detection of actual exposure and/or animal bioassay methods (see Chapter 9). Examples are Ginger Jake paralysis (Smith & Elvove, 1930), paralysis occurring in the Moroccan Episode (Smith & Spalding, 1959), Epping jaundice (Kopelman *et al.*, 1966) and the neuropathies in the the Iraq Episode (WHO, 1976). In the last three of these episodes relatively simple information was sufficient to establish the aetiology (nature of the material which contained the intoxicant, e.g. food) of the diseases from retrospective information and when the cause was isolated and exposure ceased new cases were not seen. Sometimes although the vehicle for the introduction of the intoxicant into humans is known, the nature of the contaminant may not be known (i.e. Ginger Jake paralysis) and further analytical and experimental studies are required to establish the chemical(s) responsible and later the mechanism of the toxicity.

The fourth is a prospective or cohort study which involves the choice of a particular group in the population (cohort), the members of which have different but definable characteristics, e.g. born in different years, employed in different jobs in a factory. It is possible to carry out a cohort study of people all of whom have similar exposures and to compare their fate with that of the population at large, but the best cohort studies all have internal controls. The group could be those who will be exposed to a given chemical or those taking part in a clinical trial of a potential therapeutic drug. Whatever is the nature of the cohort, a prospective study always implies that it will be observed over a period of time and that when the cohort was assembled all its members were healthy. Such studies are a powerful tool for hypothesis testing but when the group is followed up for a long time they require considerable organisation and resources. The aim in many toxicological studies will be to test the hypothesis that exposure to A leads to disease B. The selection of the healthy subjects is intended to be divorced from any direct bias of the relationship between A and B. This selection is a skilled process but there are also problems which may arise during a long-term study, e.g. some of those originally selected may fall out of the study thereby making the group unrepresentative (selection bias). Epidemiologists take immense pain to follow all the defined cohort. Lapse rates of more than 5% are undesirable and may invalidate the study.

The fifth type of study involves the random allocation of subjects into two groups. Apart from clinical medicine when new treatments are tested by randomly allocated controlled trials, experiments with random allocation are rarely possible. They have been used to investigate the cause of the common cold, but they are more often attempted to test hypotheses of trying to prevent disease, e.g. aspirin to prevent myocardial infarction, β-carotene to prevent cancer. Often there are ethical problems in such studies.

12.3 Epidemiological Methods used in Occupational Exposures

Occupational mortality statistics rely on the analysis of the data acquired from population statistics collected at the ten-yearly national census. Such data can be grouped in many ways and the cause of death related to occupation. The cause could be related to a well defined job, or a less well defined combination of jobs, those who live and work in a particular geographical region or a linked combination of occupation and particular industry. Record linkage is a more powerful probe into those with a particular occupation and prospective patterns of mortality may be followed through national records. Such data can provide a valuable basis for the generation of hypotheses for further exploration.

Collation studies are less precise in that a geographical area is divided up according to the prevalence of particular industries. The incidence of particular forms of disease (e.g forms of cancer) can then be compared between these regions.

Prospective studies would aim to take a group of healthy people in a particular area, occupation in a factory or a particular job within a factory and follow their disease pattern alongside measurement of exposure, e.g. to dust or a chemical.

The ideal conclusion from an epidemiological study is proof that a chemical or agent is the cause of a defined health defect or death. This, in a strictly logical sense, is rarely achieved. However, with confirmatory results from studies from other locations and with supporting evidence from experimental animal research, firm conclusions can be reached. Guidelines have been given about the distinction between association and causation and the aspects to be considered if the association indicates a cause–effect relationship (Hill, 1965):

1 The strength of the relationship as measured by the relative risk. The interpretation of relative risk depends on the number of cases and how common the disease is, e.g. relative risks of small magnitude need not indicate lack of causality but if the disease is relatively common then causality may be difficult to prove.

2 The consistency of the association. The case for causality is strengthened by confirmation of the findings by different investigators, in different places, circumstances and times.

3 The temporal relationship between cause and effect. Exposure must proceed illness and have been sufficiently early to have covered any latency period.

4 Biological gradient of the effect. The risk of developing the disease should be positively related to the extent and severity of the exposure (i.e. a positive dose–response relationship).

5 Specificity of the association. The association should be limited to particular sites or types of disease.

6 Biological plausibility of the association. Plausibility depends on current knowledge at the time.

7 Coherence. The causal interpretation should not conflict with the general knowledge of the natural history and biology of the disease.

8 Experiment. Changes in the conditions of exposure should change the risk of the disease.

9 Analogy. There may be other comparable examples of cause and effect.

Other more detailed sources of information about the distinction between association and causation and how to move towards proof of a causal hypothesis are Hill (1962), Hernberg (1980) and IARC (1982). No formal tests of significance can answer the question of whether there is a cause–effect relationship (Hill, 1965). Such tests provide quantitative measures of the effects of chance; beyond that they contribute nothing to the 'proof' of the hypothesis.

Conclusions about causality become more persuasive if individual exposure or, better still, internal dose is known (see section 11.3 and Figure 12.1). Even though direct measurements of dose over a long period often cannot be made, surrogates for exposure can be used. Sometimes a conclusion may not be in terms of the actual chemical, i.e. the aetiological intoxicant, but be an association of the disease with, for example, the consumption of an item of diet perhaps grown or manufactured in a particular place or stored in a defined way or even with length of service in a particular industry.

In the following examples the first two present the steps towards reaching conclusions about the association of health consequences and certain exposures. In neither case has the aetiological agent(s) been identified but both cases have provided strong (in one case unassailable) evidence that the association is causal. The last example is a study to establish if long-term and low environmental exposure can cause biological dysfunction not sufficient to be seen clinically.

12.4 Smoking and Lung Cancer

The original and now classical epidemiological studies on the relationship between smoking of cigarettes and lung cancer were begun over forty years ago and studies on other health effects of smoking are still continuing. The conclusions from these studies are of such profound toxicological and public health importance that they are one of the best examples of how to design studies to attain a conclusive answer and of reasoning in terms of causality.

The records of the Registrar-General in the UK between 1922 and 1947 showed the most striking increase in the number of deaths ascribed to cancer of the lung. Over this period the number increased fifteen-fold; similar but generally smaller changes were recorded in other countries. Suggestions that the increase was due to improved standards of diagnosis were thought unlikely because the increase was so great, persisted for so long and occurred more in men than in women. The national figure was paralleled by similar increases recorded in autopsy data in teaching hospitals.

Two hypotheses were considered (Doll & Hill, 1950). First, that the increased incidence was due to an increase in general atmospheric pollution, e.g. exhaust from cars, dust from tarred roads, gas works, industrial plants and coal fires, and secondly that it was due to the smoking of tobacco which had become much more prevalent over the previous fifty years.

In Figure 12.2a is shown the death rate of the population due to lung cancer over the period 1900–1947 compared with the amount of tobacco consumed in total or as cigarettes and averaged out from national statistics. The death rate increased markedly from 1924 and by 1947 was 11 times higher than in 1924. The consumption of tobacco and cigarettes increased over the same period approximately 1.6 and 2.6 times respectively. Before 1924 the increase in the consumption of cigarettes had, however, been much greater. Cigarettes began to be smoked widely only in the 1880s and the consump-

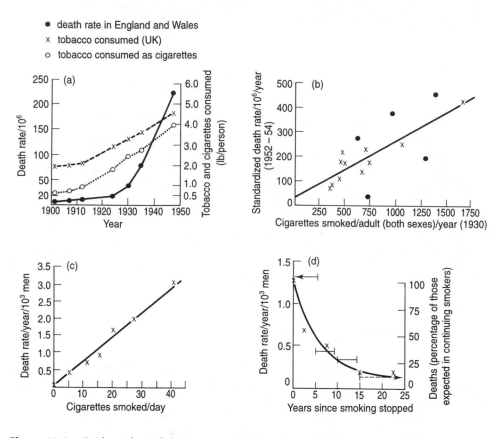

Figure 12.2 Epidemiological data concerning the relationships between smoking of cigarettes and carcinoma of the lung. (a) Death rate from cancer of the lung and the rate of consumption of tobacco in the UK. The rates are based on three-year averages for all years except 1947. (b) Relationship between lung cancer mortality and previous cigarette consumption in sixteen countries. From left to right the solid dots below the line (lower incidence) are from Japan and USA and above the line (higher incidence) from the Netherlands, Austria and England/Wales. (c) Death rate from lung cancer, standardised for age among doctors smoking different daily numbers of cigarettes. (d) Death from lung cancer among doctors who had, for differents periods, given up smoking cigarettes. ⊢────⊣ indicates data for <5, 5–9, 10–14 and >15 years since stopping smoking. (*Sources*: (a) Doll & Hill, 1950; (b) Doll *et al.*, 1959; (c) Doll & Hill, 1964; (d) Left hand vertical axis, Doll & Hill, 1964; Right hand vertical axis, Doll & Peto, 1976)

186

tion had increased three-fold between 1900 and 1924 and ten-fold between 1885 and 1924. Some of the reported increase in lung cancer was certainly due to better diagnosis but the major increase was consistent with a delay of 20–50 years in the appearance of the disease after cigarette smoking began.

In a case-control study 5,000 hospital patients were interviewed between 1948 and 1952. The hospitals were from five cities and from two rural areas. The main comparison for the study was between 1,465 patients with carcinoma of the lung and an equal number of controls with other diseases but matched for age, sex and the same hospital. From this study a strong association was found between smoking and lung cancer which, half-way through the study, had enabled the conclusion to be reached that cigarette smoking was the cause of the disease (Doll & Hill, 1950). The conclusion was not at first generally accepted but compelling evidence about the comparisons made and the absence of other hypotheses strongly supported the association with smoking (Doll & Hill, 1952, 1953). Eventually in 1957, the Medical Research Council advised the government that the conclusion should be accepted influenced by the early results of the cohort study of British doctors (see later).

A later study (Doll *et al.*, 1959; Figure 12.2b) demonstrated a relationship between the smoking of cigarettes (1930) in many countries and deaths from lung cancer (1952–54). Using all the data from sixteen countries, the regression line showed a significant correlation coefficient of 0.76. Nevertheless the rate for the USA and Japan were less affected (i.e. for a given cigarette consumption below the line) whereas the Netherlands, Austria and England/Wales were above the line. A possible explanation of the difference between USA and England/Wales was found from a study which found that a larger proportion of the cigarette was smoked in the latter: in the USA the average length of the butt was 1.65 times that in England/Wales and the higher prevalence of the use of filter tips in the USA could have been a contributory factor. This study therefore raised the possibility that some of the differences between countries could be related to the 'dose' of cigarette smoke. Other reasons for the differences were differences in the past history of consumption, e.g. the Japanese having smoked very little until after the First World War. There are still unexplained differences in national relative risks adjusted for the number of cigarettes (Forastiere *et al.*, 1993).

A prospective study was set up with a cohort of British doctors (Doll & Hill, 1954). After the collection of data for ten years a remarkable relationship was found between death rate from lung cancer and smoking habits (cigarettes smoked per day; Figure 12.2c). Such a relationship between death rate and amount smoked (an exposure–response relationship) allowed the conclusion that cigarette smoke was the aetiological agent. This was strongly supported by the results shown in Figure 12.2d. For male doctors who had given up smoking, the number of deaths due to lung cancer fell substantially. (In Figure 12.2d Doll and Hill's (1964) results were expressed as lung cancer deaths/year/1,000 men while Doll and Peto's (1976) were expressed as death as a percentage of those expected for continuing smokers). The rate continues to fall the longer smoking has been given up. This trend, which has great public health significance, is explained in terms of a diminishing risk from the previous inhalation of cigarette smoke and the curve seems to approach asymptotically that for non-smokers. These results convinced officialdom, if not all individuals, that cigarette smoking causes lung cancer. In later studies cigarette smoking has been implicated in other causes of death (Doll & Peto, 1976). Although many other groups have made substantial contributions to the detrimental health effects of cigarette smoking, the methods used by Doll and Hill over many years illustrate the successful substantiation of a hypothesis.

Epidemiological studies sometimes stimulate more research. The convincing linear exposure–response relationship (Figure 12.2c) does not indicate that all humans are equally susceptible. If the exposure (number of cigarettes smoked per day) were increased, would everyone develop lung cancer? General experience suggests the some individuals are rather resistant. Cigarette smoke is a very complex chemical mixture and the aetiological agent(s) is not known. Recent studies suggest that in tobacco smokers a high induction of a particular cytochrome P_{450} (Al) in lung and the formation of DNA adducts is associated with lung cancer risk (Bartsch *et al.*, 1992). These findings imply that whatever is the responsible chemical agent in cigarette smoke it has to be bioactivated. It is possible that the low risk of cancer in the other parts of the respiratory tract such as mouth, tongue and pharynx is due to a low activity of these bioactivating cytochrome P_{450}s, lack of induction on exposure to smoke and/or lack of delivery of the constituents of smoke, because of physical properties, to the cells containing the bioactivation system. The rapid reduction in the number of deaths due to lung cancer, i.e. the diminishing risk due to previous inhalation of smoke, for those who stop smoking (Figure 12.2d) requires further research. It is interesting that not all conditions showing an association reverse when smoking ceases (Doll & Peto, 1976).

12.5   Toxic Oil Syndrome in Spain

At the beginning of May 1981 an epidemic of respiratory disease began in Madrid and areas north-west of the capital. At least twenty thousand cases occurred over a period of 6–8 weeks and was of such severity that over three hundred died. Following this explosive outbreak accompanied by myalgia and a high eosinophil count in the circulating blood, within months a complicated multi-organ syndrome developed. This syndrome included liver damage, peripheral neuropathy, sicca syndrome, scleroderma, thrombo embolism and pulmonary hypertension. Not all those who reported to hospital with respiratory difficulties progressed to these intermediate and chronic stages but there are many who still require medical attention and some who are permanently in hospital with little hope of improvement. A unifying hypothesis is that the basic lesion is endothelial involving secondary injury in nearly every organ. This lesion is associated with many thrombotic phenomena and most of the late clinical effects can be regarded as secondary to this basic lesion. Thus the basic lesion is a non-necrotising vasculitis. For a clinical description of the disease see Martinéz-Tello *et al.*, 1982; Martinéz-Tello & Téllez in WHO, 1992; section 8.10.

Initially attention was concentrated on infective agents as the cause of the pneumonia but the spread of illness and location of the patients and insensitivity to treatment by antibiotics was not in agreement with this hypothesis. Tabuenca (1981) tested his hypothesis that it was a poisoning episode with a small epidemiological study of young children and found a strong association of the disease with the consumption of a food oil bought from door-to-door salesmen (it is now known that the distribution of the oil was much wider). Other studies showed that these oils contained aniline and aniline derivatives such as fatty acid anilides which suggested that their origin was rape seed oil imported for industrial use and denatured with 2% aniline to prevent its use as food oil. The Spanish government, in order to try to stop the epidemic, exchanged suspect oil for olive oil.

Although the 'oil hypothesis' received support from several studies and because many other hypotheses were circulating and especially while the trial of those held responsible was taking place, a more extensive epidemiological study was organised to check the association of oil containing anilides with toxic oil syndrome (Kilbourne *et al.*, 1988).

From amongst the oils which in 1981 were handed in and exchanged for olive oil, two groups were selected – one from families affected by TOS (case oils) and the other with no reported cases (control oils). Although this procedure did not follow a formal plan, there is no reason to consider that it could have introduced selection bias in the design of the study. Oil containers were further selected on the basis of a variety of factors including size and shape of the plastic container and colour of the cap; the amount of oil in the container should be sufficient for a detailed analysis but the containers should not be full. Doubts whether the containers came from families with at least one case of TOS (case oils) and doubts whether the oils were true control oils (vendor they were purchased from and, although formal diagnosis of TOS was not made, some claimed that they had had symptoms suggestive of TOS) resulted in the rejection of containers from each group. The original potential 56 case oils and 118 controls were reduced to 29 and 64 respectively. The oils were blind coded so that those carrying out the analyses had no knowledge of whether the oil was classified as coming from families with or without TOS.

The results of the analyses are shown in Table 12.1 and are grouped into three classes of constituents, (1) those expected to be specific for rape seed oil, (2) and (3) those expected to be higher and lower respectively in rape seed oil than in other oils; aniline

Table 12.1 Analysis of toxic oil syndrome (TOS) case and control oils

		Case oils (29)	Control oils (64)
	Constituents of rape seed oil	mg/g (range)	
1	Brassicasterol	0.17(0–0.55)	0.00(0–0.40)
2	Campesterol	0.66(0.15–1.77)	0.32(0.19–1.42)
	Oleic acid	389(255–511)	285(214–448)
	cis-Vaccenic acid (18 : 1)	20.8(8.8–326)	11.8(7.2–29.4)
	Gondoic acid (20 : 1)	8.4(1.4–13.2)	2.7(0.6–10.7)
3	Stigmasterol	0.13(0–0.24)	0.19(0.06–0.29)
	Palmitic acid	79(66–116)	95(70–133)
	Stearic acid	34.6(20.1–45.7)	37.0(27.0–45.4)
	Linoleic acid	215(145–422)	406(140–510)
	Aniline and fatty acid anilides	μmol/g (range)	
	Oleoyl anilide	1.01(0–3.49)	0.00(0–0.60)
	Linoleoyl anilide	0.24(0–1.12)	0.00(0–0.22)
	Palmitoyl anilide	0.12(0–0.35)	0.00(0–0.06)
	Aniline	0.0024(0–0.0064)	0.0000(0–0.0017)
	TOTAL	1.38	0.00
	ANILINE (2% v/v) IN OIL	240	Nil

The case and control oils were selected using epidemiological criteria. For details see text and Kilbourne *et al.*, 1988.
1   Constituent specific for rape seed oil.
2   Constituents at higher concentrations in rape seed oil.
3   Constituents at lower concentrations in rape seed oil.
Source: Kilbourne *et al.*, 1988.

and fatty acid anilides were also determined. Case oils contain rape seed oil shown by the presence of brassicasterol, by having a higher concentration of campesterol and certain fatty acids and a lower concentration of stigmasterol and other fatty acids than in the controls. The distribution of aniline and anilides was also almost entirely in the case oils with few control oils containing any of these substances. The association between rape seed oil and aniline and anilides and between such constituents and cases of TOS is thus very strong. When the oils are grouped with respect to oleoyl anilide concentration and the probability of cases of TOS then a straight line is obtained (Figure 12.3). Although this cannot be regarded as a formal exposure–response relationship because the amount of oil consumed by the individuals concerned is not known, it is strong evidence of a causal relationship between the disease and the consumption of oils containing rape seed oil previously 'denatured' with aniline and subsequently processed. A similar study has been done using oils collected from another district with the same result. The association of TOS and the consumption of oil purchased as food oil in the types of container described above was supported by other conventional surveys; also groups of a few cases outside the epidemic area were all found to be associated with the consumption of such oils (Kilbourne *et al.* in WHO, 1992). Examination of the raw data used in Figure 12.3 shows that there are among the 29 case oils 11 which do not contain anilides, and among the 64 control oils there are 16 containing anilides. Thus although the association of the concentration of anilide with the probability of TOS is very high, the differentiation is not absolute.

Formally oleoyl anilide cannot be regarded as the aetiological agent for the disease but only as a marker of case oils. Other constituents (Table 12.1) such as linoleoyl anilide, palmitoyl anilide and free aniline also show high odds ratios. Anilides, of all the fatty acids existing in rape seed oils, will be present but all are currently only markers of such case oils. Other aniline derivatives have also recently been shown to be markers (Hill *et al.*, 1995), but until a suitable bioassay method is available which reproduces

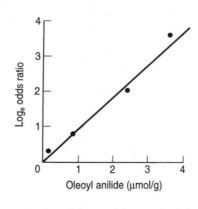

	Number of oils containing oleoyl anilide (µg/g)				Absence of anilide
	0	1–100	101–600	601–1200	1200+	(no./total)
Case oils	11	2	3	6	7	11/29
Control oils	48	6	7	3	0	48/64

Figure 12.3 The association of oleoyl anilide concentration in oils with cases of toxic oil syndrome in Spain. (*Source*: Adapted from Kilbourne *et al.*, 1988; see also Table 12.1)

all or part of the syndrome in experimental animals aniline derivatives are likely to remain only as markers (see Chapter 10) and not causes of the disease.

For a full description of the occurrence, clinical, epidemiological, chemical, experimental and immunological aspects see WHO, 1984, 1992, and Aldridge, 1992c.

In 1989 a similar disease called eosinophilia myalgia syndrome appeared in the USA and has been linked with the consumption or prescription of 1-tryptophan produced by one manufacturer. The aetiological agent causing this disease is not known (Swygert *et al.*, 1990; Slutsker *et al.*, 1990; Kilbourne *et al.*, 1991; WHO, 1991, 1993.)

12.6 Health Effects of Environmental Exposure to Cadmium

Cadmium is a toxic metal which has been much studied both experimentally in animals and in humans using clinical and epidemiological methods. Common sources of cadmium exposure are electroplating, galvanisation, manufacture of plastics, paint pigments, batteries and tobacco (cigarette smoke). Exposure of humans to dust containing cadmium may result in impairment of lung function, and long-term exposure to cadmium by inhalation or ingestion leads to its accumulation in the kidney cortex where it may cause functional and morphological change. Bone disease associated with kidney damage has occurred in several areas of Japan (Itai Itai disease) mainly in women in the 50s age group and living where drinking water and rice were contaminated with cadmium from the effluent from a lead–zinc processing plant (Friberg *et al.*, 1986). Cadmium, therefore, in addition to its effects on the lung and kidney tissues, affects the structure of bone, probably by an interference with calcium metabolism. Some have suggested that exposure to cadmium is associated with the development of hypertension although this is still controversial. Cadmium has also been implicated in various types of cancer. Although cadmium is carcinogenic in experimental animals and may enhance the occurrence of lung and prostate cancer in men exposed to airborne concentrations, there is no epidemiological or experimental evidence that exposure to cadmium via food may be associated with an increased risk of cancer (Lauwerys, 1989).

Exposure to cadmium leads to the synthesis of metallothionein which binds cadmium with very high affinity in the liver and kidney; such bound cadmium has a 10–30 year half-life (see section 5.5.4). It is widely accepted that, for the general population mainly exposed by the oral route and perhaps through inhalation of tobacco smoke, the kidney is the organ in which the first adverse effects occur. Studies of those occupationally exposed to cadmium have led to the view that if the concentration of cadmium in the renal cortex does not exceed 200 μg/g wet weight, which is associated with a urinary concentration of 10 μg/g creatinine or 10 μg/24 h, renal damage will be difficult to detect. This conclusion has, however, been based on occupationally active male subjects often exposed by inhalation and may underestimate the risks of other groups in the general population, e.g. older persons with declining renal function or others with an excessive loss of bone calcium.

Since Belgium is a major producer of cadmium and certain areas are polluted by cadmium in past emissions from non-ferrous industries, a large-scale morbidity study (Cadmibel study) was set up to assess the hypothesis that environmental pollution may lead to an increased uptake of cadmium into the human body and possibly to health effects (Lauwerys *et al.*, 1990).

A selection of four areas was made: two industrial areas one polluted with cadmium (Liege) and another not (Charleroi), and two rural areas one polluted by neighbouring non-ferrous smelters (N-Kempen) and the other not (Hechtel-Eksel). In each of these a sample of at least 200 households was randomly selected with the general aim of acquiring in the study of each area at least 300 subjects (150 males and 150 females) with 50 in each of the three age groups 20–39, 40–59 and 60–69. In fact 2,327 entered the study and the final statistical analysis was based on 1,699 subjects.

Table 12.2 shows the protocol for the field and laboratory studies. Measurements of cadmium in blood and urine were indicators that cadmium was being absorbed and were a measure of body burden/concentration in the renal cortex respectively. For environmental even more than occupational exposure, by analysing blood and urine the aim was to obtain individual data rather than population averages. The organisation of such a study and to obtain willing participation requires much effort; interest was stimulated by civil authorities and by advertisements in local newspapers and on radio and television.

Five of the variables (urinary excretion of retinol-binding protein, N-acetyl-B-glucosaminidase, β_2-microglobulin, amino acids and calcium) were significantly associated with 24 hour cadmium excretion. These associations were maintained by taking account of other possible determinants such as exposure to lead, age, sex, smoking habits, diuresis, diabetes, urinary tract diseases, consumption of analgesics and place of residence (Buchet *et al.*, 1990). With the exception of β_2-microglobulin, there was an association of the other constituents of urine with the concentration of cadmium in the 24 hour sample of urine. The population was divided into quartiles according to the 24 hour excretion of cadmium in urine and the mean values of the five associated variables standardised for other significant variables (Table 12.3). For each variable

Table 12.2 Protocol for the Cadmibel study

FIELD STUDY
Carried out over four years by ten specially trained personnel (nurses, social workers)
1 Questionnaire: medical history, current and past occupations, smoking habits, consumption of alcohol, locally grown vegetables and well water, drug intake
2 During two visits each subject was characterised by the mean of ten blood pressure measurements and by two determinations of pulse rate, height and body weight
3 During two visits two 24-hour samples of urine and a 4 ml and a 20 ml sample of venous blood were taken

CHEMICAL AND BIOCHEMICAL MEASUREMENTS

Whole blood: Cadmium, lead, selenium, zinc protoporphyrin

Serum: Zinc, calcium, magnesium
    Creatinine, cholesterol
    β_2-microglobulin, alkaline phosphatase, γ-glutamyl transferase, ferritin.

Urine: Cadmium, copper, sodium, potassium, calcium
    Aminoacids, creatinine
    Proteins (total), β_2-microglobulin[a], retinol-binding protein[b], albumin[c], N-acetyl-β-glucosaminidase[d]

[a,b] Bernard & Lauwerys, 1981.
[c] Bernard *et al.*, 1979; Gompertz *et al.*, 1983.
[d] Kawada *et al.*, 1989.
Source: Lauwerys *et al.*, 1990.

Table 12.3 Association between cadmium excretion and the mean values of five significant variables

Component excreted in 24 h	Urinary excretion of cadmium (μg/24 h)			
	0.00–0.51	0.52–0.89	0.90–1.40	1.41–8.00
Retinol binding protein (μg)	119 (413) A	132 (419) B	145 (416) C	153 (421) C
N-acetyl-β-glucosaminidase (IU)	1.53 (413) A	1.70 (419) B	1.75 (416) B	1.89(420) C
β_2-Microglobulin (μg)	99 (402) A	101 (407) A	107 (401) A,B	117 (404) B
Aminoacids (mg a–N)	195 (402) A	213 (408) B	211 (401) B	229 (405) C
Calcium (mmol)	1.54 (403) A	1.90 (410) B	2.02 (403) B	2.55 (408) C

Note: The results are expressed as the antilog of the geometric mean (number of subjects) A, B, C indicating significance. Significance was determined by analysis of variance; from left to right means with the same letter do not differ significantly. Since data were missing for some subjects the totals are not 1,699.
Source: Data from Buchet *et al.*, 1990.

there was a significant dose-effect relationship. Other statistical analysis allowed the estimate to be made that more than 10% of values would be abnormal when the cadmium excretion rate exceeded 2.87 μg/24 h for retinol-binding protein, 2.74 μg/24 h for N-acetyl-B-glucosaminidase, 3.05 μg/24 h for β_2-microglobulin, 4.27 μg/24 h for aminoacids and 1.92 μg/24 h for calcium.

This study shows that in people aged 20–80 years who have never been occupationally exposed to cadmium, the body burden (estimated on the basis of 24 hour urinary cadmium excretion) may be associated with changes in proximal tubular function and with a higher urinary excretion of calcium. This conclusion differs from previous studies on adult male workers (age 20–55) in whom the cadmium excretion showing no detectable effects was about 10 μg/24 h corresponding to a concentration of cadmium in the renal cortex of 200 μg/g wet weight. This difference is usually ascribed to the healthy worker effect that usually operates in industrial populations, leading to underestimates of the health risk for the general population. From the Cadmibel study the health significance of the renal dysfunction associated with a cadmium body burden lower than that usually considered critical in adult male workers is still unknown. In other research it has been shown that, in subjects occupationally exposed to cadmium, the presence of renal dysfunction more pronounced than that seen in the Cadmibel study may be predictive of subsequent development of some degree of renal insufficiency (Roels *et al.*, 1989).

For full account of this study see Lauwerys *et al.*, 1990, 1991, and Buchet *et al.*, 1990.

12.7 Discussion

The selective choice of three epidemiological studies illustrate the difficulties of organising studies which lead to conclusions regarding causality. For the toxic oil syndrome it has been established with reasonable certainty that consumption of food oils containing rape seed oil and aniline derivatives is the cause of the disease. Fatty acid anilides are only markers of TOS case oils and may not be regarded as the aetiological agent(s). Without the development of an experimental model of whole or part of the syndrome so that a bioassay system may be used alongside fractionation of the oils to isolate and identify the causative agent it is difficult to envisage how the problem will be solved.

For smoking and carcinoma of the lung there can be no doubt that cigarette smoke contains the aetiological agent(s). Such smoke is a highly complex chemical mixture but, again, suitable experimental animal models have proved difficult to find. Even though it is proving possible to isolate adducts derived from bioactivated polycyclic hydrocarbons other adducts have been isolated such as hydroxyethyl derivative of *N*-terminal valine (presumably derived from ethene in tobacco smoke; Tornqvist *et al.*, 1986). Thus even though the nature of some of the (internal) dose is known, the identity of causative agent(s) is not. It is possible that several substances are carcinogenic and that certain subgroups of the population are capable of bioactivating or initiating the disease. These considerations refer to the question of why only some smokers develop lung cancer and detracts nothing from knowledge of the broad spectrum of ill effects of tobacco.

For the Cadmibel study there is a huge background of information on cadmium both from epidemiological studies on occupationally exposed workers and on the toxicokinetics of cadmium in experimental animals and in humans. The biology of the response is also well worked out and early markers of renal insufficiency are known. With this background information the Cadmibel study could be undertaken and results be obtained which indicate that environmental exposure of the general population in Belgium can lead in some people to evidence of absorption, accumulation of cadmium and consequential renal dysfunction. The relationship of such renal changes to possible development of ill health such as renal insufficiency or loss of bone calcium cannot be assessed at present.

All three studies illustrate that if a dose–response relationship can be established then associations are more certain. The development of biomonitoring techniques utilising non-invasive methods help in reaching this desirable situation. With few exceptions most of epidemiological studies on the health effects of environmental pollutants have attempted to assess the relationships between various external indicators of exposure (presence of emission sources, results of environmental monitoring) and morbidity (clinical signs and/or mortality data). This approach has many limitations. Current and/or past exposure to pollutants can usually only be estimated on a population basis and diagnosed clinical entities are late indicators of previous functional/pathological processes. The main disadvantage is that the identification of the aetiology can only be achieved when exposure is overwhelming by comparison with other factors (e.g. aging) or when the time interval between exposure and diagnosis is not too long. These difficulties can be overcome if assessment of exposure is carried out on an individual basis by the use of biological (dose) monitoring (see Chapter 11) and if early biological effects can be detected as predictors of future ill health.

The Cadmibel study could not have been attempted without the use of biological monitoring methods. Although this study may be a special case – because of the availability of measurements of current (cadmium in blood) and integrated exposure (cadmium in urine) and knowledge of early changes detectable long before renal insufficiency – the general principles should apply to all epidemiological studies of the toxicity of chemicals (see section 12.2 and Figure 12.1).

The difficulty of establishing causality between exposure to a particular chemical and toxicity by epidemiological studies is not unique. Similar problems arise in trying to establish the mechanism of initiation of disease, i.e. the causal relationship between reaction with a component of a particular cell and the subsequent biological changes. For both, the demonstration of an exposure– or dose–response relationship is a vital part of substantiation – for epidemiological studies this is the association between absorbed dose and biological effect, and for mechanistic studies it is the association between the dose delivered to the affected cell and the biological events leading to clinical signs.

The three studies discussed in this chapter were chosen because they have led to strong associations between exposure and biological effect. They illustrate the finesse in design and the size and number of studies required to reach firm conclusions. As in most branches of scientific investigation, strong association and high probability often fall short of proof of causality and, in toxicology, identity of the aetiological agent. Proof moves nearer if support is available from experiments showing similar effects in animals. Mechanistic studies leading to common measurements in animals and humans may round the circle.

12.8 Summary

1 Epidemiology is the study of factors determining the frequency and distribution of disease, injury and other health-related effects and their cause in defined populations.

2 When a chemical is suspected of causing disease the aim is to establish first the vehicle (food, water, air) for and then the nature of the aetiological agent.

3 When large numbers are affected in a rapid outbreak of disease the identification of the vehicle for the poison may be relatively easy. The chemical identity of the agent usually follows when an experimental model of the disease is established (bioassay).

4 When exposure is to complex mixtures for a long time and there is considerable background incidence of the disease the identity of the causative agent(s) may be difficult to establish.

5 The choice of the control (unexposed) population and the establishment of an exposure–response relationship are the most important features which determine cause–effect, i.e. that exposure to A leads to disease B.

6 The availability of biomarkers for dose and effect monitoring reduces variation, particularly in individual exposure.

7 The Hill (1965) guidelines define important aspects to be addressed when establishing if an association between events indicates a cause–effect relationship.

13

Environmental and Ecotoxicology

13.1 Introduction

Ecotoxicology is concerned with the adverse impact of chemicals on ecosystems. In addition, by common usage, it has come to include the study of how chemicals reach man through the environment. It is difficult for us, by our humanocentric mode of thought, to consider or concede what is good for the environment; decisions depend on judgements we are probably unable to make, i.e. criteria for normality, non-human risk–benefit assessment and derived from it what are tolerable changes.

The recent history of the biological world is mainly that of its exploitation by humans. The 'balance of nature' has been changed and is still changing not least by continually developing agriculture. Catastrophic volcanic eruptions cause enormous changes in the local biology but also influence far afield as a result of the dissemination of dust and smoke. Studies after such disasters are illuminating in the rapidity of repopulation by plants and animals. Sometimes in the light of such happenings the potential effects of man-made chemicals seem slight and perhaps trifling.

An ecosystem includes countless number of organisms from micro-organisms to plants and animals that interact dynamically in complex ways among themselves and with their physical environment. Many factors affect the dynamics of an ecosystem and hence the balance within it, e.g. light, temperature, energy and nutrient supplies, competition, predation (including agricultural practice), pollution and disease. The most important property of an ecosystem is its robustness, e.g. the way it can withstand or adapt to changes which affect the dynamics of the system. Included in this robustness is the ability to return to 'normal' after the cessation of the stimulus to which it is sensitive. Organisms in the environment, e.g. in soil, water, plants and animals, possess an array of enzyme systems capable of detoxifying many chemical intoxicants (Bumpus *et al.*, 1985; Sandermann, 1992; Ghiorse & Wilson, 1988).

The possibility of irreversible change which will reduce biological diversity is most worrying. In recent years there has been a growing appreciation that the world is finite and that it is, in essence, a large ecosystem which should be in some kind of state which cycles about an 'equilibrium' position. Probably the most serious aspects influencing world biology away from such a position are the large factors resulting from increasing population and its striving for physical comfort and protection. Human beings using their ingenuity to develop technology have extracted from the earth oil and minerals and by this utilisation have distributed them on a huge scale (e.g. lead, cadmium, etc. and combustion products such as carbon dioxide, nitrogen oxides, polycyclic hydro-carbons). Other chemicals designed for specific technological purposes, e.g. halo-hydro-carbons for refrigerants, polyhalogenated aromatics as insulating fluids for transformers, are coincidentally extremely stable to biological attack; their release into the environment has led to their widespread dissemination. The release of long-lived radioactive isotopes raises the same sorts of question concerning persistence and non-dilution out from certain ecosystems. The task of the ecotoxicologist is to design procedures to prevent such contamination not only in use but during their disposal, to design predictive tests to prevent undesirable new compounds being used and, if they are released, to determine whether they are having any effect (eco-epidemiology).

13.2 Polychlorinated Biphenyls

The industrial production of the polychlorinated biphenyls began over sixty years ago and, worldwide, it is estimated that over one million tons have been produced. Their commercial advantage was based on their high chemical stability, low aqueous solu-bility, non-inflammability and high insulating properties. This range of properties made them excellent as heat transfer fluids in transformers and capacitors, as flame retar-dants and in lubricating and hydraulic oils.

Polychlorinated biphenyls are synthesised by the substitution of chlorine atoms into the biphenyl core of the molecule. Different amounts of chlorine may be substituted and the chlorine content in commercial products has ranged from 20% to 70%. The basic structure (Figure 13.1) has the empirical formulae $C_{12}H_{10-n}Cl_n$ and although 209 different structures are possible not all are formed in the chlorination process. Products are available under a variety of trade names; perhaps for the experimental toxicolo-gist the most common is Aroclor with a range of chlorine contents from 21% to 60%.

In their initial use, polychlorinated biphenyls escaped not only via leakage from transformers (by the dumping of large quantities in obsolescent equipment) but also by their use in open systems such as paint, rubber, carbonless copy paper and wood preservatives. Although the use of these materials in open systems is now restricted and regulations for their disposal are in place, we are left with the legacy of their early dispersal. The properties which make the polychlorinated biphenyls so technologically useful are those which ensure its stability and spread in the environment. They are

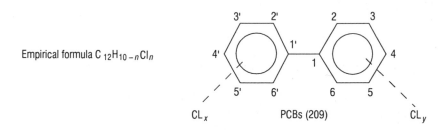

Figure 13.1 Structural formulae of polychlorinated biphenyls

very lipophilic with a very low solubility in water and are only slowly degraded. Thus if released into the environment their properties ensure partition into the lipids of all organisms they contact. Analytical methods are available for their identification and determination in small amounts; they have been found in plants and animals in the oceans, in birds, in terrestrial animals and in human adipose tissue. Thus these lipid-soluble and stable compounds are now globally distributed to places where they have never been produced or used. Analyses of surface sea water in the North Pacific indicate concentrations as low as 0.3 ng/litre with intermediate concentrations in plankton and fish and, at the end of the food chain, 3,700 μg/kg in striped dolphin – a bioaccumulation of over ten million.

The signs and symptoms of poisoning in both animals and humans are varied and indicate profound changes in normal physiology (Table 13.1). There are some notable differences between species. The skin manifestations which seem to be due to systemic disturbances to which human are very sensitive cannot be produced in rodents (except for a hyperkeratotic and acne-like lesion in rabbit ear) but have been seen in cattle and rhesus and marmoset monkeys. An early finding in cattle following exposure to chlorinated naphthalenes was a rapid decline of blood vitamin A levels. Further experiments have shown that after the administration of polychlorinated biphenyls to a variety of experimental animals (rabbit, rat, mice, Japanese quail and monkeys) there are falls in hepatic and/or serum vitamin A levels. These findings and a resemblance between

Table 13.1 Toxic responses of rodents, sub-human primates and humans to polychlorinated biphenyls

Signs and symptoms	Rat/mouse	Monkey	Humans	Vitamin A deficiency (rat)
General (body weight loss, loss of appetite	+	+	+	+
Skin (chloracne, hyperpigmentation, hair loss)	−	+	+	−
Periocular (eyelid swelling, cysts, hyperpigmentation)	−	+	+	+
Ocular (night blindness)				+
Liver (parenchymal lesions)	+	−	+	+
Polyneuropathy	+	−	+	+
Endocrinological (irregular cycles)	+	−	+	
Metabolic disorders (porphryia, hyperlipidaemia)	+	+	+	
Immune defects (thymus depletion, suppression of T cells)	+	−		+
Gastro-intestinal tract (hyperplasia, ulcers)	+	+	+	
Reproductive (low birth rate, testicular degeneration)	+	+		+
Teratogenic	+	+		+

Source: Data from Kimbrough, 1980; Reggiani, 1983; McLaren, 1978.

the signs and symptoms of poisoning and vitamin A deficiency led to a hypothesis that interference in distribution, disposal and mechanism of action of retinol could be involved in the mechanism of toxicity of polychlorinated biphenyls.

Vitamin A is transported from the liver to its peripheral target cells such as the testis, liver, kidney, retina, dermis and epidermis mainly as the alcohol, retinol, bound to a specific carrier protein known as retinol binding protein (RBP). This protein is synthesised in the liver parenchymal cells and has a molecular weight of about 20,000 and binds one molecule of retinol to one molecule of RBP. In plasma, RBP interacts with transthyretin (TTR), a thyroxin-binding protein, and this complex circulates as a 1 : 1 RBP–TTR complex. RBP is delivered in this form to the target cells. The target cells contain low molecular weight intracellular proteins which bind retinol, retinoic acid or retinal depending on which is the active form. The production and secretion of RSP by the liver is controlled by the vitamin A status of the animal; in deficient states less is secreted and with adequate supplies more (Goodman, 1980; Chytil & Ong, 1978; Stubbs *et al.*, 1979). The mechanism whereby vitamin A (or its metabolites) exerts its influence on biological processes such as growth, reproduction and epithelial differentiation is not understood in any detail. This situation has its parallel with knowledge about the mechanism of toxicity of chemicals.

Research, initially on rats and using the pure isomer 3,3',4,4'-tetrachlorobiphenyl, has indicated a mechanism whereby the transport of both retinol and thyroxine is affected. This isomer is metabolised to the 5-hydroxy derivative by cytochrome $P_{450}1A1$; this hydroxy derivative has a structural resemblance to thyroxine, has an 2.5-fold higher affinity for transthyretin than l-thyroxine and causes a rapid loss of thyroxine from the circulation. The attachment of the 5-hydroxy derivative to transthyretin is postulated to cause a conformational change so that subsequent complex formation with RBP is prevented. The RBP not bound to transthyretin is small enough to pass through the glomerular membrane causing a loss of retinol (Figure 13.2; Brouwer *et al.*, 1988, 1990). These findings have been expanded in two directions. The first is to determine structural requirements for binding to transthyretin and the second to compare responses of other animal species (Table 13.2). Metabolism of polychlorinated biphenyls is required for effects on the retinol-binding system and occurs when either the 5-hydroxy or 4-hydroxy derivative is formed from tetra chlorobiphenyls. In some cases induction of the requisite P_{450} enhances this metabolism; such induction occurs via interaction of the parent compounds with the Ah (aryl hydroxylase) receptor (Safe, 1984, 1990) so much studied in the context of the mode of action of TCDD (dioxin; Poland & Knutson, 1982). Many but not all species show reductions of plasma retinol and l-thyroxine after experimental exposure to 3,4,3',4'-TCB (Table 13.2). After high field exposure of cormorants to PCBs, only plasma l-thyroxine was reduced (Brouwer, 1991).

In the harbour seal both parameters are affected; if the original hypothesis is correct – that interference in the functions of vitamin A is the cause of at least some of the signs and symptoms of poisoning by polychlorinated biphenyls – then plasma retinol/thyroxine concentrations should be an effect biomarker. Fish from the Whadden Sea were more contaminated with PCBs and pp'-DDE than fish caught in the north-west Atlantic. Seals fed with fish contaminated with high concentrations of polychlorinated biphenyls (daily intake 1.5 mg PCBs and 0.4 mg pp'-DDE) had lower retinol and thyroxine levels in the plasma than those fed with lower concentrations (daily intake 0.22 mg PCBs and 0.13 mg pp'-DDE) When those fed on the high concentrations were fed with the less contaminated fish for six months, plasma retinol and thyroxine returned to normal (Brouwer *et al.*, 1989).

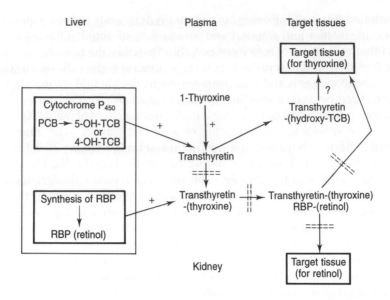

Figure 13.2 The transport pathways for retinol and thyroxine and interference by hydroxy metabolites of polychlorinated biphenyls (TCBs). TCB = tetrachlorobiphenyl; RBP = retinol-binding protein; transthyretin = carrier protein for thyroxine. The rate of pathways crossed by double dashed lines is reduced by reaction of transthyretin with hydroxy-TCBs; this leads to reductions in the circulating concentration of the thyroxine complex and in the transport of retinol

Table 13.2 Tetrachlorinated biphenyls (TCBs) and their effects on retinol and thyroxine transport systems. (a) Competitive potency of ^{125}I-thyroxine binding by 3,4,3',4'-TCB and its hydroxy derivatives. (b) Effects of 3,4,3',4'-TCB on plasma levels of retinol and thyroxine in different species

(a)

Compound	50% Inhibition (nM)	Relative potency
1-Thyroxine	59	100
3,4,3',4'-TCB	≫1,000	≪1
3,4,3',4'-TCB, 2-OH	111	53
3,4,3',4'-TCB, 4-OH	23	256
3,4,3',4'-TCB, 5-OH	22	268
3,4,3',4'-TCB, 6-OH	980	6

(b)

Species (strains)	Dose (mg/kg)	Plasma thyroxine (%)	Plasma retinol (%)
Mouse (BL)	50 (S)	66	42
Mouse (D$_2$)		44	31
Rat (W)	50 (S)	5	45
Marmoset monkey	3 (R)	3	67
Herring gull	50 (S)	105	95
Eider duck	50 (S)	105	110

(S) single intraperitoneal, (R) oral twice/week for 18 weeks.
Sources: (a) Data from Brouwer *et al.*, 1990. (b) Data from Brouwer, 1991.

These studies illustrate the interplay among fundamental research on mechanisms of toxicity, basic biology and practical problems in the environment. Interference in the pathways involved in the action of vitamin A could produce the complicated syndrome described for PCBs. It seems possible that the syndrome is the consequence of action on more than one system perhaps by different chemical structures in the original technical material and/or produced by metabolism *in vivo*.

13.3 Toxic Chemicals produced by Cyanobacteria (Algae)

In many countries bloom-forming cyanobacteria (blue-green algae) have grown in abnormal amounts in inland lakes and coastal waters (Anderson, 1994). The cause of the excessive growth is almost certainly an excess of nutrients in water run-off following the increased use of fertilisers in agriculture and forestry and also the discharge of effluents into lakes, rivers and coastal waters; the association of these factors with good summers is a powerful stimulus to explosive growth. Many of these organisms produce, in addition to lipopolysaccharide endotoxin, other compounds which are highly toxic to many animals (Codd, 1984; Carmichael *et al.*, 1985; Carmichael, 1992; Persson *et al.*, 1984). Since surface waters are a frequent source of drinking water, the health significance of the growth of blue-green algae is of concern; liver damage in humans in Australia due to *Microcystis aeruginosa* in the local water has been reported (Falconer *et al.*, 1983). It is not known what are the factors that influence the differing amounts of toxin produced by the same organism at different times.

Hepatotoxicity is a frequent consequence of consumption of lake water by animals or of the administration of extracts of the algae to experimental animals. The signs of poisoning in mice after intraperitoneal injection are piloerection, paresis of the hindlimbs, tachypnea (rapid shallow breathing), pallor and cold peripheries. At autopsy the liver is engorged with blood and much larger than normal, and histological examination indicates large haemorrhages and distortion of the normal sinusoidal architecture with early signs of necrosis. The kidney shows minimal damage with little or no change in other organs.

Different strains of cyanobacteria species from different genera, e.g. *Microcystis, Anabaema, Oscillatoria, Nodularia*, produce similar but not identical peptides. The toxins are cyclic heptapeptides of molecular weight about 1,000 and contain an unusual β-aminoacid (Adda; see Figure 13.3a; Botes *et al.*, 1984; Sivonen *et al.*, 1992; Lanarus *et al.*, 1991). The part of the molecule necessary for toxicity is not known. The current hypothesis is that the mechanism of toxicity involves changes in the cytoskeletal elements, e.g. actin, shown by blebbing on the surface of the cell (Hooser *et al.*, 1991; Eriksson *et al.*, 1987, 1990). Protein phosphatase is inhibited by concentrations as low as 2–6 nM of the toxin from Microcystin LR; such an inhibition could influence the degree of phosphorylation of a functionally important protein (Eriksson *et al.*, 1990; Nishiwaki-Matsushima *et al.*, 1991).

These hepatotoxins are interesting from a mechanistic point of view. They are also potentially important since they are lethal to mammals, birds and other animals at low concentrations. Health significance to humans and the adequacy of water treatment processes requires attention. The ecological significance is difficult to assess but there is evidence that some organisms (e.g. mussels) can accumulate the peptides without toxic effects, and thus they enter the food chains.

Recently a neurotoxin produced by *Anabaena flos-aqua*, a cyanobacteria, has been

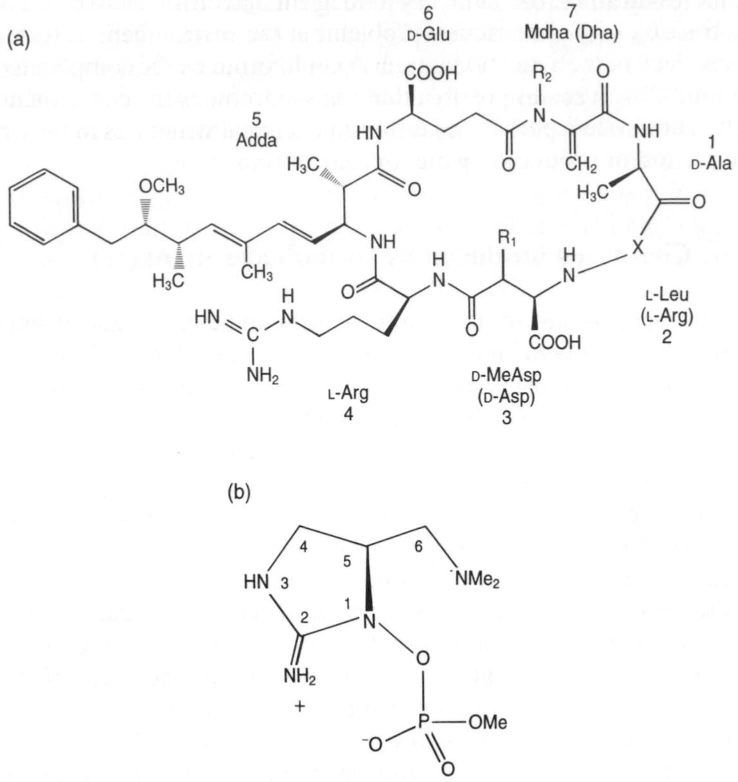

(a)

(b)

Figure 13.3 The general structure of (a) hepatotoxins produced by various cyanobacteria and (b) the anti-acetylcholinesterase produced by *Anabaema flos-aqua*. (a) In different strains the structures vary: X can be l-leucine or l-arginine and R_1 and R_2 can be methyl or a hydrogen atom (Sivonen *et al.*, 1992). (b) For structural analysis see Matsunaga *et al.*, 1989

identified as an organophosphate (Hyde & Carmichael, 1991; see Table 1.1 and Figure 13.3b). This compound is toxic to large and small mammals (signs of toxicity to rats at $20 \mu g/kg$) and the signs of poisoning are those expected from an anti-acetyl-cholinesterase action. The primary structure contains an ionised hydroxyl attached to the phosphorus atom. Organophosphates with such a negative charge are not normally powerful inhibitors of acetylcholinesterase but in this case the negative charge is neutralised by the formation of a zwitterion with the ionised NH_2.

13.4 Methylmercury: Minamata and Niigata Episodes

From 1953 to 1965 in Japan an unusual disease was observed in the peasant fishermen and their families. The symptoms were paresthesia, numbness of the hands, feet, lips and tongue (sensory) and ataxia, gait and speech impediments (motor). Constriction of the visual fields was also a common symptom. The signs and symptoms were clearly neuropathic and, since cats were also affected, it seemed probable that it was due to an exogenous toxin rather than to an infective agent. Those affected lived at the mouths of rivers and it was subsequently established that the origin of the toxin was effluent containing mercury which had been discharged into the rivers from industrial plants. Initially around 170 cases were reported but this has now risen to approximately 1,200 (Table 13.3). Fishermen, their families and cats were affected because the major part of their diet was fish containing high concentrations of methylmercury. The known neurotoxicity of methylmercury would therefore explain the disease and its distribution among the population. There have been many other episodes of neurotoxicity poisoning particularly in Iraq; the overall total of cases is probably between nine and ten thousand (Table 13.3; see also section 11.5).

The sensory disturbances of methylmercury poisoning are probably due to patchy demyelination in the sensory nerves which affects the whole length of the nerve (see section 8.8). The origin of the long-lasting motor disturbances is partially due to cell necrosis, particularly in the cerebellum. Involuntary movements (tremor, myoclonic jerks and muscle twitching) were also seen and the severe clinical picture was similar to cerebral palsy. In less severely affected adults some gradual improvement was seen in muscle power, ataxia and dysarthia (speech defects) but the visual changes were slowest to improve with in many cases no recovery and complete and permanent blindness. Previous research had shown that the rat is a suitable experimental model and established the cellular basis of the toxicity. The detailed molecular mechanism is as yet unknown and although it is accepted that the mercury is absorbed and distributes as methylmercury it is not known for certain if the local toxic effects in the nervous system are due to this form or to the demethylated mercuric form slowly released from it (Vahter *et al.*, 1994).

The release of mercury into the aqueous environment can lead to the accumulation of methylmercury in the food chain and especially in fish. Mercury had been used as a fungicide in paper production from wood pulp and in some countries the consumption of fish caught in the adjoining lakes has been restricted. Many micro-organisms can methylate many metals (germanium, tin, lead, arsenic, antimony, mercury; Craig & Glockling, 1988). For several years it was assumed that the pathway from the industrial plants in Japan to the methylmercury in the fish was caused by the biological methy-

Table 13.3 Outbreaks of methylmercury poisoning

Source of exposure	Location and date of outbreak	Number of cases
Fish	Minamata, 1953–60	>700
Fish	Niigata, 1964–65	>500
Seed grain	Iraq, 1956	>100
Seed grain	Iraq, 1960	1,022
Seed grain	Pakistan, 1969	100
Seed grain	Guatemala, 1963–65	45
Seed grain	Ghana, 1967	144
Seed grain	Iraq, 1971	6,530
		TOTAL >9,100

For information about these outbreaks see Bakir *et al.*, 1973; Clarkson *et al.*, 1976; Skerfving & Vostal, 1972; Tsubaki & Irukayama, 1977; WHO, 1976.

lation of mercury released in the effluent; the synthesis of acetaldehyde from acetylene used inorganic mercury as a catalyst. However later analysis of the effluents has shown that it contains methylmercury produced as a by-product in the above reaction. It is now agreed that the major part of the methylmercury in the fish originated from its presence in the effluent. Absorption of methylmercury by mammals is efficient by the oral route and owing to its high affinity for thiols it accumulates (see section 11.5). These episodes of poisoning in Minamata and Niigata have been reviewed by Tsubaki & Irukayama (1977).

13.5 Chlorinated Mutagenic Agents in Drinking Water

The Castner–Kellner process has ensured a cheap and plentiful supply of chlorine. Not only has this influenced the production of many bioactive organochlorine compounds but also chlorine, hypochlorous acid as sodium hypochlorite and other oxychlorine compounds are used for bleaching and for water purification. Chlorine has been widely used to ensure satisfactory disinfection of drinking water and has many advantages: it is toxic to many micro-organisms, it is cheaper than many other disinfectants, if required it can be prepared at the waterworks, and is not critically sensitive to the range of pH and temperature normally encountered. Disinfection can occur before and after the water leaves the waterworks. Chlorine persists in the water for some time and ensures that bacterial growth does not occur in the distribution network. Although widely used, chlorination came under attack twenty years ago after trihalomethanes were detected in drinking water sometimes at concentrations exceeding 1,000 μg/l. More recently, the finding that drinking water treated with chlorine is mutagenic by the Ames test has stimulated much research in many countries (Meier, 1988).

For the following reasons research in Finland will be described. First, about one-half of the population drinks processed surface water. Secondly, Finnish research has been very active in the detection and identification of mutagenic agents and other polutants containing chlorine. Thirdly, Finland has a large wood pulp industry which discharges effluent into the surface water. Fourthly, some of the lakes or interconnecting systems of lakes contain high concentrations of humus (complex macromolecules formed from the decomposition of plant materials and containing polymeric phenolic structures). Fifthly, the inhabitants have lived in the same area for a long time. Sixthly, the Finnish cancer register is one of the most comprehensive and has been in operation for many years, and lastly, a method has been found to estimate retrospectively the concentration of one mutagenic agent in drinking water in areas of high and low total organic carbon content.

Some chlorinated drinking waters in Finland are mutagenic and the mutagenic agent can be concentrated for testing by extraction with organic solvents after acidification (Vartiainen & Liimatainen, 1986). A highly active mutagen has been identified and shown to account for at least one-half of the total mutagenicity of the water. This compound is 3-chloro-4-(dichloromethyl)-5-hydroxy-2(5H)-furanone, often called MX and exists in three geometric isomers in equilibrium with each other (Holmbom *et al.*, 1984; Vartiainen and Liimatainen, 1986; Figure 13.4). The mutagenic activity by the Ames salmonella testing procedure is very high and the number of revertants depends on the type of strain of salmonella (Ames *et al.*, 1975b). Strain T100, suitable for detecting base-pair substitution mutations, was the most sensitive

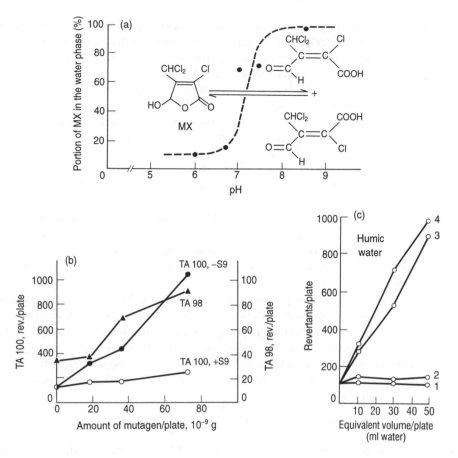

Figure 13.4 Properties of MX and its mutagenicity, and the production of mutagens by different treatments of humic waters. (a) Distribution of MX between ethylacetate and water at different pH. (*Source*: Adapted from Holmbom *et al.*, 1984 and Kronberg & Vartiainen, 1988). (b) Mutagenicity of MX tested on salmonella strains TA100 (± rat liver S-9 fraction) and TA98. (*Source*: Adapted from Holmbom *et al.*, 1984). (c) Mutagenicity of humic water treated with (1) ozone, (2) chlorine dioxide, (3) chlorine, (4) ozone/chlorine tested on salmonella strain TA100. (*Source*: Adapted from Backlund *et al.*, 1985)

and metabolic activation was not necessary; indeed it greatly reduced the number of revertants (Figure 13.4b). Strain T98, effective for frameshift mutagens, was at least ten times less effective but T97 was almost as sensitive as T100 (Vartiainen *et al.*, 1987). The mutagenicity of extracts of drinking water showed a linear relationship to MX concentration (Kronberg & Vartiainen, 1988). Treatment of humus containing water with ozone or chlorine dioxide did not result in enhanced mutagenicity whereas chlorine treatment with or without ozone resulted in a high activity (Figure 13.4c; Backlund *et al.*, 1985). In addition to the reaction between chlorine and the constituents of humic waters, MX is present in the effluent from wood pulp processing plants together with many other compounds including chlorinated phenols and chloroacetones (Holmbom *et al.*, 1984).

MX is a mutagenic compound and as such would be expected to react with proteins and nucleic acids. The complex reaction between proteins and MX appears to be mainly reversible with the regeneration of the parent compound on dissociation. The microsomal fraction from induced rat liver decreases the mutagenic activity in the Ames type test (Figure 13.4b) and it seems probable that MX will be destroyed fairly rapidly in mammals. It is difficult to assess the significance of such detoxification because many potent electrophilic carcinogens are also rapidly destroyed *in vivo*.

The health significance of the consumption of MX is of considerable interest. The current view that the initiation of cancer is a mutagenic event indicates that both animal experimentation and human epidemiology are necessary. Methods are available for the determination of MX in current drinking water. MX has been synthesised so that experimental research on animals may be undertaken. Administration of MX to rats at oral doses of 30 and 45–75 mg/kg 5 days a week for 14–18 weeks caused a significant increase in sister-chromatid exchanges in both sexes. Dose-related increases were also found after incubation of cultured rat peripheral lymphocytes with concentrations of 20–60 μg/ml for 44 hours (Jansson *et al.*, 1993). At present there is no means of comparison of the dose–response of these two findings. The results of two-year carcinogenicity studies are not yet available.

Retrospective estimation of previous concentration of MX now seems possible because of a strong correlation between the concentration of organic matter as measured by colour or the permanganate oxidation test and the concentration of MX produced by chlorination (Kronberg & Vartiainen, 1988). Using the following relationship a good correlation has been found between actual measured mutagenicity and that calculated from the total organic carbon and chlorine for both the prechlorination and postchlorination treatment:

$$\text{Mutagenicity in TA100} = A(1 - e^{-kc(R)} + A(1 - e^{-kc(D)})$$

in which TOC = total organic carbon, $c = [\text{TOC}][\text{Cl}_2]$, R refers to the parameters for prechlorination and D to the parameters for postchlorination of the drinking water, and A and k are constants (Vartiainen *et al.*, 1988). The first study using this method of retrospective estimation of mutagenicity and data from the Finnish Cancer Registry indicates a statisically significant exposure–response association between the mutagenicity of drinking water and the incidence of bladder, kidney and stomach cancers. In a town using chlorinated surface water for drinking with a mutagenicity of 3,000 revertants per litre the relative risk was 1.2 for bladder and 1.2–1.4 for kidney cancer compared with towns where non-mutagenic water was consumed (Kolvusalo *et al.*, 1994).

13.6   Discussion

The view that the balance of nature should not be allowed to change is unrealistic. However, vigilance is required to avoid long-term, perhaps permanent, changes being brought about by chemical contamination; our knowledge of the long-term consequences of such changes is rudimentary. Humans have continually altered and, at an increasing pace, will continue to alter the balance of nature to provide for their own comfort, protection from disease and ease of movement. With continual increase in population the possibility of continual slow build-up of chemical residues must be kept under review. Generalised contamination can come about by metals such as lead, stable radioactive isotopes and by stable lipophilic molecules such as chlorinated hydrocarbons. Such materials may accumulate in food chains causing toxicity not only for humans but also for other organisms. The view is now accepted that stable chemicals should not be released into the environment (although prevention is difficult) and that the cost/benefit ratio of the use of some chemicals is different in different parts of the world (see Chapter 14 on risk). Pesticides now must be shown to be degradable in the environment to low toxicity material, i.e. by chemical, light, micro-organisms, etc.

Contamination of local environments by chemicals are frequent occurrences, e.g. intentional or accidental release into rivers. Undesirable as such contamination is, experience has shown that ecosystems are very resilient and recovery does usually take place. Nevertheless, information must be collected and research conducted after large episodes. For this purpose staff and facilities must be available quickly and capable of the generation and assessment of information relevant to medical, veterinary and zoological sciences. Most important is the involvement of those with expertise in analytical and experimental toxicology. More knowledge may lead to improvements in predictive tests and better decision-taking which balance public concern, economic reality and biological facts. Sometimes events themselves show that information was available and could have been used to predict ecotoxicity. An example is tri *n*-butyltin compounds; sufficient was known about the lipophilic properties of the chloride, its biocidal properties, its stability in the environment and its high biological activity against energy conservation systems to predict that closed areas such as marinas might become sterile when, to prevent the attachment and growth of barnacles, boats were treated with varnish containing high concentrations of the tin compound.

Research must establish whether hypotheses about the effects of a chemical in the environment have a firm base. The main questions are:

1 Is the chemical there or has it been there?
2 Does the chemical penetrate and/or concentrate in the organism?
3 Do experimental studies confirm the proposed aetiology?
4 What is the mechanism of the toxic effect?

Epidemiological research on exposure of humans to MX via drinking water (section 13.5) is of general interest. The development of simple *in vitro* tests to detect and determine the potency of mutagenic substances has shown that many are consumed, particularly in cooked food (Sugimura & Wakabayashi, 1991). The health significance of these observations is not known. The mutagenic MX in drinking water has presented an opportunity with defined populations and using retrospective exposure to assess the magnitude of the problem.

13.7 Summary

1 Ecotoxicology is concerned with adverse impacts on ecosystems; it may be of direct relevance to humans, to the population balance between species or species diversity.
2 A cause–effect relationship may be relatively easy to establish if the contamination is local and high.

3   When exposure is to a low concentration of complex mixtures for a long time, a cause–effect relationship may be difficult to prove.

4   Contamination may arise from effluent, changes in nutrients which influence the growth of toxic organisms and by water treatments.

5   Although cause–effect relationship may be established for an exposure, the identification of the aetiological agent will require other information, e.g. is the chemical there or has it been there, does it penetrate and/or concentrate in the organism, do experimental studies confirm the aetiology and indicate a plausible mechanism?

14

Reflections, Research and Risk

14.1 Reflections

Intoxication classified by clinical diagnosis, morphological change or change in physiological function is mediated by selective action on specific cells and induced by specific interactions between the intoxicant and components of the cells. The component(s) thus modified are called targets. This is the central theme of mechanisms of toxicity (stage 3 in Figure 2.1). The whole process of induction of toxicity by chemicals involves other chemical-related events which modify the dose of intoxicant reaching the target (stages 1 and 2) and other biology related events (stage 4) which influence the final expression of toxicity (stage 5). The ability of a chemical to intoxicate is determined by the structural relationship between the intoxicant and the target: they must possess a 'lock and key' complementarity which ensures interaction and sometimes the formation of a covalent bond between them.

The description and understanding of living matter has progressed from morphological definition of the shape and form suitable for carrying out physiological functions to the chemical structure of the macromolecules making up this structure. The basic unit is the cell, and this has many different morphological forms which are also composed of different macromolecules. The chemical nature of the cellular structures show that most are not inert materials solely for containment or compartmentation; cells possess areas of chemical specificity such as channels for specific ions, receptors for small and large molecular weight chemical messengers and unique tertiary structures in enzymes which catalyse essential energy-supplying and energy-using functions. The organism is well protected by enzyme systems capable of converting to innocuous materials potentially toxic endogenous by-products and exogenous natural substances to which the organism is exposed via air, food and water. All of these functions, together with the control systems to maintain homeostasis, are brought about by the chemistry of interaction of large and small molecules at particular chemical tertiary structures on or within macromolecules. The whole system works by virtue of a kind of steady state between all the competing chemical interactions. From knowledge of genetic variants in humans it is clear that modification of only one key component can cause either death or ill health or be silent sometimes waiting for an external stimulus to illuminate the defect. Thus the chemical structure of living matter can be modified by mutations or by interaction with chemicals and still be able to carry out its normal functions in a normal manner.

Notwithstanding the above it seems obvious that there must be almost limitless possibilities for the discovery of new chemical structures which can interact with essential chemical structures (targets) within mammals to cause perturbation of homeostasis. These chemicals can arise from those synthesised in the laboratory or from natural compounds synthesised by other organisms. The large scope considered in this book can also be widened to include large molecular weight compounds (say over 1,000) and toxicity to organisms other than mammals. The study of higher molecular weight natural compounds is sometimes called toxinology but the same principles govern those compounds' mechanisms of action as govern chemicals and there is much common ground between pharmacology and toxicology. Both are dependent upon and involved with the advancement of knowledge of the biological sciences. Claude Bernard expressed this very clearly in 1875 (see Preface) but a slightly updated version is:

> the poison becomes an instrument which dissociates and analyses the special properties of different living cells; by establishing their mechanism in causing cell death or changes in cell function we can learn indirectly much about the relation between molecular structure and the physiological process of life. (Aldridge, 1981)

Toxicology is an interdisciplinary subject and uses as well as contributes to developments in these disciplines. New procedures are required to encourage collaboration between basically monodisciplinary departmental structures (see Figure 1.1). Departments for interdisciplinary and chiefly postgraduate subjects such as toxicology, nutrition, engineering, history of science, etc., should have both the same status as the primary undergraduate departments and the responsibility of developing teaching and research geared to cross-fertilisation across the disciplines.

14.2 Research

There is often confusion about what is research in the context of mechanistic studies in toxicology. The essence is that mechanistic studies are designed to establish relationships between different observations and establish cause and effect in developing toxicity. Experimental conditions are continually modified in trying to create conditions which will enable results to be more accurately interpreted, hypotheses confirmed, modified or disproved and new ones proposed. Such an approach contrasts with the acquisition of data through the use of tests with rigid protocols, for example, many testing methods required by the regulatory authorities. However, unexpected findings from such tests may be the starting point of research on the mechanism of a new mode of toxicity or may necessitate a change in current views on other mechanisms. The essence of this research process is that for a well designed and carefully executed experiment an unexpected negative result is as valuable as a positive one.

> Truth is more likely to come out of error, if this is clear and definite, than out of confusion, and my experience teaches me that it is better to hold a well-understood and intelligible opinion, even if it should turn out to be wrong, than be content with a muddle-headed mixture of conflicting views, sometimes called impartiality, and often no better than no opinion at all. (Bayliss, 1920)

The criterion of the scientific basis of theory (mechanism, concept) is its falsifiability or refutability or testability. (Popper, 1974)

It is often implicitly assumed that the flow of information in science is from the basic or pure studies to the practical. In most areas this is not the case. Himsworth (1970) presents a convincing case that, historically, the development of particular areas of science has followed from the need and/or desire to understand some natural phenomenon. The usual analogy for the development of knowledge is the tree of knowledge, the trunk being the general science out from which develop, via the branches, the more specialised sciences. Himsworth considers that this is misleading and develops an analogy which is based on diametrically opposite principles. The model he puts forward is that of a vast globe of primitive ignorance, around which there is a whole series of problems prompting humans to seek understanding. In this model these problems provide the specialised questions in total contrast to the 'tree of knowledge' analogy. A quotation illustrates his extension of his globe concept:

> I have been emboldened to suggest a different concept of structure: that of a vast globe of ignorance from the surface of which at many different places enquiries are being driven centrally to deeper levels where they tend increasingly to coalesce and to produce subjects that come to underline, not one, but several such penetrations. These penetrations I have called provinces of natural knowledge and I conceive of each forming a smooth continuum of inter-related subjects from its specialised periphery to the more unspecialised depths of its pene-tration. It is within the perspective of such provinces that the individual scientific subjects find their intellectual context and larger significance. (Himsworth, 1970)

This concept applies generally across the whole spectrum of science but the relevance of this view to toxicology is obvious. The drive to understand mechanisms, prompted by the specialised requirements of the use of hazardous chemicals leads to the development of information of value for the solution of many problems. Not least, the drive to understand the problems thrown up by the practical questions, throw light on hitherto little understood areas of biological science. In no other science is this more true than in the study of toxicity. An interpretation of this globe concept applied to toxicology is illustrated in Figure 14.1; it explains the meaning of specialised and unspecialised knowledge, its significance following from research penetrating to deeper and more unspecialised information for a wider range of problems and the difference between the hard logic required in problem solving and the gaining of new insights by lateral thinking. Because of the intellectual relationship between subjects within the 'provinces of knowledge' it is possible to devise, on the basis of genuine scientific considerations, a comprehensive research policy for further development. As emphasised above, progress depends on cross-fertilisation and collaboration within many different disciplines.

In research to understand mechanisms of toxicity the ultimate aim is to define the molecular basis of the initiating reactions, but important advances arise from information which is certainly not molecular. For example, a radical change in thinking may be necessitated when it is shown that within a series of chemical homologues two types of clinical sign or syndrome can be distinguished and the homologues divided into two groups. In experimental research designed to test a hypothesis about mechanisms, a firm view of what result is expected from an experiment is vital so that a hypothesis may be confirmed or, more importantly, rejected or modified if expectations are not fulfilled. In practice the areas which often lead to the modification of mechanisms of

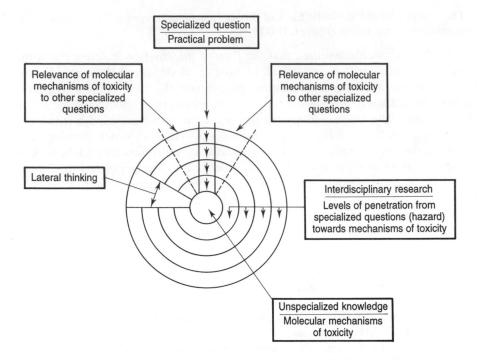

Figure 14.1 Diagrammatic representation of Himsworth's globe applied to toxicological research. This diagram summarizes the route for the progress of interdisciplinary research starting with specialised (often practical) problems and moving towards the basic and unspecialised mechanisms of toxicity

Table 14.1 Current research problems in toxicology. The central aim, if it can be attempted, should be towards identification of the initiating targets, a study of their properties and definition of the biological consequences

OVERALL RESEARCH

1 Immunotoxicity: stimulation and suppression
2 Neurotoxicity: parameters involved in the selective vulnerability to intoxicants of cells in the nervous system
3 Inflammatory reactions
4 Necrosis and apoptosis
5 Selective toxicity: different species and strains
6 Reproductive toxicity: teratology, male and female effects
7 Biomonitoring: susceptibility, dose and effect
8 Chemical carcinogenesis and mutagenesis
9 *In vitro* techniques

RESEARCH OF DIRECT RELEVANCE TO HUMANS

1 Therapeutic procedures
2 Biomonitoring: non-invasive methods in accessible tissue for susceptibility, dose and effects
3 Accident follow-up: accidental and intentional poisoning

concepts are dose–response and structure–activity relationships, comparison of effective doses in *in vitro* and *in vivo* experiments.

Although the framework for the acquisition and organisation of scientific knowledge applies to all research areas with no differences in priority, choices of areas for research must be made. Table 14.1 sets out the author's current view of priority areas for research. The list is by no means comprehensive and is likely to be altered or extended at any time owing to advances in biological science or the discovery of an intoxicant causing unexpected clinical signs or syndrome. The origin of chemicals with interesting biological properties range from unexpected side-effects of drugs (postmarketing surveillance), toxicity testing of new chemical structures in industry (many reports stay locked up in files) to the discovery of new natural toxins (fungi, plants, etc.). The primary academic and practical need is identification of initiating targets and the relation of their modification to the unfolding changes (biochemical, physiological, morphological) affecting biological function and leading to intoxication.

14.3   Risk

The following definitions (Royal Society Study Group, 1992) apply to parts of the process of the translation of information from toxicity testing protocols to an assessment if a chemical poses a risk to exposed populations. The definitions are given in general terms covering human injury or damage to the environment but are restricted to exposure to chemicals.

> *Hazard* is a situation of exposure which could occur and has a potential for human injury or damage to the environment.
> *Risk* is the chance, in quantitative terms, of a defined hazard occurring.
> *Risk assessment* is an integrated analysis of the risks inherent in exposure to a chemical.
> *Risk management* is the process whereby decisions are made to accept a known or assessed risk and/or its implementation.

The process of risk assessment and research leading to fundamentals of toxicology (mechanisms and concepts) exist in a symbiotic relationship to one another. New discoveries of different toxicological responses or of new structures which cause the same response as other intoxicants necessitate research. Practical decisions are more certain when there is a firm base of knowledge about cellular specificity, delivery of the intoxicant to its site of action, exposure and/or dose– and structure–response and structure–activity relationships. Risk assessment and its dependence upon many factors is shown in Figure 14.2. For new chemicals with unexpected toxicity the only information available is from studies using experimental animals. For chemicals which have been in use for a long time reassessments may be required about acceptable exposure risks when new information about human exposure becomes available from measurements of biomarkers for dose and effect. Risk assessment of many chemicals can be definitive when there are fundamental reasons for the existence of a threshold and more tentative when current hypotheses are that there may be no threshold and an acceptable risk (say 1 in 10^6) has to be quantified. Most of the processes relevant to the estimation of acceptable risk have been considered in previous chapters.

At the risk management stage the decisions are implemented using the best science that can be brought to bear on the process. At this stage many other factors have to be considered in the broad area of risk and benefit. Included is the economic risk: a

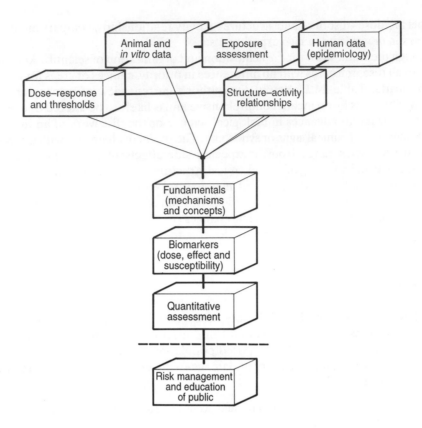

Figure 14.2 Steps in the assessment of risk of exposure to chemicals

comparison of the cost of implementation of the precautions with the benefit of the product. One of the difficult and unpredictable areas is public perception of the risk. It is not too long ago that a product was manufactured or a material was mined if an industrial need was perceived. The precautions undertaken depended on the degree of sophistication of the country with little control exercised by central government. Problems arose, e.g. asbestosis, pneumoconiosis, lead poisoning, etc., and then action was taken to improve the working conditions. Now society demands, before a product is on the market, that information is available to ensure that the product is safe. Safety is the freedom of unacceptable risk of personal harm and as such is ill defined – there is no such thing as absolute safety (see Jukes, 1983). The public's perception of what is acceptable differs with the uses of the particular chemical. When the chemical is for the treatment of disease then a reasonable risk–benefit judgement can be made by patients. Even so, when an unexpected and unpredictable form of toxicity appears in a few out of many patients after long administration of the drug, the patients' response, taken up by the organs of modern publicity, is often extreme. When exposure is involuntary, such as chemicals in drinking water then many campaign for zero exposure – consider the years of protest about the addition of fluoride to drinking water to prevent dental caries. Attitudes to exposure at work are, in general, intermediate between these two extremes, and naturally attitudes vary in countries at different stages of their development.

Experience with the use of DDT has taught us many lessons. Even though DDT was synthesised in 1874 it was 1939 before its insecticidal properties were known and realised by direct dusting of humans for the control of lice and other insects during the Second World War. It seemed to be a 'miracle' pesticide: very active and very stable with no undesirable effects in humans. At this time regulatory testing of pesticides was not necessary. Such desirable properties encouraged its overuse and unregulated disposal of excess spraying dispersions. Excessive use, however, did lead to environmental problems which were publicised in *Silent Spring* by Rachel Carson (1962) and, as a result, even the safety of its regulated use was questioned. Gradually four problems came into focus:

1 The desirable stability became a defect because its intense lipophilic nature meant that it was taken up by organisms and moved up the food chains. It became clear with the availability of sensitive analytical methods that DDT sprayed in one place moved to others far away; this movement was initially overemphasised because the earliest analyses were not specific and did not distinguish between DDT and other chlorinated compounds such as the polychlorinated biphenyls (see section 13.2).

2 Effects on wildlife were due both to excessive use and the above movement up the food chains.

3 Development of resistance in insects became serious and more insecticide was needed for the necessary insect kill.

4 In experimental studies tumours were induced in rodent liver.

Problems 1 and 2 could perhaps be attributed to overuse especially in agriculture, but DDT was proving to be very effective in the control of vectors responsible for the infection of humans with various diseases and especially malaria. Although the use of DDT was banned in the USA after the chemical was shown to induce tumours in rodents, elsewhere there was some scepticism about the relevance to human health of carcinogenesis seen only in rodents. DDT, like phenobarbitone, causes liver enlargement and both cause tumours in rat liver. There was no evidence that DDT was carcinogenic to humans after its intensive use in many countries as a pesticide or after occupational exposure during its manufacture (Hayes, 1982); also there was no evidence that the use of phenobarbitone as an anticonvulsant for the treatment of epilepsy caused an increase in the incidence of liver or other cancer (Clemmesen *et al.*, 1974). Since resistance could be contained, the World Health Organization has always taken the view that in certain circumstances the use of DDT should be allowed in public health programmes. Even so the prohibition of its use in the USA persuaded some tropical countries to stop using it; the result was a resurgence of malaria resulting in many deaths.

Other classes of insecticide have been developed, e.g. organophosphorus compounds, carbamates and pyrethroids. These are all more expensive, less stable and more likely to cause problems in their application. The use of organophosphorus compounds and carbamates requires supervision to avoid serious toxicity. Pyrethroids are very active insecticides and are used at high dilution; in use, the only problem is a short-lasting but unpleasant local paresthesia following contamination of the skin. WHO now approves the use of DDT only for in-house spraying of walls to protect the occupants against mosquitoes during the night.

Two recent epidemiological studies have claimed links between previous exposure to DDT and human cancer. Twenty-eight cases of pancreatic cancer in employees of a company over the period 1948–88 (Garabant *et al.*, 1992, 1993; Malats *et al.*, 1993) were claimed to be associated with exposure to DDT even though not only DDT but also related compounds and many other chemicals had been manufactured. The probability (odds ratio) of such an association being causal are reduced because the definition of exposure is necessarily vague and exposure will have been to many chemicals. An association between exposure to DDT and breast cancer in 58 American women has been deduced on the basis of an increase in the concentration of DDE in blood taken six months before the positive diagnosis compared with 171 controls (Wolff *et al.*, 1993). Before acceptance of this as a causal relationship more studies are required to establish the significance of the small differences between case and controls (11.0 ± 9.1 and 7.7 ± 6.8, a difference of 42%) and to develop a sound dose–response curve. The study must also be judged against the increasing incidence of breast cancer in the Western world irrespective of the introduction or banning of the use of DDT.

The case in favour of the localised use of DDT includes efficacy, low cost, local persistence, evidence of slow degradation in soil, on hut walls and little movement from the locality. The weight given in developed and developing countries to the various factors will obviously vary. Opinions vary about the interpretation of positive carcinogenicity tests in rodents for prediction of hazard and/or risk to humans. It may seem reasonable for Western countries to insist that pesticides used should not persist in the environment or be present in harvested food and this attitude is now accepted by all pesticide manufacturers. However, developing countries struggling to contain huge problems in the proportion of their health budgets spent on treating vector transmitted diseases, are willing to take perhaps a little more risk to attain considerably more benefit.

Balancing of different risks seems almost impossible, e.g. compare the risk of the use of pesticides and the use of the motor car in the UK. For a general discussion of these issues see British Medical Association (1987) and the Royal Society (1992). Safety, when considered by regulatory bodies, is one of predicted low incidence; however an ill person (or the relatives) who perceive that the illness arose from exposure to a particular chemical is unlikely to be convinced by a statistical argument about incidence. Public interest in possible health effects of chemicals (but only for man-made chemicals, rarely for natural intoxicants) has become more intense as longevity increases. The example of DDT shows that opinions about acceptable risk may be radically different when lifespans are much lower and changes to other, more expensive insecticides may overwhelm health budgets mainly devoted to malaria. Gaps in perception between manufacturers, governments and the public will probably never be bridged; gradual improvement in the public's perception of the likelihood of harm from exposure to low concentrations of chemicals may come about by education to increase the proportion of the population who can appreciate the general principles of biology and toxicology with special emphasis on dose–response. All that can be done is to do the best we can to promote more understanding of mechanisms and concepts, leading to better and cheaper testing procedures while avoiding chasing the illusory panacea of absolute safety.

> Men can only be safe when they do not assume that the object of life is safety.
>
> With apologies to George Orwell (1944)

14.4 Summary

1 Advancing knowledge of the chemical structures in organisms essential for an ordered life indicate that there must be almost limitless possibilities for chemicals to perturb biological systems.

2　The study of the way in which chemicals perturb physiological systems advances both toxicology and physiology.

3　Collaboration of many disciplines in research on mechanisms of toxicity is essential. As molecular biology advances a chemical/biochemical approach becomes generally feasible and rewarding.

4　Research in toxicology aims to establish relationships between different observations and to establish the mechanisms involved in cause and effect in developing toxicity.

5　Testing for toxicity (and therefore safety) aims to acquire data through the use of testing procedures with rigid protocols; continual interplay between research and testing is essential.

6　As knowledge of mechanisms of toxicity advance towards molecular explanations, hypotheses generated become increasingly relevant to other problems.

7　Hazard, risk, risk assessment and risk management are sequential stages in decision-taking about the safety and sometimes the consequences and acceptable risks of exposure of populations to chemicals.

References

ADAMSON, I.Y.R., BOWDEN, D.H., CÔTÉ, M.G. & WITSCHI, H.P. (1977) Lung injury induced by butylated hydroxytoluene: cytodynamic and biochemical studies in mice. *Laboratory Investigations*, 36, 26–32.

AHLSTEDT, S., EKSTROM, B., SVARD, P.O. *et al.* (1980) New aspects on antigens in penicillin allergy. *CRC Critical Reviews in Toxicology*, 7, 219–277.

ALAJOUANINE, T., DEROBERT, L. & THIEFFRY, S. (1958) Etude clinique d'ensemble de 210 cas d'intoxication par les sels organiques d'etain. *Revues neurologique*, 98, 85–96.

ALBERT, A. (1985) *Selective Toxicity: The Physicochemical Basis of Therapy*. Chapman and Hall, London.

ALDERSON, M. (1983) *An Introduction to Epidemiology*. Macmillan, Basingstoke.

ALDRIDGE, W.N. (1953) The inhibition of erythrocyte cholinesterase by triesters of phosphoric acid: 3. The nature of the inhibitory process. *Biochemical Journal*, 54, 442–448.

(1954) Tricresyl phosphates and cholinesterase. *Biochemical Journal*, 56, 185–189.

(1976a) Chronic toxicity as an acute phenomena. In *The Prediction of Chronic Toxicity from Short-term Studies* (eds W.A.M. Duncan, B.J. Leonard & B. Brunaud). Proceedings of the European Society of Toxicology, Vol. 17, pp. 5–6. Excerpta Medica, Amsterdam.

(1976b) The influence of organotin compounds on mitochondrial functions. *Advances in Chemistry Series*, 157, 186–196.

(1980) Acetyl cholinesterase and other esterase inhibitors. In *Enzyme Inhibitors as Drugs* (ed. M. Sandler), pp. 115–125. Macmillan, Basingstoke.

(1981) Mechanisms of toxicity: new concepts are required in toxicology. *Trends in Pharmacology*, 2, 228–231.

(1986) The biological basis and measurement of thresholds. *Annual Reviews in Pharmacology and Toxicology*, 26, 39–58.

(1987) Toxic disasters with food contaminants. In *Attitudes to Toxicology in the European Economic Community* (ed. P.L. Chambers), pp. 57–71. Wiley, Chichester.

(1989a) Cholinesterase and esterase inhibitors and reactivators of organophosphorus inhibited esterases. In *Design of Enzyme Inhibitors as Drugs* (eds M. Sandler & H.J. Smith), pp. 294–313. Oxford University Press, Oxford.

(1989b) The advisory subgroup in toxicology of the European Medical Research Councils. *Archives of Toxicology*, 63, 253–256.

(1990) An assessment of the toxicological properties of pyrethroids and their neurotoxicity. *CRC Critical Reviews in Toxicology*, 21, 89–104.

218

(1992a) Chemistry in relation to toxicity and to risks, of exposure to organotin compounds. In *Chemistry and Technology of Silicon and Tin* (eds V.G. Kumar Das, N.G. Seik Weng & M. Geilen), pp. 78–92. Oxford University Press, Oxford.

(1992b) Selective neurotoxicity: problems in establishing the relevance of *in vitro* data to the *in vivo* situation. In *Tissue-specific Toxicity: Biochemical Mechanisms* (eds W. Dekant & H.G. Neumann), pp. 15–31. Academic Press, London.

(1992c) The toxic oil syndrome (TOS, 1981): from the disease towards a toxicological understanding of its chemical aetiology and mechanism. *Toxicology Letters*, 64/65, 59–70.

(1993) Postscript to the symposium on organophosphorus compound induced delayed neuropathy. *Chemico-Biological Interactions*, 87, 463–466.

(1995a) Aspects of selectivity and mechanisms in neurotoxicity. In *Molecular Mechanisms of Toxicity*, (eds F. DeMatteis and L.L. Smith), pp. 3–17. CRC Press, Boca Raton, Florida.

(1995b) Defining thresholds in occupational and environmental toxicology. *Toxicology Letters*, 77, 109–118.

ALDRIDGE, W.N. & BARNES, J.M. (1961) Neurotoxic and biochemical properties of some triaryl phosphates. *Biochemical Pharmacology*, 6, 177–188.

ALDRIDGE, W.N. & BROWN, A.W. (1988) The biological properties of methyl and ethyl derivatives of tin and lead. In *The Biological Alkylation of Heavy Metals* (eds P.J. Craig & F. Glockling), pp. 147–163. Special Publication No. 66, Royal Society of Chemistry, London.

ALDRIDGE, W.N. & CONNORS, T.A. (1985) Chemical accidents and toxicology. *Human Toxicology*, 4, 477–479.

ALDRIDGE, W.N. & LOVATT EVANS, C. (1946) The physiological effects and fate of cyanogen chloride. *Quarterly Journal of Experimental Physiology*, 33, 241–266.

ALDRIDGE, W.N. & REINER, E. (1972). *Enzyme Inhibitors as Substrates: Interaction of Esterases with Esters of Organophosphorus and Carbamic Acids*. North-Holland, Amsterdam.

ALDRIDGE, W.N. & STREET, B.W. (1970) Oxidative phosphorylation: the specific binding of trimethyltin and triethyltin to rat liver mitochondria. *Biochemical Journal*, 118, 171–179.

ALDRIDGE, W.N., MILES, J.W., MOUNT, D.L. & VERSCHOYLE, R.D. (1979) The toxicological properties of impurities in malathion. *Archives of Toxicology*, 42, 95–106.

ALDRIDGE, W.N., DINSDALE, D., NEMERY, B. & VERSCHOYLE, R.D. (1987) Toxicology of impurities in malathion: potentiation of malathion toxicity and lung toxicity caused by trialkyl phosphorothioates. In *Selectivity and Molecular Mechanisms of Toxicity* (eds F. De Matteis & E.A. Lock), pp. 265–294. Macmillan, Basingstoke.

ALDRIDGE, W.N., STREET, B.W. & SKILLETER, D.N. (1977) Halide-dependent and halide-independent effects of triorganotin and triorganolead compounds on mitochondrial functions. *Biochemical Journal*, 168, 353–364.

ALDRIDGE, W.N., STREET, B.W. & NOLTES, J.G. (1981) The action of 5-coordinate triorganotin compounds on rat liver mitochondria. *Chemico-Biological Interactions*, 34, 223–232.

AMES, B.N., DURSTAN, W.E., YAMASAKI, E. & LEE, F.D. (1975a) Carcinogens are mutagens: a simple test system combining liver homogenates for activation and bacteria for detection. *Proceedings of the National Academy of Sciences*, 70, 2281–2285.

AMES, B.N., McCANN, J. & YAMASAKI, E. (1975b) Methods for detecting carcinogens and mutagens with the Salmonella/mammalian-microsome mutagenicity test. *Mutation Research*, 31, 347–364.

AMOS, H.E., BRIGDEN, W.D. & McKERRON, R.A. (1975) Untoward effects associated with practolol: demonstration of antibody binding to epithelial tissue. *British Medical Journal*, 1, 598–600.

ANDERS, M.W. ed. (1985) *Bioactivation of Foreign Compounds*. Academic Press, Orlando.

ANDERSEN, M.E., CLEWELL, H.J. III, GARGAS, M.L., SMITH, F.A. & REITZ, R.H. (1987) Physiologically based pharmacokinetics and the risk assessment process for methylene chloride. *Toxicology and Applied Pharmacology*, 87, 185–205.

ANDERSON, D., ed. (1990) Male-mediated F_1 abnormalities. *Mutation Research*, 103–247.

ANDERSON, D.M. (1994) Red tides. *Scientific American*, 271, 52–58.

APOSHIAN, H.V. & APOSHIAN, M.M. (1990) Meso-2,3-dimercaptosuccinic acid: chemical, pharmacological and toxicological properties of an orally effective metal chelating agent. *Annual Reviews of Pharmacology and Toxicology*, 30, 279–306.

ASHBY, J. & PATON, D. (1993) The influence of chemical structure on the extent and sites of carcinogenesis for 522 rodent carcinogens and 55 different human carcinogen exposures. *Mutation Research*, 3–74.

ASHBY, J. *et al.* (1994) Mechanistically-based human hazard assessment of peroxisome proliferator-induced hepatocarcinogenesis. *Human and Experimental Toxicology*, 13 (suppl.), S1–S117.

AXELSON, O., ANDERSSON, K., HUYSTEDT, C., *et al.* (1978) A cohort study on trichlorethylene exposure and cancer mortality. *Journal of Occupational Medicine*, 20, 194–196.

BACKLUND, P., KROMBERG, L., PENSAR, G. & TIKKANEN, L. (1985) Mutagenic activity in humic water and alum flocculated humic water treated with alternative disinfectants. *The Science of the Total Environment*, 47, 257–264.

BAER, R.L., RAMSEY, D.L. & BONDI, E. (1973) The most common contact allergens. *Archives of Dermatology*, 108, 74–78.

BAILEY, E., FARMER, P.B., BIRD, I., LAMB, J.H. & PEAL, J.A. (1986) Monitoring exposure to acrylamide by the determination of S-(2-carboxyethyl) cysteine in hydrolysed haemoglobin by gas chromatography–mass spectrometry. *Analytical Biochemistry*, 157, 241–248.

BAKER, E.L., ZACK, M., MILES, J.W., *et al.* (1978) Epidemic malathion poisoning in Pakistan malaria workers, *Lancet*, 1, 31–33.

BAKIR, F., DAMLIJI, S.F., AMIN-ZAKI, L., *et al.* (1973) Methylmercury poisoning in Iraq. *Science*, 181, 230–241.

BALDWIN, R.C., PASI, A., MACGREGOR, J.C. & HINE, G.H. (1975) The rates of radical formation from dipyridilium herbicides, paraquat, diquat and morphamquat in homogenates of lung, kidney and liver: an inhibitory effect of carbon monoxide. *Toxicology and Applied Pharmacology*, 32, 298–304.

BALLANTYNE, B. & MARRS, T.C., eds (1992) *Clinical and Experimental Toxicology of Organophosphates and Carbamates*, pp. 1–641. Butterworth/Heinemann, Oxford.

BARNES, J.M. (1970) Observations on the effects on rats of compounds related to acrylamide. *British Journal of Industrial Medicine*, 27, 147–149.

BARNES, J.M. & DENZ, F.A. (1953) Experimental demyelination with organophosphorus compounds. *Journal of Pathology and Bacteriology*, 65, 597–605.

BARTSCH, H., CASTEGNARO, M., ROJAS, M., *et al.* (1992) Expression of pulmonary p4501A1 and carcinogen DNA adduct formation in high risk subjects for tobacco-related lung cancer. *Toxicology Letters*, 64/65, 477–483.

BAYLISS, W.M. (1920) *Principles of General Physiology (Preface)*. Longman, Green & Co., London.

BEAUMONT, J.J. & BRESLOW, N.E. (1981) Power considerations in epidemic studies of vinyl chloride workers. *American Journal of Epidemiology*, 114, 725–734.

BELAND, F.A. & POIRIER, F.C. (1993) Significance of DNA adduct studies in animal models for cancer molecular dosimetry and risk assessment. *Environmental Health Perspectives*, 99, 5–10.

BERENBLUM, I. (1974) *Carcinogenesis as a Biological Problem*. pp. 1–376. North-Holland, Amsterdam.

BERGMARK, E., CALLEMAN, C.J. & COSTA, L.G. (1991) Formation of haemoglobin adducts of acrylamide and its epoxide metabolite glycidamide in the rat. *Toxicology and Applied Pharmacology*, 111, 352–363.

BERGMARK, E., CALLEMAN, C.J., HE, F. & COSTA, L.G. (1993) Determination of haemoglobin adducts in humans occupationally exposed to acrylamide. *Toxicology and Applied Pharmacology*, 120, 45–54.

BERNARD, C. (1875) *La Science Experimentale*. Baillière, Paris.

BERNARD, A. & LAUWERYS, R. (1981) Retinol-binding protein in urine: a more practical index than urinary β_2-microglobulin for the screening of renal tubular function. *Clinical Chemistry*, 27, 1781–1782.

BERNARD, A., BUCHET, J.P., ROELS, H. *et al.* (1979) Renal excretion of proteins and enzymes in workers exposed to cadmium. *European Journal of Clinical Investigation*, 9, 11–22.

BERNARD, A., ROELS, H., BUCHET, J.P. & LAUWERYS, R. (1992) Decrease in serum Clara cell protein in smokers. *Lancet*, 339(1), 1620.

BERNDT, W.O. & MEHENDALE, H.M. (1979) Effects of hexachlorobutadiene (HCBD) on renal function and renal organic ion transport in the rat. *Toxicology*, 14, 55–65.

BIBBO, M., GILL, W., AZIZI, F., *et al.* (1977) Follow-up study of male and female offspring of DES-exposed mothers. *Obstetrics and Gynaecology*, 49, 1–8.

BIDSTRUP, P.L., BONNELL, J.A. & BECKETT, A.G. (1953) Paralysis following poisoning by a new organophosphorus insecticide. *British Medical Journal*, 1, 1068–1072.

BIGGAR, J.W., DUTT, G.R. & RIGGS, R.L. (1967). Predicting and measuring the solubility of p,p'DDT in water. *Bulletin of Environmental and Contaminant Toxicology*, 2, 90–100.

BISCHOFF, K.B. & BROWN, R.H. (1966) Drug distribution in mammals. *Chemical Engineering Progress Symposium Series*, 62, 33–45.

BISHOP, J.M. (1991) Molecular themes in oncogenesis. *Cell*, 64, 235–248.

BLACK, R.M. & UPSHALL, D.G. (1988) Assessing the danger. *Chemistry in Britain* (special issue), *Chemical Defence*, 659–662.

BLACKBURN, D.M., GRAY, A.J., LLOYD, S.C., SHEARD, C.M. & FOSTER, P.D.M. (1988) A comparison of the effects of the three isomers of dinitrobenzene on the testis of the rat. *Toxicology and Applied Pharmacology*, 92, 54–64.

BOEKELHEIDE, K. (1987) 2,5-Hexanedione alters microtubule assembly. 1: Testicular atrophy, not nervous system toxicity, correlates with enhanced tubulin polymerisation. *Toxicology and Applied Pharmacology*, 88, 370–382.

(1988) Rat testis during 2,5-hexanedione intoxication and recovery. 1: Dose–response and the reversibility of germ cell loss. *Toxicology and Applied Pharmacology*, 92, 18–27.

BOEKELHEIDE, K. & EVELETH, J. (1988) The rate of 2,5-hexanedione intoxication, not total dose, determines the extent of testicular injury and altered microtubule assembly in the rat. *Toxicology and Applied Pharmacology*, 94, 76–83.

BOTES, D.P., TUINMAN, A.A., WESSELS, P.L., *et al.* (1984) The structure of cyanoginosin-LA, a cyclic heptapeptide from the cyanobacterium *Microcystis aeruginosa*. *Journal of the Chemical Society, Perkins Transactions*, 1, 2311–2318.

BOULDIN, T.W. and CAVANAGH, J.B. (1979a) Organophosphorus neuropathy. 1: A teased fiber study of the spatio-temporal shred of axonal degeneration. *American Journal of Pathology*, 94, 241–252.

(1979b) Organophosphorus neuropathy. 2: A fine structural study of the early stages of axonal degeneration. *American Journal of Pathology*, 94, 253–270.

BOULDIN, B.W., GOINES, N.D., BAGNELL, C.R. & KRIGMAN, M.R. (1981) Pathogenesis of trimethyltin neuronal toxicity: ultrastructural and cytochemical observations. *American Journal of Pathology*, 104, 237–249.

BOUMA, J.M.W. & SMIT, M.J. (1989) Gadolinium chloride selectively blocks endocytosis by Kupffer cells. In *Cells of the Hepatic Sinusoid* (eds E. Wisse, D.L. Knook and K. Decker), pp. 132–133. Kupffer Cell Foundation, Rijswijk, The Netherlands.

BREMNER, I. (1979) Mammalian absorption, transport and excretion of cadmium. In *The Chemistry, Biochemistry and Biology of Cadmium* (ed. M. Webb), pp. 175–193. Elsevier/North-Holland, Amsterdam.

BRENNER, B.B. & RECTOR, F.C. Jr, eds (1976) *The Kidney*. Vols 1 and 2, (3rd edn). W.B. Saunders, Philadelphia.

BRIDGES, J.W., DAVIES, D.S. & WILLIAMS, R.T. (1967) The fate of ethyltin and diethyltin derivatives in the rat. *Biochemical Journal*, 105, 1261–1267.

BRITISH MEDICAL ASSOCIATION (1987) *Living with Risk*. Wiley, Chichester.

BRODIE, M.E. & ALDRIDGE, W.N. (1982) Elevated cerebellar cyclic GMP levels during the deltamethrin-induced syndrome. *Neurobehavioural Toxicology and Teratology*, 4, 109–111.

BRODIE, M.E., OPACKA-JUFFRY, J., PETERSEN, D.W. & BROWN, A.W. (1990) Neurochemical changes in hippocampal and caudate dialysates associated with early trimethyltin neuro-toxicity in rats. *Neurotoxicology*, 11, 35–46.

BROUWER, A. (1991) Role of biotransformation in PCB-induced alterations in vitamin A and thyroid hormone metabolism in laboratory and wildlife species. *Biochemical Society Transactions*, 19, 731–737.

BROUWER, A., BLANER, W.S., KUKLER, A. & VAN DEN BERG, K.J. (1988) Study on the mechanism of interference of 3,4,3',4'-tetrachlorobiphenyl with the plasma retinol-binding proteins in rodents. *Chemico-Biological Interactions*, 68, 203–217.

BROUWER, A., REIJNDERS, P.J.H. & KOEMAN, J.H. (1989) Polychlorinated biphenyl (PCB)-contaminated fish induces vitamin A and thyroid hormone deficiency in the common seal (*Phoca vitulina*). *Aquatic Toxicology*, 15, 99–106.

BROUWER, A., KLASSEN-WEHLER, E., BOKDAM, M., MORSE, D.C. & TRAAG, W.A. (1990) Competitive inhibition of thyroxine binding to transthyretin by monohydroxy metabolites of 3,4,3',4'-tetrachlorobiphenyl. *Chemosphere*, 20, 1257–1262.

BROWN, A.W., ALDRIDGE, W.N. & VERSCHOYLE, R.D. (1979) The behavioural and neuropathologic sequelae of intoxication by trimethyltin compounds in the rat. *American Journal of Pathology*, 97, 59–81.

BROWN, A.W., CAVANAGH, J.B., VERSCHOYLE, R.D., et al. (1984) Evolution of the intracellular changes in neurons caused by trimethyltin. *Neuropathology and Applied Neurobiology*, 10, 267–283.

BRUGGEMAN, I.M., TEMMINK, J.H.M. & VAN BLADEREN, P.J. (1986) Glutathione and cysteine mediated cytotoxicity of allyl and benzyl isothiocyanate. *Toxicology and Applied Pharmacology*, 83, 349–359.

BUCHET, J.P., LAUWERYS, R., ROELS, H., et al. (1990) Renal effects of cadmium body burden of the general population. *Lancet*, 336, 699–702.

BUMPUS, J.A., TIEN, M., WRIGHT, D. & AUST, D. (1985) Oxidation of persistent environmental pollutants by white rot fungus. *Science*, 228, 1434–1436.

BUS, J.S., CAGEN, S.Z., OLGAARD, M. & GIBSON, J.E. (1976) A mechanism of paraquat toxicity in mice and rats. *Toxicology and Applied Pharmacology*, 35, 501–513.

CAPORASO, N.E., TUCKER, M.A., HOOVER, R.N., et al. (1990) Lung cancer and the debrisoquine metabolic phenotype. *Journal of the National Cancer Institute*, 82, 1264–1272.

CARAFOLI, E. (1987) Intracellular Ca^{2+} homeostasis. *Annual Reviews of Biochemistry*, 56, 395–433.

CAROLDI, S., LOTTI, M. & MASUTTI, A. (1984) Intraarterial injection of diisopropylfluorophosphate or phenylmethanesulphonyl fluoride produces unilateral neuropathy or protection, respectively, in hens. *Biochemical Pharmacology*, 33, 3213–3217.

CARMICHAEL, W.W. (1992) Cyanobacteria secondary metabolites – the cyanotoxins. *Journal of Applied Bacteriology*, 72, 445–459.

CARMICHAEL, W.W., JONES, C.L.A., MAHMOOD, N.A. & THEISS, W.C. (1985) Algal toxins and water based diseases. *Critical Reviews in Environmental Control*, 15, 275–313.

CARSON, R. (1962) *Silent Spring*. Houghton Mifflin, Boston.

CASIDA, J.E., KIMMEL, E.C., HOLM, B. & WIDMARK, G. (1971) Oxidative dealkylation of tetra, tri and di-alkyltins and tetra and trialkyllead by liver microsomes. *Acta Chemical Scandinavica*, 25, 1497–1499.

CAVANAGH, J.B. (1964) The significance of the 'dying-back' process in experimental and human neurological disease. *International Reviews and Experimental Pathology*, 3, 219–267.

(1973) Peripheral neuropathy caused by toxic agents. *CRC Critical Reviews in Toxicology*, 2, 365–417.

(1982a) Mechanisms of axon degeneration in three toxic 'neuropathies': organophosphorus, acrylamide and hexacarbon compared. *Recent Advances in Neuropathology*, 2, 213–242.

(1982b) The pathokinetics of acrylamide intoxication: a reassessment of the problem. *Neuropathology and Applied Neurobiology*, 8, 315–336.

CHANG, L.W., TIEMEYER, T.M., WENGER, G.R., MCMILLAN, D.E. & REULL, K.R. (1982)

Neuropathology of trimethyltin intoxication. II: Electron microscopic study on the hippocampus. *Environmental Research*, 29, 445–458.

CHANG, L.W., TIERMEYER, T.M., WENGER, G.R. & MCMILLAN, D.E. (1983) Neuropathology of trimethyltin intoxication. III: Changes in brainstem neurones. *Environmental Research*, 30, 399–411.

CHAPIN, R.E., DUTTON, S.L., ROSS, M.D., SUMRELL, B.M. & LAMB, J.C. (1984) The effects of ethylene glycol monomethylether on testicular histology in F344 rats. *Journal of Andrology*, 5, 369–380.

CHAPIN, R.E., DUTTON, S.L., ROSS, M.D. & LAMB, J.C. (1985) Effects of ethylene glycol monomethyl ether (EGME) on mating performance and epididymal sperm parameters in F344 rats. *Fundamental and Applied Toxicology*, 5, 182–189.

CHENG, K.K. (1956) Experimental studies on the mechanism of zonal distribution of beryllium liver necrosis. *Journal of Pathology and Bacteriology*, 71, 265–276.

CHOLERTON, S., DALY, A.K. & IDLE, J.R. (1992) The role of individual human cytochromes P-450 in drug metabolism and clinical response. *Trends in Pharmacological Sciences*, 13, 434–439.

CHRISTIAN, M.S., ed. (1985) Cancer and the environment: possible mechanisms for thresholds for carcinogens and other toxic substances. *Journal of the American College of Toxicology*, 2, 1–321.

CHU, F.S. (1974). Studies on ochratoxins. *Critical Reviews in Toxicology*, 2, 499–524.

CHYTIL, F. & ONG, D.E. (1978) Cellular vitamin A binding proteins. *Vitamin and Hormones*, 36, 1–32.

CICERO, T.J., COWAN, W., MOORE, B.W. & SUNTZEFF, V. (1970) The cellular localisation of the two brain specific proteins, S-100 and 14-3-2. *Brain Research*, 18, 25–31.

CLARK, D.G., MCELLIGOTT, T.F. & HURST, E.W. (1966) The toxicity of paraquat. *British Journal of Industrial Medicine*, 23, 126–132.

CLARKE, D.O., ELSWICK, B.A., WELSCH, F. & CONOLLY, R.B. (1993) Pharmacokinetics of 2-methoxyethanol and 2-methoxyacetic acid in the pregnant mouse: a physiologically based mathematical model. *Toxicology and Applied Pharmacology*, 121, 239–252.

CLARKSON, T.W., AMIN-ZAKI, L. & AL-TIKRITI, S.K. (1976) An outbreak of methylmercury poisoning due to consumption of contaminated grain. *Federated Proceedings*, 35, 2395–2399.

CLARKSON, T.W., MAGOS, L., COX, C., *et al.* (1981) Tests of efficacy of antidotes for removal of methylmercury in human poisoning during the Iraq outbreak. *Journal of Pharmacology and Experimental Therapeutics*, 218, 74–83.

CLEMMESEN, J., FUGLSANG-FREDERIKSEN, V. & PLUM, C.M. (1974) Phenobarbitone, liver tumours and thorotrast, *Lancet*, 1, 37–38.

CLEWELL, H.J., III & ANDERSEN, M.E. (1989) Improving toxicity testing protocols using computer simulation. *Toxicology Letters*, 49, 139–158.

CODD, G.A. (1984) Toxins of freshwater cyanobacteria. *Microbiological Science*, 1, 48–52.

COHEN, A.J. & GRASSO, P. (1981) Review of the hepatic response to hypolipidaemic drugs in rodents and assessment of its toxicological significance to man. *Food and Cosmetic Toxicology*, 19, 585–605.

COHEN, G.M., MACFARLANE, M., FEARNHEAD, H.O., SUN, X.M. & DINSDALE, D. (1995) Mechanisms of cell death, with particular reference to apoptosis, In *Molecular Mechanisms of Toxicity* (eds F. DeMatteis & L.L. Smith), pp. 185–205. CRC Press, Boca Raton, Florida, USA.

COHEN, J.J. & DUKE, R.C. (1984) Glucocorticoid activation of a calcium dependent endonuclease in thymocyte nuclei leads to cell death. *Journal of Immunology*, 132, 38–42.

COHEN, S.M. & ELLWEIN, L.B. (1991) Genetic errors, cell proliferation and carcinogenesis. *Cancer Research*, 51, 6493–6505.

COLLINS, M.K.L. & RIVAS, A.L. (1993) The control of apoptosis in mammalian cells. *Trends in Biochemical Sciences*, 18, 307–309.

COLLINS, R.C., KIRKPATRICK, J.B. & MCDOUGAL, D.B. (1970) Some regional and metabolic consequences in mouse brain of pyrithiamine-induced thiamine deficiency. *Journal of Neuropathology and Experimental Neurology*, 29, 57–69.

CONNING, D.M., FLETCHER, K. & SWAN, A.A.B. (1969) Paraquat and related bipyridyls. *British Medical Bulletin*, 25, 245–249.

CONOLLY, R.B. & ANDERSEN, M.E. (1991) Biologically based pharmacodynamic models: tools for toxicological research and risk assessment. *Annual Reviews of Pharmacology and Toxicology*, 31, 503–523.

COOK, W.O., DELLINGER, J.A., SINGH, S.S., *et al.* (1989) Regional brain cholinesterase activity in rats injected intraperitoneally with anatoxin-a(S) or paraoxon. *Toxicology Letters*, 49, 29–34.

COOPER, A.J.L. & ANDERS, M.W. (1990) Glutamine transaminase K and cysteine conjugate β-lyase. *Annals of the New York Academy of Sciences*, 585, 118–127.

CORCORAN, G.B., FIX, L., JONES, D.P., *et al.*, (1994) Apoptosis: molecular control point in toxicity. *Toxicology and Applied Pharmacology*, 128, 169–181.

COURI, D. & MILKS, M. (1982) Toxicity and metabolism of the neurotoxic hexacarbons *n*-hexane, 2-hexanone and 2, 5-hexanedione. *Annual Review of Pharmacology and Toxicology*, 22, 145–166.

CRAIG, P.J. & GLOCKLING, F., eds (1988) *The Biological Alkylation of Heavy Metals*, pp. 1–298. Special Publication No. 66, Royal Society of Chemistry, London.

CREASEY, D.M. & FOSTER, P.M.D. (1984) The morphological development of glycol ether-induced testicular atrophy in the rat. *Fundamental and Molecular Pathology*, 40, 169–176.

CREECH, J.L. & JOHNSON, M.N. (1974) Angiosarcoma of the liver in the manufacture of PVC. *Journal of Occupational Medicine*, 16, 150–151.

CREMER, J.E. (1958) The biochemistry of organotin compounds: the conversion of tetraethyltin into triethyltin. *Biochemical Journal*, 68, 685–692.

(1959) Biochemical studies on the toxicity of tetraethyllead and other organolead compounds. *British Journal of Industrial Medicine*, 16, 191–199.

CREMER, J.E. & CALLAWAY, S. (1961) Furthur studies on the toxicity of some tetra- and tri-alkyllead compounds. *British Journal of Industrial Medicine*, 18, 277–282.

CREMER, J.E., CUNNINGHAM, V.J., RAY, D.E. & GURCHURAN, S. (1980) Regional changes in brain glucose utilisation in rats given a pyrethroid insecticide. *Brain Research*, 194, 278–282.

CRUICKSHANK, J.M. & PRICHARD, T. (1988) *Beta-blockers in Clinical Practice*. Churchill Livingstone, Edinburgh.

CRUMP, K.S., HOEL, D.G., LANGLEY, C.H. & PETO, R. (1976) Fundamental carcinogenic processes and their implications for low-dose risk assessment. *Cancer Research*, 36, 2973–2979.

CUNNINGHAM, V.J. & CREMER, J.E. (1985) Current assumptions behind the use of PET for measuring glucose utilisation in brain. *Trends in Neurosciences*, 8, 96–99.

DAHL, A.R. & HADLEY, W.H. (1991) Nasal cavity enzymes involved in xenobiotic metabolism: effects on the toxicity on inhalants. *Critical Reviews in Toxicology*, 21, 345–372.

DAVIS, A. & BAILEY, D.R. (1969) Metrifonate in urinary schistosomiasis. *Bulletin of the World Health Organization*, 41, 209–224.

DEAN, J.H., MURRAY, M.J. & WARD, E.C. (1986) Toxic responses of the immune system. In *Toxicology: The Basic Science of Poisons*, (eds C.D. Klassen, M.O. Amdur & J. Doull), pp. 245–285. Macmillan, New York.

DEANGELO, A.B., DANIEL, F.B., MCMILLAN, L., WERNSING, P. & SAVAGE, R.E. (1989) Species and strain sensitivity to the induction of peroxisome proliferation by chloracetic acids. *Toxicology and Applied Pharmacology*, 101, 285–298.

DEARFIELD, K.L., ABERNATHY, C.O., OTTLEY, M.S., BRANSTON, J.H. & HAYES, P.F. (1988) Acrylamide: its metabolism, developmental and reproductive effects, genotoxicity and carcinogenicity. *Mutation Research*, 195, 45–77.

DECAPRIO, A.P. (1985) Molecular mechanisms of diketone neurotoxicity. *Chemico-Biological Interactions*, 54, 257–270.

(1987) Hexane neuropathy: studies in experimental animals and man. In *Selectivity and Molecular Mechanisms of Toxicity* (eds F. De Matteis & E.A. Lock), pp. 249–263. Macmillan, Basingstoke.

DeCAPRIO, A.P. & O'NEILL, E.A. (1985) Alterations in rat axonal cytoskeletal proteins induced by *in vitro* and *in vivo* 2, 5-hexanedione exposure. *Toxicology and Applied Pharmacology*, 78, 235–247.

DeDUVE, C. & BAUDHUIN, P. (1966) Peroxisomes (microbodies and related particles). *Physiological Reviews*, 46, 319–375.

DEKANT, W., BERTHOLD, K., VAMVAKAS, S. & HENSCHLER, D. (1988) Thioacylating agents as ultimate intermediates in the β-lyase catalysed metabolism of S-(pentachlorobutadienyl)-1-cysteine. *Chemico-Biological Interactions*, 67, 139–148.

DEKANT, W., VAMVAKAS, S. & ANDERS, M.W. (1992) The kidney as a target organ for xenobiotics bioactivated by glutathione conjugation. In *Tissue Specific Toxicity: Biochemical Mechanisms* (eds W. Dekant & H-G. Neumann), pp. 163–194. Academic Press, London.

DE MATTEIS, F. & ALDRIDGE, W.N., eds (1978) *Heme and Hemoproteins*. Springer-Verlag, Berlin.

DEVONSHIRE, A.L. & MOORE, G.D. (1984) Different forms of insensitive acetylcholinesterase in insect-resistant house flies (*Musca domestica*). *Pesticide Biochemistry and Physiology*, 21, 336–340.

DEWAR, A.J. & MOFFETT, B.J. (1979) Biochemical methods for detecting neurotoxicity – short review. *Pharmacology and Therapeutics*, 5, 545–562.

DINSDALE, D., SKILLETER, D.N. & SEAWRIGHT, A.A. (1981) Selective injury to rat liver Kupffer cells caused by beryllium phosphate: an explanation of reticuloendothelial blockade. *British Journal of Experimental Pathology*, 62, 383.

DiVINCENZO, G.D., KAPLAN, C.J. & DEDINAS, J. (1976) Characterisation of the metabolites of methyl *n*-butyl ketone, methyl iso-butyl ketone and methyl ethyl ketone in guinea pig serum and their clearance. *Toxicology and Applied Pharmacology*, 36, 511–522.

DiVINCENZO, G.D., KRASAVAGE, W.J. & O'DONOGHUE, J.L. (1980) Role of metabolism in hexacarbon neuropathy. In *The Scientific Basis of Toxicity Assessment* (ed. H.P. Witschi), pp. 183–200. Elsvier/North-Holland, Amsterdam.

DIXON, M. & WEBB, E.C. (1966) *Enzymes*. Longman, Green & Co, London.

DODDS, P.F. (1991) Incorporation of xenobiotic carboxylic acids into lipids. *Life Sciences*, 49, 629–649.

DOEGLAS, H.M.G., HERMANS, E.H. & HUISMAN, J. (1961) The margarine disease. *American Medical Association Archives of Dermatology*, 83, 837–843.

DOLL, R. & HILL, A.B. (1950) Smoking and carcinoma of the lung. *British Medical Journal*, 2, 739–748.

(1952) A study of the aetiology of carcinoma of the lung. *British Medical Journal*, 2, 1271–1286.

(1953) Smoking and lung cancer. *British Medical Journal*, 1, 505–506.

(1954) Mortality of doctors in relation to their smoking habits. *British Medical Journal*, 1, 1451–1455.

(1964) Mortality in relation to smoking: ten years observations of British doctors. *British Medical Journal*, 1, 1399–1410 & 1460–1467.

DOLL, R. & PETO, R. (1976) Mortality in relation to smoking: 20 years observation of male British doctors. *British Medical Journal*, 1, 1525–1536.

(1978) Cigarette smoking and bronchial carcinoma: dose and time relationships among regular smokers and life long non-smokers. *Journal of Epidemiology and Community Health*, 32, 303–313.

(1981) The causes of cancer: quantitative estimates of avoidable risks of cancer in the United States today. *Journal of the National Cancer Institute*, 66, 1191–1308.

DOLL, R., HILL, A.B., GRAY, P.G. & PARR, E.A. (1959) Lung cancer mortality and length of cigarette ends. *British Medical Journal*, 1, 3233–3232.

References

DONNINGER, C. (1971) Species specificity of phosphate triester anticholinesterases. *Bulletin of the World Health Organization*, 44, 265–268.

DORMAN, D.C., DYE, J.C., NASSISE, M.P., *et al.* (1993) Acute methanol toxicity in the minipig. *Fundamental and Applied Toxicology*, 20, 341–347.

DRIVER, H.E., WHITE, I.N.H. & BUTLER, W.H. (1987) Dose–response relationships in chemical carcinogenesis: renal mesenchymal tumours induced in the rat by single dose dimethylnitrosamine. *British Journal of Experimental Pathology*, 68, 133–143.

DUNCKEL, A.E. (1975). An updating on the polybrominated biphenyl disaster in Michigan. *Journal of the American Veterinary Medical Association*, 167, 838–848.

EDSALL, J.T. & WYMAN, J. (1958) *Biophysical Chemistry*, Vol. 1. Academic Press, New York.

EDWARDS, M.J., KELLER, B.J., KAUFFMAN, F.C. & THURMAN, R.G. (1993) The involvement of Kupffer cells in carbon tetrachloride toxicity. *Toxicology and Applied Pharmacology*, 119, 275–279.

EDWARDS, P.M. (1975) Neurotoxicity of acrylamide and its analogues and the effects of these analogues and other agents on acrylamide neuropathy. *British Journal of Industrial Medicine*, 32, 31–38.

EHRENBERG, L. & TORNQVIST, M. (1992) Use of biomarkers in epidemiology: quantitative aspects. *Toxicology Letters*, 64/65, 485–492.

EHRENBERG, L., HIESCHE, K.D., OSTERMAN-GOLKAR, S. and WENNBERG, I. (1974) Evaluation of genetic risks of alkylating agents: tissue doses in the mouse from air contaminated with ethylene oxide. *Mutation Research*, 24, 83–103.

ELCOMBE, C.R. (1985) Species differences in carcinogenicity and peroxisome proliferation due to trichlorethylene: a biochemical human hazard assessment. *Archives of Toxicology*, suppl. 8, 6–17.

ELDER, G.H. (1978) Porphyria caused by hexachlorobenzene and other polyhalogenated aromatic hydrocarbons. In *Heme and Hemoproteins* (eds F. De Matteis & W.N. Aldridge), pp. 157–200. Springer-Verlag, Berlin.

ELFARRA, A.A. & ANDERS, M.W. (1984) Renal processing of glutathione conjugates: role in nephrotoxicity. *Biochemical Pharmacology*, 33, 3729–3732.

ELING, T.E., THOMPSON, D.C., FOUREMAN, G.L., CURTIS, J.F. & HUGHES, M.F. (1990) Prostaglandin H synthase and xenobiotic oxidation. *Annual Reviews of Pharmacology and Toxicology*, 30, 1–45.

ELLIOTT, B.M. & ALDRIDGE, W.N. (1977) Binding of triethyltin to cat haemoglobin and modification of the binding sites by diethylpyrocarbonate. *Biochemical Journal*, 163, 583–589.

ELLIOTT, B.M., ALDRIDGE, W.N. & BRIDGES, J.M. (1979) Triethyltin binding to cat haemoglobin: evidence for two chemically distinct sites and a role for both histidine and cysteine residues. *Biochemical Journal*, 177, 461–470.

ELLIOTT, M. (1971) The relationships between the structure and the activity of pyrethroids. In *Alternative Insecticides for Vector Control*, pp 315–324. World Health Organization, Geneva. (1979) Progress in the design of pesticides. *Chemistry and Industry*, pp. 757–768.

ERIKSSON, J.E., HAGERSTRAND, H. & ISOMAA, B. (1987) Cell selective toxicity of a peptide toxin from the cyanobacterium *Microcystis aeruginosa*. *Biochimica et Biophysica Acta*, 930, 304–310.

ERIKSSON, J.E., TOIVOLA, D., MERILNOTO, J.A., *et al.* (1990) Hepatocyte deformation induced by cyanobacterial toxins reflects inhibition of protein phosphatase. *Biochemical and Biophysical Research Communications*, 173, 1347–1353.

ETO, M., CASIDA, J.E. & ETO, T. (1962) Hydroxylation and cyclisation reaction involved in the metabolism of tri o-cresyl phosphate. *Biochemical Pharmacology*, 11, 337–352.

ETO, M. ABE, M. & TAKAHARA, H. (1971) Metabolism of tri p-ethylphenyl phosphate and neurotoxicity of the metabolites. *Agricultural and Biological Chemistry*, 35, 929–940.

EVANS, C.H. (1990) *Biochemistry of the Lanthanides*, pp. 1–444, Plenum, New York.

EVANS, D.A.P., MANLEY, K.A. & MCKUSICK, V.A. (1960) Genetic control of isoniazid metabolism in man. *British Medical Journal*, 2, 485–491.

EXON, J.H., MATHER, G.G., BUSSIERE, J.L., OLSON, D.P. & TALCOTT, P.A. (1991) Effects of subchronic exposure of rats to 2-methoxyethanol or 2-butoxyethanol: thymic atrophy and immunotoxicity. *Fundamental and Applied Toxicology*, 16, 830–840.

FALCONER, I.R., BERESFORD, A.M. & RUNNEGAR, M.T.C. (1983) Evidence for liver damage by toxin from a bloom of the blue–green alga, *Microcystis aeruginosa. Medical Journal of Australia*, 1, 511–514.

FARBER, E. (1971) Biochemical pathology. *Annual Review of Pharmacology*, 11, 71–96.

FARMER, P.B. (1994) Carcinogen adducts: use in diagnosis and risk assessment. *Clinical Chemistry*, 40, 1438–1443.

FARMER, P.B., BAILEY, E., GORF, S.M., *et al.* (1986) Monitoring human exposure to ethylene oxide by determination of haemoglobin adducts using gas chromatography–mass spectrometry. *Carcinogenesis*, 7, 637–640.

FARMER, P.B., NEUMANN, H.G. & HENSCHLER, D. (1987) Estimation of exposure of man to substances reacting covalently with macromolecules. *Archives of Toxicology*, 60, 251–260.

FARMER, P.B., BAILEY, E., NAYLOR, S., *et al.* (1993) Identification of endogenous electrophiles by means of mass spectrometric determination of protein and DNA adducts. *Environmental Health Perspectives*, 99, 19–24.

FARRINGTON, J.A., EBERT, M., LAND, E.J. & FLETCHER, K. (1973) Bipyridilium quaternary salts and related compounds. V: Pulse radiolysis studies on the reaction of paraquat radical with oxygen. Implications for the mode of action of bipyridilium herbicides. *Biochimica et Biophysica Acta*, 314, 372–381.

FARRIS, F.F., DEDRICK, R.L., ALLEN, P.V. & SMITH, J.C. (1993) Physiological model for the pharmacokinetics of methylmercury in the growing rat. *Toxicology and Applied Pharmacology*, 119, 74–90.

FEARS, R. (1985) Lipophilic xenobiotic conjugates: the pharmacological and toxicological consequences of the participation of drugs and other foreign compounds as substrates in lipid biosynthesis. *Progress in Lipid Research*, 24, 177–195.

FELIX, R.H., IVE, F.A. & DAHL, M.D.C. (1974) Skin reaction to practolol. *British Medical Journal*, 2, 321–324.

FENWICK, G.R., HEANEY, R.K. & MULLIN, W.J. (1983) Glucosinolates and their breakdown products in food and food plants. *Critical Reviews in Food Science and Nutrition*, 18, 123–201.

FERGUSON, J.S. & ALARIE, Y. (1991) Long term pulmonary impairment following a single exposure to methyl isocyanate. *Toxicology and Applied Pharmacology*, 107, 253–268.

FIELD, E.A., PRICE, C.J., SLEET, R.B., *et al.* (1990) Developmental toxicity evaluation of acrylamide in rats and mice. *Fundamental and Applied Pharmacology*, 14, 502–512.

FINGL, E. & WOODBURY, D.M. (1966) General principles. In *Pharmacological Basis of Therapeutics* (ed. L.S. Goodman & A. Gilman), pp. 1–36. Macmillan, New York.

FISH, R.H., KIMMEL, E.C. & CASIDA, J.E. (1976a) Bioorganotin chemistry: biological oxidation of organotin compounds. In *Organotin Compounds: New Chemistry and Applications*, pp. 197–203. Advances in Chemistry Series No. 157, American Chemical Society, Washington, DC.

(1976b) Bioorganotin chemistry: reactions of tributyltin derivatives with a cytochrome P-450 dependent monooxygenase enzyme system. *Journal of Organometal Chemistry*, 118, 41–54.

FLEISCHNER, G., ROBBINS, J. & ARIAS, I.M. (1972) Immunological studies of Y-protein – a major cytoplasmic organic anion binding protein in rat liver. *Journal of Clinical Investigation*, 51, 677–684.

FORASTIERE, F., PERUCCI, C.A., ARCÀ, M. & AXELSON, O. (1993) Indirect estimates of lung cancer death rates in Italy not attributable to active smoking. *Epidemiology*, 4, 489–492 & 502–510.

FORSHAW, P.J., LISTER, T. & RAY, D.E. (1993) Inhibition of a neuronal voltage dependent chloride channel by the type II pyrethroid, deltamethrin. *Neuropharmacology*, 32, 105–111.

FRIBERG, L. (1959). Studies on the metabolism of mercuric chloride and methyl mercury dicyandiamide. *Archives of Industrial Health*, 20, 42–49.

FRIBERG, L., ELINDER, C.G., LJELLSTROM, T. & NORDBERG, G.F. (1986) *Cadmium and Health: A Toxicological and Epidemiological Appraisal*, volume 2. CRC Press, Boca Raton, Florida.

FRIEDBERG, T., SIEGERT, P., GRASSOW, M.A., BARTLOMOWICZ, B. & OESCH, F. (1990) Studies on the expression of the cytochrome P450IA, P450IIB and P450IIC gene family in extra-hepatic and hepatic tissues. *Environmental Health Perspectives*, 88, 67–70.

FULLERTON, P.M. & BARNES, J.M. (1966) Peripheral neuropathy in rats produced by acrylamide. *British Journal of Industrial Medicine*, 23, 210–221.

GAGE, J.C. (1953) A cholinesterase inhibitor derived from *OO*-diethyl-*O*-*p*-nitrophenyl thio-phosphate *in vivo*. *Biochemical Journal*, 54, 426–430.

(1964) Distribution and excretion of methyl and phenyl mercury salts. *British Journal of Industrial Health*, 21, 197–202.

(1968) The action of paraquat and diquat on the respiration of liver cell fractions. *Biochemical Journal*, 109, 757–761.

GAINES, B. (1969) Acute toxicity of pesticides. *Toxicology and Applied Pharmacology*, 14, 515–534.

GALJAARD, H. (1986) Biochemical diagnosis of genetic disease. *Experientia*, 42, 1075–1085.

GARABANT, D.H., HELD, J., LANGHOLZ, B., PETERS, J.M. & MACK, T.M. (1992) DDT and related compounds and risk of pancreatic cancer. *Journal of the National Cancer Institute*, 84, 764–771.

GARABANT, D.H., HELD, J. & HOMA, D. (1993) Response to 'DDT and pancreatic cancer'. *Journal of the National Cancer Institute*, 85, 328–329.

GAVRILESCU, N. & PETERS, R.A. (1931) Biochemical lesions in vitamin B deficiency. *Biochemical Journal*, 25, 1397–1409.

GEHRING, P.J., WATANABE, P.G. & PARK, C.N. (1978) Resolution of dose–response toxicity data for chemicals requiring metabolic activation: example vinyl chloride. *Toxicology and Applied Pharmacology*, 44, 581–591.

GENTER ST. CLAIR, M.B., AMARNATH, V., MOODY, M.A., *et al.* (1988) *Chemical Research in Toxicology*, 1, 179–185.

GHIORSE, W.C. & WILSON, J.T. (1988) Microbial ecology of the terrestrial subsurface. *Advances in Applied Microbiology*, 33, 107–172.

GIBSON, G.G. & SKETT, P. (1994) *Introduction to Drug Metabolism*. Chapman and Hall, London.

GILGER, A.P. & POTTS, A.M. (1955) Studies on the visual toxicity of methanol. V: The role of acidosis in methanol poisoning. *American Journal of Opthamology*, 39, 63–86.

GILLETTE, J.R. (1982) The problem of chemically reactive metabolites. *Drug Metabolism Reviews*, 13, 941–961.

GLEICHMANN, E., KIMBER, I. & PURCHASE, I.F.H. (1989) Immunotoxicology: suppressive and stimulatory effects of drugs and environmental chemicals on the immune system. *Archives of Toxicology*, 63, 257–273.

GLOWAZ, S.L., MICHNIKA, M. & HUXTABLE, R.J. (1992) Detection of a reactive pyrrole in the hepatic metabolism of the pyrollizidine alkaloid, monocrotaline. *Toxicology and Applied Pharmacology*, 115, 168–173.

GOMPERTZ, D., FLETCHER, J.G., PERKINS, J., *et al.* (1983) Renal dysfunction in cadmium smelters: relation to *in vivo* liver and kidney cadmium concentrations. *Lancet*, 1, 1185–1187.

GONZALEZ, F.J. (1989) The molecular biology of cytochrome P450's. *Pharmacological Reviews*, 40, 243–288.

(1992) Human cytochromes P-450: problems and prospects. *Trends in Pharmacological Sciences*, 13, 346–352.

GOODMAN, D.S. (1980) Plasma retinol-binding protein in lipoprotein structure. *Annals of the New York Academy of Sciences*, 348, 378–390.

GOTTSCHALK, C.W. (1964) Osmotic concentration and dilution of urine. *American Journal of Medicine*, 36, 670–685.

GRAHAM, D.G. (1980) Hexane polyneuropathy: a proposal for the pathogenesis of a hazard of occupational exposure and inhalant abuse. *Chemico-Biological Interactions*, 32, 339–345.

GRAHAM, D.G., SZAKAL-QUIN, G., PRIEST, J.W. & ANTHONY, D.G. (1984) *In vitro* evidence that covalent crosslinking of neurofilaments occurs in γ-diketone neuropathy. *Proceedings of the National Academy of Sciences*, 81, 4979–4982.

GRASSO, P., SHARRATT, M. & COHEN, A.J. (1991) Role of persistent, non-genotoxic tissue damage in rodent cancer and relevance to humans. *Annual Reviews of Pharmacology and Toxicology*, 31, 253–287.

GRAY, T.J.B. (1986) Testicular toxicity *in vitro*: sertoli-germ cell co-cultures as a model system. *Food and Chemical Toxicology*, 6/7, 601–605.

GRAY, T.J.B., MOSS, E.J., CREASEY, D.M. & GANGOLLI, S.D. (1985) Studies on the toxicity of some glycol ethers and alkoxyacetic acids in primary testicular cell cultures. *Toxicology and Applied Pharmacology*, 79, 490–501.

GREEN, S., TUGWOOD, J.D. & ISSEMANN, I. (1992) The molecular mechanism of peroxisome proliferator action: a model for species differences and mechanistic risk assessment. *Toxicology Letters*, 64/65, 131–139.

GRIEG-SMITH, P.W. (1993) Killing with care – can pesticides be environmentally friendly? *Biologist*, 40, 132–136.

GRIFFIN, J.W., PRICE, D.L., KUETHE, D. & GOLDBERG, A.M. (1980) Neurotoxicity of misonidazole in rats. *Neurotoxicology*, 1, 653–666.

GRIMMER, H. & JOSEPH, A. (1959) An epidemic of infectious erythema in Germany. *American Medical Association Archives of Dermatology*, 80, 283–285.

GUENGERICH, F.P. (1990) Enzymic oxidation of xenobiotic chemicals. *Critical Reviews in Biochemistry and Molecular Biology*, 25, 97–153.

(1991) Reactions and significance of cytochrome P450 enzymes. *Journal of Biological Chemistry*, 266, 10019–10022.

GUPTA, R.C. (1985) Enhanced sensitivity of the $[^{32}p]$-post labelling assay for aromatic carcinogen–DNA adducts. *Cancer Research*, 51, 6470–6491.

GURTNER, H.P. (1979) Pulmonary hypertension, 'Plexogenic Pulmonary Arteriopathy' and the appetite depressant drug aminorex: post or propter. *Bulletin Europien Physiopathologique Respiratoire*, 15, 897–923.

GUTFREUND, H. (1965) *An Introduction to the Study of Enzymes*. Blackwell Scientific, Oxford.

HABIG, W.H., PABST, M.J., FLEISCHNER, G., *et al.* (1974) The identity of glutathione S-transferase B with ligandin, a major binding protein of the liver. *Proceedings of the National Academy of Science, USA*, 71, 3879–3882.

HALL, E.S., HALL, S.J. & BOEKELHEIDE, K. (1992) Sertoli cells isolated from adult 2, 5-hexanedione exposed rats exhibit atypical morphology and actin distribution. *Toxicology and Applied Toxicology*, 117, 9–18.

HANNA, P.E. & BANKS, R.B. (1985) Arylhydroxylamines and arylhydroxamic acids: conjugation reactions. In *Bioactivation of foreign compounds* (ed. M.W. Anders), pp. 375–402. Academic Press, Orlando.

HARD, G.C. & BUTLER, W.H. (1970a) Cellular analysis of renal neoplasia: induction of renal tumours in dietary conditioned rats by dimethylnitrosamine, with a reappraisal of morphological characteristics. *Cancer Research*, 30, 2796–2805.

(1970b) Cellular analysis of renal neoplasia: light microscopic study of the development of interstitial lesions induced in the rat kidney by a single carcinogenic dose of dimethylnitrosamine. *Cancer Research*, 30, 2806–2815.

(1971a). Ultrastructural study of the development of interstitial lesions leading to mesenchymal neoplasia induced in the rat renal cortex by dimethylnitrosamine. *Cancer Research*, 31, 337–347.

(1971b) Ultrastructural analysis of renal mesenchymal tumour induced in the rat by dimethylnitrosamine. *Cancer Research*, 31, 348–365.

(1971c) Ultrastructural aspects of renal adenocarcinoma induced in the rat by dimethylnitrosamine. *Cancer Research*, 31, 366–372.

HASCHEK, W.M. & WITSCHI, H. (1979) Pulmonary fibrosis – a possible mechanism. *Toxicology and Applied Pharmacology*, 51, 475–487.

References

HASHIMOTO, K. & ALDRIDGE, W.N. (1970) Biochemical studies on acrylamide, a neurotoxic agent. *Biochemical Pharmacology*, 19, 2591–2604.

HASHIMOTO, K., HAYASHI, M., TANTI, H. & SAKAMOTO, J. (1988) Toxicological aspects of acrylamide neuropathy. *Journal of the Union of Occupational and Environmental Hygiene*, 10, 209–218.

HASSALL, K.A. (1990) *The Biochemistry and Uses of Pesticides*. Macmillan, Basingstoke.

HATEFI, Y. (1985) The mitochondrial electron transport and oxidative phosphorylation system. *Annual Reviews in Biochemistry*, 54, 1015–1069.

HAWKINS, J.M., JONES, W.E., BONNER, F.W. & GIBSON, G.G. (1987) The effect of peroxisome proliferators on microsomal and mitochondrial enzyme activities in the liver and kidney. *Drug Metabolism Reviews*, 18, 441–515.

HAYES, W.J., Jr (1982) *Pesticides Studied in Man*. Williams & Wilkins, Baltimore.

HE, F., WANG, S., LIU, L., CHEN, S., ZHANG, Z. & SUN, J. (1989) Clinical manifestations and diagnosis of acute pyrethroid poisoning. *Archives of Toxicology*, 63, 54–58.

HEIN, D.W., RUSTAN, T.D., DOLL, M.A., *et al.* (1992) Acetyltransferases and susceptibility to chemicals. *Toxicology Letters*, 64/65. 123–130.

HEINDEL, J.J., GULATI, D.K., MOUNCE, R.C., RUSSELL, S.R. & LAMB, J.C. (1989) Reproductive toxicity of three phthalic esters in a continuous breeding protocol. *Fundamental and Applied Toxicology*, 12, 508–518.

HENSCHLER, D. (1987) Mechanisms of genotoxicity of chlorinated aliphatic hydrocarbons. In *Selectivity and Molecular Mechanisms of Toxicity* (eds F. De Matteis & E.A. Lock), pp. 153–181. Macmillan, Basingstoke.

HERBST, A.L., COLE, P., COLTON, T., ROBBOY, S. & SCULLY, R. (1977) Age-incidence and risk of diethylstilboestrol-related clear cell adenocarcinoma of the vagina and cervix. *American Journal of Obstetrics and Gynaecology*, 128, 43–50.

HERNBERG, S. (1980) Evaluation of epidemiological studies in assessing the long-term effects of occupational noxious agents. *Scandinavian Journal of Work and Environmental Health*, 6, 163–169.

HEYLINGS, J.R. (1991) Gastro-intestinal absorption of paraquat in the isolated mucosa of the rat. *Toxicology and Applied Pharmacology*, 107, 482–493.

HIGGINSON, J. & MUIR, C.S. (1979) Environmental carcinogenesis: misconception and limitations to cancer control. *Journal of the National Cancer Institute*, 63, 1291–1298.

HILL, A.B. (1962) *Statistical Methods in Clinical and Preventative Medicine*. Oxford University Press, Oxford.

——— (1965) The environment and disease. *Proceedings of the Royal Society of Medicine*, 58, 295–300.

HILL, R.H., SCHURZ, H.H., POSADA, M., *et al.* (1995) Possible etiological agents for Toxic Oil Syndrome: fatty acid esters of 3-(N-phenylamino)-1,2-propanediol. *Archives of Environmental Contamination & Toxicology*, 28, 259–264.

HIMSWORTH, II. (1970) *The Development of Organisation of Scientific Knowledge*. Heinemann, London.

HINSEN, J.A. (1980) Biochemical toxicology of acetaminophen. *Reviews in Biochemical Toxicology*, 2, 103–129.

HIRANO, S., KODAMA, N., SHIBATA, K. & SUZUKI, K.T. (1993) Metabolism and toxicity of injected yttrium chloride in rats. *Toxicology and Applied Pharmacology*, 121, 224–232.

HODGKIN, A.L. & HUXLEY, A.F. (1952) A quantitative description of membrane current and its application to conduction and excitation in nerve. *Journal of Physiology*, 117, 500–544.

HOFER, W. (1981) Chemistry of Metrifonate and Dichlorvos. *Acta Pharmacologica et Toxicologica*, 49 (suppl. V), 7–14.

HOLAN, G. (1971) Rational design of insecticides. *Bulletin of the World Health Organization*, 44, 355–362.

HOLMBOM, B., VOSS, R.H., MORTIMER, R.D. & WONG, A. (1984) Fractionation, isolation and characterisation of Ames mutagenic compounds in kraft chlorination effluents. *Environmental Science and Technology*, 18, 333–337.

HOLMSTEDT, B. (1980) Prolegomena to Seveso. *Archives of Toxicology*, 44, 211–230.

HOLMSTEDT, B. & LILJESTRAND, G. (1963) *Readings in Pharmacology*. Pergamon, Oxford.

HOLMSTEDT, B., NORDGREN, I., SANDOZ, M. & SUNDWALL, A. (1978) Metrifonate: summary of toxicological and pharmacological information available. *Archives of Toxicology*, 41, 3–29.

HOOK, J.B. & HEWITT, W.R. (1986) Toxic responses of the kidney. In *Toxicology: The Basic Science of Poisons* (eds C.D. Klaasson, M.O. Amdur & J. Doull), pp. 310–329. Macmillan, New York.

HOOK, J.B., ROSE, M.S. & LOCK, E.A. (1982) The nephrotoxicity of hexachloro-1, 3-butadiene in the rat: studies of organic anion and cation transport in renal slices and the effect of monooxygenase inducers. *Toxicology and Applied Pharmacology*, 65, 373–382.

HOOK, J.B., ISHMAEL, J. & LOCK, E.A. (1983) Nephrotoxicity of hexachloro-1,3-butadiene in the rat: the effect of age, sex and strain. *Toxicology and Applied Pharmacology*, 67, 121–131.

HOOSER, S.B., BEASLEY, B.R., WAITE, L.L., *et al.* (1991) Actin filament alterations in rat hepatocytes induced *in vivo* and *in vitro* by microcystin-LR, a hepatotoxin from the blue green algae *Microcystis aeruginosa*. *Veterinary Pathology*, 28, 259–266.

HORTON, V.L., SLEET, R.B., JOHN-GREEN, J.A. & WELSCH, F. (1984) Developmental stage-specific and dose-related teratogenic effects of ethylene glycol monomethyl ether in CD-1 mice. *Toxicology and Applied Pharmacology*, 80, 108–118.

HORVATH, J.J., WITMER, C.M. & WITZ, G. (1992) Nephrotoxicity of the 1 : 1 acrolein–glutathione adduct in the rat. *Toxicology and Applied Pharmacology*, 117, 200–207.

HUANG, J., SHIBATA, E., KATO, K., ASEADA, N & TAKEUCHI, Y. (1992) Chronic exposure to a *n*-hexane induces changes in nerve-specific marker proteins in the distal peripheral nerve of the rat. *Human and Experimental Toxicology*, 11, 323–327.

HUTSON, D.H. (1982) Formation of lipophilic conjugates of pesticides and other xenobiotic compounds. *Progress in Pesticide Biochemistry*, 2, 171–184.

HUTSON, D.H. & HATHWAY, D.E. (1967) Toxic effects of chlorfenvinphos in dogs and rats. *Biochemical Pharmacology*, 16, 949–962.

HUTSON, D.H. & MILLBURN, P. (1991) Enzyme-mediated selective toxicity of an organophosphate and a pyrethroid: some examples from a range of animals. *Biochemical Society Transactions*, 19, 737–740.

HUTSON, D.H. & WRIGHT, A.S. (1980) The effect of hepatic microsomal monooxygenase induction on the metabolism and toxicity of the organophosphorus insecticide chlorfenvinphos. *Chemico-Biological Interactions*, 31, 93–101.

HUXTABLE, R.J. (1990) Activation and pulmonary toxicity of pyrrolizidine alkaloids. *Pharmacology and Therapeutics*, 47, 371–389.

HYDE, E.G. & CARMICHAEL, W.W. (1991) Anatoxin-a(S), a naturally occurring organophosphate, is an irreversible active site-directed inhibitor of acetylcholinesterase (EC 3.1.1.7). *Journal of Biochemical Toxicology*, 6, 195–201.

IARC (1982) Some industrial chemicals and dyestuffs. *IARC Monograph on the Evaluation of Carcinogenic Risk of Chemicals to Humans*. International Agency for Cancer Research, Lyon, France.

INGRAM, A.J. & GRASSO, P. (1985) Nuclear enlargement: an early change produced in mouse epidermis by carcinogenic chemicals applied topically in the presence of a promoter. *Journal of Applied Toxicology*, 5, 53–60.

(1987) Nuclear enlargement produced in mouse skin by carcinogenic mineral oils. *Journal of Applied Toxicology*, 7, 289–295.

INSTITUTE OF MEDICAL ETHICS (1991) *Lives in the Balance: The Ethics of Using Animals in Biomedical Research* (eds J.A. Smith & K.M. Boyd). Oxford University Press, Oxford.

IOANNIDES, C. & PARKE, D.V. (1990) Cytochrome P450 I family of microsomal haemoproteins and their role in the metabolic activation of chemicals. *Drug Metabolism Reviews*, 22, 1–85.

ISHIKAWA, T. (1992) The ATP-dependent glutathione S-conjugate export pump. *Trends in Biochemical Sciences*, 17, 463–468.

References

JACOBS, J.M. & FORD, W.C.L. (1981) The neurotoxicity and antifertility properties of 6-chloro-6-deoxyglucose in the mouse. *Neurotoxicology*, 2, 405–417.

JAFFE, D.R., HASSEL, C.D., BRENDEL, K. & GANDOLFI, A.J. (1983) *In vivo* and *in vitro* nephrotoxicity of the cysteine conjugate of hexachlorobutadiene. *Journal of Toxicology and Environmental Health*, 11, 857–867.

JAKOBY, W.R. (1978) The glutathione-S-transferases: a group of multifunctional detoxification proteins. *Advances in Enzymology*, 46, 383–414.

JAKOBY, W.B. & ZIEGLER, D.M. (1990) The enzymes of detoxification. *Journal of Biological Chemistry*, 265, 20715–20718.

JAKOBY, W.B., KETTERER, B. & MANNERVIK, B. (1984) Glutathione transferase: nomenclature. *Biochemical Pharmacology*, 33, 2539–2540.

JANSSON, K., MAKI-PAAKKANEN, J., VAITTINEN, S-L., *et al.* (1993) Cytogenetic effects of 3-chloro-4-(dichloromethyl)-5-hydroxy-2(5H)-furanone (MX) in rat peripheral lymphocytes *in vitro* and *in vivo*. *Mutation Research*, 229, 25–28.

JENCKS, W.P. (1969) *Catalysis in Chemistry and Enzymology*. McGraw-Hill, New York.

JENNER, P. & MARSDEN, C.D. (1987) Parkinsonian syndrome caused by 1-methyl-4-phenyl-1,2,3,6-tertahydropyridine (MPTP) in man and animals. In *Selectivity and Molecular Mechanisms of Toxicity* (eds F. De Matteis and E.A. Lock), pp. 213–248. Macmillan, Basingstoke.

JOHNSON, M.K. (1975a) The delayed neuropathy caused by some organophosphorus esters: mechanism and challenge. *CRC Critical Reviews in Toxicology*, 3, 289–316.

(1975b) Organophosphorus esters causing delayed neurotoxic effects: mechanism of action and structure/activity studies. *Archives of Toxicology*, 34, 259–288.

(1982) The target for initiation of delayed neurotoxicity by organophosphorus esters: biochemical studies and toxicological applications. *Reviews in Biochemical Toxicology*, 4, 141–212.

(1993) Symposium introduction: retrospect and prospects for neuropathy target esterase (NTE) and the delayed polyneuropathy (OPIDP) induced by some organophosphorus esters. *Chemico-Biological Interactions*, 87, 339–346.

JOHNSON, M.K. & SAFI, J.M. (1993) The R−(+) isomer of O-n-hexyl S-methyl phosphorothioamidate causes delayed neuropathy in hens after generation of a form of inhibited neuropathy target esterase (NTE) which can be reactivated *ex vivo*. *Chemico- Biological Interactions*, 87, 443–448.

JONES, H.B. & CAVANAGH, J.B. (1983a) Distortions of the nodes of Ranvier from axonal distension by filamentous masses in hexacarbon intoxication. *Journal of Neurocytology*, 12, 439–458.

(1983b) Cytochemical staining characteristics of peripheral nodes of Ranvier in hexacarbon intoxication. *Journal of Neurocytology*, 12, 459–473.

JUKES, J.H. (1983) Chasing a receeding zero: impact of the zero threshold concept on action of the regulatory officials. *Journal of the American College of Toxicology*, 2, 147–160.

KADAR, T., COHEN, G., SAHAR, R., ALKALIE, D. & SHAPIRA, S. (1992) Long term study of brain lesions following Soman, in comparison to DFP and Metrazol poisoning. *Human and Experimental Toxicology*, 11, 517–523.

KAGI, J.H.R. & VALLEE, B.L. (1960). Metallothionein: a cadmium and zinc-containing protein from equine renal cortex. *Journal of Biological Chemistry*, 235, 3460–3465.

KAGI, J.H.R., HIMMELHOCH, S.R., WHANGER, P.D., BETHUNE, J.L. & VALLEE, B.E. (1974). Equine hepatic and renal metallothioneins. *Journal of Biological Chemistry*, 249, 3537–3542.

KALOW, W. (1962) *Pharmacogenetics: Heredity and the Response to Drugs*. W.B. Saunders, Philadelphia.

KAMAT, S.R., MAHASHUR, A.A., TIWARI, A.K.B., *et al.* (1985a) Early observations on pulmonary changes and clinical morbidity due to the isocyanate gas leak in Bhopal. *Journal of Postgraduate Medicine*, 31, 63–72.

KAMAT, S.R., PATEL, M.H., KOLHATHKAR, V.P., DAVE, A.A. & MAHASHUR, A.A. (1985b). Sequential respiratory changes in those exposed to the gas leak in Bhopal. *Indian Journal of Medical Research*, 82(suppl.), 20–38.

KAMATAKI, T., LIN, M.C.M.L., BELCHER, D.H. & NEAL, R.A. (1976) Studies of the metabolism of parathion with an apparently homogeneous preparation of rabbit liver cytochrome P450. *Drug Metabolism and Disposition*, 4, 180–189.

KAMINSKY, L.S. (1985) Benzene and substituted benzenes. In *Bioactivation of Foreign Compounds* (ed. M.W. Anders), pp. 157–175. Academic Press, Orlando.

KAMINSKY, L.S. & FASCO, M.J. (1992) Small intestinal cytochrome P450. *Critical Reviews in Toxicology*, 21, 407–422.

KAO, C.Y. (1966) Tetrodotoxin, saxitoxin and their significance in the study of excitation phenomena. *Pharmacological Reviews*, 18, 997–1049.

KAVET, R. & NAUSS, K.M. (1990) The toxicity of inhaled methanol vapors. *CRC Critical Reviews in Toxicology*, 21, 21–50.

KAWADA, T., KOYAMA, H. & SUZUKI, S. (1989) Cadmium, NAG activity and β_2-microglobulin in the urine of cadmium pigment workers. *British Journal of Industrial Medicine*, 46, 52–55.

KEAYS, R., HARRISON, P.M., WENDON, J.A., *et al.* (1991) Intravenous acetylcysteine in paracetamol-induced fulminant hepatic failure: a prospective controlled trial. *British Medical Journal*, 303, 1026–1029.

KEDDERIS, L.B., MILLS, J.J., ANDERSEN, M.E. & BIRNBAUM, L.S. (1993) A physiologically based pharmacokinetic model for 2,3,7,8-tetrabromodibenzo-*p*-dioxin (TBDD) in the rat: tissue distribution and CYP1A induction. *Toxicology and Applied Pharmacology*, 121, 87–98.

KEELING, A.K., PRATT, I.S., ALDRIDGE, W.N. & SMITH, L.L. (1981) The enhancement of paraquat toxicity in rats by 85% oxygen: lethality and cell-specific lung damage. *British Journal of Experimental Pathology*, 62, 643–654.

KEELING, P.L., SMITH, L.L. & ALDRIDGE, W.N. (1982) The formation of mixed disulphides in rat lung following paraquat administration: correlation with changes in intermediary metabolism. *Biochimica Biophysica Acta*, 716, 249–257.

KENNEDY, A.L., SINGH, G., ALARIE, Y. & BROWN, W.E. (1993) Autoradiographic analyses of guinea pig airway tissue following inhalation exposure to ^{14}C-labelled methyl isocyanate. *Fundamental and Applied Pharmacology*, 20, 57–67.

KETLEY, J.N., HABIG, W.H. & JAKOBY, W.B. (1975) Binding of non-substrates ligands to the glutathione transferases. *Journal of Biological Chemistry*, 250, 8670–8673.

KILBOURNE, E.M., BERNERT, J.T., POSADA DE LA PAZ, M., *et al.* (1988) Chemical correlates of pathogenicity of oils related to the toxic oil syndrome epidemic in Spain. *American Journal of Epidemiology*, 127, 1210–1227.

KILBOURNE, E.M., POSADA DE LA PAZ, M., ABAITUA BORDA, I. *et al.* (1991) Toxic Oil Syndrome: a current clinical and epidemiological summary, including comparisons with the eosinophilia–myalgia syndrome. *Journal of the American College of Cardiology*, 18, 711–717.

KIMBROUGH, R, D. (1980) Occupational exposure. In *Halogenated Biphenyls, Terphenyls, Naphthalenes, Dibenzodioxins and Related Compounds* (ed. R.D. Kimbrough), pp. 373–397. Elsevier/North-Holland, Amsterdam.

KIMBROUGH, R.D. and GAINES, T.B. (1971) Hexachlorophene effects on the rat brain. *Archives of Environmental Health*, 23, 114–118.

KIMMEL, E.C., FISH, R.H. & CASIDA, J.E. (1976) Bioorganotin chemistry: metabolism of organotin compounds in microsomal monooxygenase systems and in mammals. *Journal of Agricultural and Food Chemistry*, 25, 1–9.

KLAASSEN, C.D. (1986) Distribution, excretion and absorption of toxicants. In *Casarett and Doull's Toxicology: The Basic Science of Poisons* (eds C.D. Klaassen, M.O. Amdur & J. Doull), pp. 33–63. Macmillan, New York.

KLAASSEN, C.D. & WATKINS, J.B. (1984) Mechanisms of bile formation, hepatic uptake and biliary secretion. *Pharmacological Reviews*, 36, 1–67.

KLAASSEN, C.D., EATON, D.L. & CAGEN, S.Z. (1981) Hepatobiliary disposition of xenobiotics. In *Progress in Drug Metabolism* (eds J.W. Bridges & L.F. Chasseaud), Vol. 6, pp. 1–75. Wiley, Chichester.

References

KOELLE, G.B., ed. (1963) *Cholinesterases and Anticholinesterase Agents*. Springer-Verlag, Berlin.

KOIVUSALO, M., JAAKKOLA, J.J.K., VARTIAINEN, T., *et al.* (1994) Drinking water mutagenicity and gastrointestinal and urinary tract cancers: an ecological study in Finland. *American Journal of Public Health*, 8, 1233–1228. See also 8, 1211–1213.

KOMULAINEN, H. & BONDY, S.C. (1988) Increased free intracellular Ca^{2+} by toxic agents: an index of potential neurotoxicity? *Trends in Pharmacological Sciences*, 9, 154–156.

KOPELMAN, H., ROBERTSON, M.H., SANDERS, P G. & ASH, I. (1966) The Epping jaundice. *British Medical Journal*, 1, 514–516.

KRAGH-HANSEN, U. (1981) Molecular aspects of ligand binding to serum albumin. *Pharmacological Reviews*, 33, 17–53.

KRASAVAGE, W.J., O'DONOGHUE, J.L., DIVINCENZO, G.D. & TERHAAR, C.J. (1980) The relative neurotoxicity of methyl-*n*-butyl ketone, *n*-hexane and their metabolites. *Toxicology and Applied Pharmacology*, 52, 433–441.

KRONBERG, L. & VARTIAINEN, T. (1988) Ames mutagenicity and concentration of the strong mutagen 3-chloro-4-(dichloromethyl)-5-hydroxy-2(5H)-furanone and its geometric isomer E-2-chloro-3-(dichloromethyl)-4-oxo-butenoic acid in chlorine treated tap waters. *Mutation Research*, 206, 177–182.

KUPERMAN, A.G. (1958) Effects of acrylamide on the central nervous system of the cat. *Journal of Pharmacology and Experimental Therapeutics*, 123, 180–192.

LADU, B.N. (1972) Pharmacogenetics: defective enzymes in relation to reaction to drugs. *Annual Review of Medicine*, 23, 453–468.

LAIDLER, K.J. (1958) *The Chemical Kinetics of Enzyme Action*. Oxford University Press, Oxford.

LAKE, B.G., GRAY, T.J.B., PELS RIJCKEN, W.R., BEAMAND, J.A. & GANGOLLI, S.D. (1984) The effect of hypolipidaemic agents of peroxisomal β-oxidation and MFO activities in primary cultures of rat hepatocytes: relationship between induction of palmitoyl-CoA oxidation and lauric acid hydroxylation. *Xenobiotica*, 14, 269–276.

LANARUS, T., COOK, C.M., ERIKSSON, J.E., MERILNOTO, J.A. & HOTOKKA, M. (1991) Computer modelling of the 3-dimensional structure of the cyanobacterial hepatotoxin microcystin-LR and nodularin. *Toxicon*, 29, 901–906.

LANGSTONE, J.W., FORNO, L.S., REBERT, C.S. & IRWIN, I. (1984) Selective nigral toxicity after systemic administration of 1-methyl-4-phenyl-1,2,3,6-tetrahydropyridine (MPTP) in the squirrel monkey. *Brain Research*, 292, 390–394.

LARSON, J.L. & BULL, R.J. (1992) Species differences in the metabolism of trichloroethylene to the carcinogenic metabolites trichloroacetate and dichloroacetate. *Toxicology and Applied Pharmacology*, 115, 278–285.

LARSSON, A., ORRENIUS, S., HOLMGREN, A. & MANNERVIK, B. (1983) *Functions of Glutathione: Biochemical, Physiological, Toxicological and Clinical Aspects*. Raven, New York.

LAUWERYS, R.R. (1986) Occupational toxicology. In *Toxicology: The Basic Science of Poisons* (eds C.D. Klaassen, M.O. Amdur & J. Doull), pp. 902–915. Macmillan, New York.

  (1989) Metals – epidemiological and experimental evidence for carcinogenicity. *Archives of Toxicology* 13 (suppl.), 21–27.

LAUWERYS, R. & LOIS-FERDINAND (1984) The need for closer collaboration between clinical and experimental toxicologists. *Human Toxicology*, 3, 61–62.

LAUWERYS, R., AMERY, A., BERNARD, A., *et al.* (1990) Health effects of environmental exposure to cadmium: objectives, design and organisation of the Cadmibel study: a cross sectional morbidity study carried out in Belgium from 1985–1989. *Environmental Health Perspectives*, 87, 283–289.

LAUWERYS, R., BERNARD, A., BUCHET, J.P., *et al.* (1991) Does environmental exposure to cadmium represent a health risk? Conclusions from the Cadmibel study. *Acta Clinica Belgica*, 46, 219–225.

LAZARO, W.P. (1978) Rat liver peroxisomes catalyse the β-oxidation of fatty acids. *Journal of Biological Chemistry*, 253, 1522–1528.

LAZARO, W.P.L. & FUJIKI, Y. (1985) Biogenesis of peroxisomes. *Annual Reviews of Cell Biology*, 1, 489–530.

LEADBEATER, L. (1988) When all else fails. (Chemical Defence). *Chemistry in Britain*, 24, 683–688.

LEBLOND, C.P. & CLERMONT, Y. (1952) Definition of the stages of the cycle of the seminiferous epithelium in the rat. *Annals of the New York Academy of Science*, 55, 548–573.

LEVINE, R.R. & STEINBERG, G.M. (1966) Intestinal absorption of pralidoxime and other aldoximes. *Nature (London)*, 209, 269–271.

LIEBER, C.S. (1990) Mechanism of ethanol-induced hepatic injury. *Pharmacology and Therapeutics*, 46, 1–41.

LIEBERMAN, M.W., VERBIN, R.S., LANDAY, M., *et al.* (1970) A probable role for protein synthesis in intestinal epithelial cell damage induced *in vivo* by cytosine arabinoside, nitrogen mustard or X-irradiation. *Cancer Research*, 30, 942–951.

LIJINSKY, W., LOO, J. & ROSS, A.E. (1968) Mechanism of alkylation of nucleic acids by nitrosodimethylamine. *Nature (London)*, 218, 1174–1175.

LILLIE, R.D. & SMITH, M.I. (1932) The histopathology of some neurotoxic phenyl esters. *USA Public Health Reports*, 47, 54–64.

LINDAMOOD, G. (1991) Xenobiotic transformation. In *Hepatotoxicity* (eds R.G. Meeks, S.D. Harrison & R.J. Bull), pp. 139–180. CRC Press, Boca Raton, Florida.

LITWACK, G., KETTERER, B. & ARIAS, I.M. (1971) Ligandin: a hepatic protein which binds steroids, bilirubin, carcinogens and a number of exogenous organic anions. *Nature (London)*, 234, 466–467.

LOCK, E.A. & ISHMAEL, J. (1979) The acute toxic effects of hexachloro-1,3-butadiene on the rat kidney. *Archives of Toxicology*, 43, 47–57.

LOCK, E.A., MITCHELL, A.M. & ELCOMBE, C.R. (1989) Biochemical mechanisms of induction of hepatic peroxisome proliferation. *Annual Reviews in Pharmacology and Toxicology*, 29, 145–163.

LOTTI, M. (1987) Organophosphorus-induced delayed neuropathy in man and perspectives for biomonitoring. *Trends in Pharmacological Sciences*, 8, 176–177.

(1992) The pathogenesis of organophosphorus polyneuropathy. *Critical Reviews in Toxicology*, 21, 465–488.

LOTTI, M. & JOHNSON, M.K. (1980) Repeated small doses of a neurotoxic organophosphate: monitoring of neurotoxic esterase in brain and spinal cord. *Archives of Toxicology*, 45, 263–271.

LOTTI, M., BECKER, C.E. & AMINOFF, M.J. (1984) Organophosphate polyneuropathy: pathogenesis and prevention. *Neurology*, 34, 658–662.

LOTTI, M., CAROLDI, S., CAPODICASA, E. & MORETTO, A. (1991) Promotion of organophosphorus-induced delayed polyneuropathy by phenylmethanesulfonyl fluoride. *Toxicology and Applied Pharmacology*, 108, 234–241.

LOTTI, M., MORETTO, A., CAPODICASA, E., *et al.* (1993) Interactions between neuropathy target esterase and its inhibitors and the development of polyneuropathy. *Toxicology and Applied Pharmacology*, 122, 165–171.

LUSTER, M.I. & DEAN, J.H. (1982) Immunological hypersensitivity resulting from environmental or occupational exposure to chemicals: a state-of-the-art workshop summary. *Fundamental and Applied Toxicology*, 2, 327–330.

LUSTER, M.I., BLANK, J.A. & DEAN, J.H. (1987) Molecular and cellular basis of chemically induced immunotoxicity. *Annual Review of Pharmacology and Toxicology*, 27, 23–49.

MAGEE, P.N. (1956) Toxic liver injury: the metabolism of dimethylnitrosamine. *Biochemical Journal*, 64, 676–682.

MAGEE, P.N. & BARNES, J.M. (1956) The production of malignant primary hepatic tumours in the rat by feeding dimethylnitrosamine. *British Journal of Cancer*, 10, 114–122.

(1967) Carcinogenic nitroso compounds. *Advances in Cancer Research*, 10, 163–246.

MAGEE, P.N. & FARBER, E. (1962). Toxic liver injury and carcinogenicity: methylation of rat liver nucleic acids by dimethylnitrosamine. *Biochemical Journal*, 83, 114–124.

MAGOS, L. (1976) The effects of dimercaptosuccinic acid on the excretion and distribution of mercury in rats and mice treated with mercuric chloride and methylmercury chloride. *British Journal of Pharmacology*, 56, 479–484.

(1981) Metabolic factors in the distribution and half time of mercury after exposure to different mercurials. In *Industrial and Environmental Xenobiotics* (eds I. Gut, M. Cikrt & G.L. Plaa), pp. 1–15. Springer-Verlag, Berlin.

MAKAR, A.B., TEPHLY, T.R., SAHIN, G. & OSWEILER, G. (1990) Formate metabolism in young swine. *Toxicology and Applied Pharmacology*, 105, 315–320.

MALATS, N., REAL, F.X. & PORTA, M. (1993) DDT and pancreatic cancer. *Journal of the National Cancer Institute*, 85, 328.

MALI, J.W.H. & MALTEN, K.E. (1966) An epidemic of polymorph toxic erythema in the Netherlands in 1960. *Acta Dermatol-Venereol*, 46, 123–135.

MANNERVIK, B., AWASHTHI, I.C., BOARD, P.G., et al. (1992) Nomenclature for human glutathione transferases. *Biochemical Journal*, 282, 305–308.

MARGOSHES, M. & VALLEE, B.L. (1957) A cadmium protein from equine kidney cortex. *Journal of the American Chemical Society*, 79, 4813–4814.

MARON, D.M. & AMES, B.N. (1983) Revised methods for the *Salmonella* mutagenicity test. *Mutation Research*, 113, 173–215.

MARSELOS, M. & TOMATIS, L. (1992) I. Pharmacology, toxicology and carcinogenicity in humans. *European Journal of Cancer*, 28A, 1182–1189.

MARTIN, C.N. and GARNER, R.C. (1977) Aflatoxin B_1-oxide generated by chemical or enzymic oxidation of aflatoxin B_1 causes guanine substitution in nucleic acids. *Nature (London)*, 267, 863–865.

MARTIN-AMAT, G., MCMARTIN, K.E., HAYREH, S.S., HAYREH, M.S. & TEPHLY, T.R. (1978) Methanol poisoning: ocular toxicity produced by formate. *Toxicology and Applied Pharmacology*, 45, 201–208.

MARTINÉZ-TELLO, F.J., NAVAS-PALACIOS, J.J., RICOY, J.R., et al. (1982) Pathology of a new toxic syndrome caused by ingestion of adulterated oil in Spain. *Virchows Archives (A)*, 397, 261–285.

MATSUNAGA, S., MOORE, R.E., NIEMCZURA, W.P. & CARMICHAEL, W.W. (1989) Anatoxin-a(S), a potent anticholinesterase from *Anabaena flos-aquae*. *Journal of the American Chemical Society*, 111, 8021–8023.

MATTOCKS, A.R. (1968) Toxicity of pyrollizidine alkaloids. *Nature (London)*, 217, 723–728.

(1986) *Chemistry and Toxicology of Pyrrolizidine Alkaloids*. Academic Press, London.

MATTOCKS, A.R., LEGG, R.F. & JUKES, R. (1990) Trapping of short-lived electrophilic metabolites of pyrrolizidine alkaloids escaping from perfused rat liver. *Toxicology Letters*, 54, 93–99.

MCCONKEY, D.J., HARTZELL, P., DUDDY, S.K., HAKANSSON, H. & ORRENIUS, S. (1988) 2,3,7,8-Tetrachlorodibenzo-*p*-dioxin kills immature thymocytes by Ca^{2+}-mediated endonuclease activation. *Science*, 242, 256–259.

MCCONKEY, D.J. & ORRENIUS, S. (1989) 2,3,7,8-Tetrachlorodibenzo-*p*-dioxin (TCDD) kills glucocorticoid-sensitive thymocytes *in vivo*. *Biochemical and Biophysical Research Communications*, 160, 1003–1008.

MCLAREN, D.S. (1978) Nutritional deficiencies in animals and man: vitamin A. In *Effect of Nutrient Deficiencies in Man: Handbook Series in Nutrition and Food*. (ed. M. Recheigl), Vol. 3, pp. 107–116. CRC Press, Boca Raton, Florida.

MCLEAN, E.K. (1970) The toxic action of pyrrolizidine (Senecio) alkaloids. *Pharmacological Reviews*, 22, 429–483.

MCLEMORE, T.L., ADELBERG, S., LIU, M.C., et al. (1990) Expression of CYP1A1 gene in patients with lung cancer: evidence for cigarette smoke-induced expression in normal lung tissue and for altered gene regulation in primary pulmonary carcinomas. *Journal of the National Cancer Institute*, 82, 1333–1339.

MEBUS, C.A., CLARKE, D.A., STEDMAN, D.B. & WELSCH, F. (1992) 2-Methoxyethanol metabolism in pregnant CD-1 mice and embryos. *Toxicology and Applied Pharmacology*, 112, 87–94.

MEDAWAR, P. (1986) *Memoir of a Thinking Radish – An Autobiography*. Oxford University Press, Oxford.

MEEHAN, A.P. (1984) *Rats and Mice: Their Biology and Control*, pp. 1–383. Rentokil Ltd, East Grinstead. UK.

MEIER, J.R. (1988) Genotoxicity activity of organic chemicals in drinking water. *Mutation Research*, 196, 211–245.

MEISTER, A. & ANDERSON, M.E. (1983) Glutathione. *Annual Review of Biochemistry*, 52, 432–435.

MEREDITH, C. & JOHNSON, M.K. (1988) Neuropathy target esterase: rates of turnover *in vivo* following covalent inhibition with phenyl di *n*-pentylphosphinate. *Journal of Neurochemistry*, 51, 1097–1101.

MESNIL, R.T., TESTA, B. & JENNER, P. (1985) Arylhydrocarbon hydroxylase in rat brain microsomes. *Biochemical Pharmacology*, 34, 435–436.

MILATOVIC, D. & JOHNSON, M.K. (1993) Reactivation of phosphorodiamidated acetyl-cholinesterase (AChE) and neuropathy target esterase (NTE) by treatment of inhibited enzyme with potassium fluoride. *Chemico-Biological Interactions*, 87, 425–430.

MILLER, M.S. & SPENCER, P.S. (1985) The mechanisms of acrylamide axonopathy. *Annual Reviews in Pharmacology and Toxicology*, 25, 643–666.

MILLER, R.R., HERMANN, E.A., LANGVARDT, P.W., McKENNA, M.J. & SCHWETZ, B.A. (1983) Comparative metabolism and disposition of ethylene glycol monomethyl ether and propylene glycol monomethyl ether in male rats. *Toxicology and Applied Pharmacology*, 67, 229–237.

MINCHIN, R.F. & BOYD, M.R. (1983) Localisation of metabolic activation and deactivation systems in the lung: significance to the pulmonary toxicity of xenobiotics. *Annual Reviews of Pharmacology and Toxicology*, 23, 217–238.

MINN, A., GHERSI-EGEA, J.F., PERRIN, R., LEININGER, B. & SIEST, G. (1991) Drug metabolising enzymes in the brain and cerebral micro-vessels. *Brain Research Reviews*, 16, 65–82.

MORETTO, A., CAPODICASA, E., PERIACA, M. & LOTTI, M. (1991) Age sensitivity to organophosphate-induced delayed polyneuropathy. *Biochemical Pharmacology*, 41, 1497–1504.

MORETTO, A., CAPODICASA, E. & LOTTI, M. (1992) Clinical expression of organophosphate-induced delayed polyneuropathy in rats. *Toxicology Letters*, 63, 97–102.

MORGAN, K.T., GROSS, E.A., LYGHT, O. & BOND, J.A. (1985) Methodological and biochemical studies of a nitrobenzene-induced encephalopathy in rats. *Neurotoxicology*, 6, 105–116.

MOORHOUSE, K.G., LOGAN, C.J., HUTSON, D.H. & DODDS, P.F. (1990) The incorporation of 3-phenoxybenzoic acid and other xenobiotic acids into xenobiotic lipids by enzymes of the monoacylglycerol pathway in microsomes from adult and neonatal tissues. *Biochemical Pharmacology*, 39, 1529–1536.

MOORHOUSE, K.G., DODDS, P.F. & HUTSON, D.H. (1991) Xenobiotic triacylglycerol formation in isolated hepatocytes. *Biochemical Pharmacology*, 41, 1179–1185.

MOSS, E.J., THOMAS, L.V., COOK, M.W., *et al.* (1985) The role of metabolism in methoxyethanol-induced testicular toxicity. *Toxicology and Applied Pharmacology*, 79, 480–489.

MULDER, G.J. (1992) Pharmacological aspects of drug conjugates: is morphine 6-glucuronide an exception? *Trends in Pharmacological Sciences*, 13, 302–304.

MURRAY, R.E. & GIBSON, J.E. (1972) A comparative study of paraquat intoxication in rats, guinea pigs and monkeys. *Experimental and Molecular Pathology*, 17, 317–325.

NARAHASHI, T. (1990) Occurrence and mechanism of action of marine neurotoxins. In *Basic Science in Toxicology* (eds G.N. Volans, J. Sims, F.M. Sullivan & P. Turner), pp. 580–595. Taylor & Francis, London.

(1992) Nerve membrane Na$^+$ channels as targets of insecticides. *Trends in Pharmacological Sciences*, 13, 236–241.

References

NASH, J.A., KING, L.J., LOCK, E.A. & GREEN, T. (1984) The metabolism and disposition of hexachloro-1,3-butadiene in the rat and its relevance to nephrotoxicity. *Toxicology and Applied Pharmacology*, 73, 124–137.

NATIONAL RESEARCH COUNCIL/NATIONAL ACADEMY OF SCIENCE. (1982) *Diet, Nutrition and Cancer*. National Academy Press, Washington, DC.

NELSON, B.K., SETZER, J.B., BRIGHTWELL, W.S., *et al.* (1984) Comparative inhalation teratology of four glycol ether solvents and an amino derivative in rats. *Environmental Health Perspectives*, 57, 261–271.

NELSON, D.R., KAMATAKI, T., WAXMAN, D.J., *et al.* (1993) The P450 superfamily: update on new sequences, gene mapping, accession numbers, early trivial names of enzymes and nomenclature. *DNA and Cell Biology*, 12, 1–51.

NEMERY, B. & ALDRIDGE, W.N. (1988a) Studies on the metabolism of the pneumotoxin O,S,S,-trimethyl phosphorodithioate. 1: Lung and liver microsomes. *Biochemical Pharmacology*, 37, 3709–3715.

(1988b) Studies of the metabolism of the pneumotoxin O,S,S,-trimethyl phosphorodithioate. 2: Lung and liver slices. *Biochemical Pharmacology*, 37, 3717–3722.

NEMERY, B., DINSDALE, D., SPARROW, S. & RAY, D.E. (1985). Effects of methylisocyanate on the respiratory tract of rats. *British Journal of Industrial Medicine*, 42, 799–805.

NEUMANN, H.G. (1980) Dose–response relationship in the primary lesion of strong electrophilic carcinogens. *Archives of Toxicology* (Suppl. 3), 69–77.

NISHIWAKI-MATSUSHIMA, R., OHTA, T., NISHIWAKI, S., *et al.* (1991) Liver tumour promotion by the cyanobacterial cyclic peptide toxin microcystin-LR. *Journal of Cancer Research and Clinical Oncology*, 118, 420–424.

NORDGREN, I., BERGSTROM, M., HOLMSTEDT, B. & SANDOZ, M. (1978) Transformation and action of metrifonate. *Archives of Toxicology*, 41, 31–41.

NUYTS, G.D., ROELS, H.A., VERPOOTEN, G.F., *et al.* (1992) Intestinal-type alkaline phosphatase in urine as an indicator of mercury induced effects on the S3 segment of the proximal tubule. *Nephrology, Dialysis and Transplantation*, 7, 225–229.

O'BRIEN, R.D., TRIPATHI, R.K. & HOWELL, L.L. (1978) Substrate preferences of wild mutant housefly acetylcholinesterase and a comparison with bovine erythrocyte enzyme. *Biochimica Biologica Acta*, 526, 129–134.

ORRENIUS, S., MCCABE, M.J. & NICOTERA, P. (1992) Ca^{2+}-dependent mechanisms of cytotoxicity and programmed cell death. *Toxicology Letters*, 64/65, 357–364.

ORRENIUS, S, , MCCONKEY, D.J., BELLOMO, G. & NICOTERA, P. (1989) Role of Ca^{2+} in toxic cell killing. *Trends in Pharmacological Sciences*, 10, 281-285.

ORRENIUS, S. & MOLDEUS, P. (1984) The multiple role of glutathione in drug metabolism. *Trends in Pharmacological Sciences*, 5, 432–435.

ORWELL, G. (1944) Essay No. 68, Arthur Koestler. In *The Collected Essays, Journalism and Letters of George Orwell, Volume 3, 1943–1945*, pp. 270–282. Penguin, London.

OSTERMAN-GOLKAR, S., FARMER, P.B., SEGERBACK, D., *et al.* (1983) Dosimetry of ethylene oxide in the rat by quantitation of alkylated histidine in haemoglobin. *Teratogen Carcinogen and Mutagen*, 3, 395–405.

PADDLE, G.M. (1983) Incidence of liver cancer and trichloroethylene manufacture: joint study by industry and a cancer registry. *British Medical Journal*, 286, 846–847.

PARACELSUS, THEOPHRASTUS BOMBASTUS VON HOHENHEIM GEN. (1538) *Epistola dedicatora St. Veit/Karnten; Sieben Defensionen oder Sieben Schutz- Schirm- und Trutzreden. Drit Defension*.

PARKE, D.V. (1968) *The Biochemistry of Foreign Compounds*. Chapman and Hall, Oxford.

PATEL, J.M., WOOD, J.C. & LEIBMAN, K.C. (1980) The biotransformation of alkyl alcohol and acrolein in rat liver and lung preparations. *Drug Metabolism and Disposal*, 8, 305–308.

PATON, W. (1994) *Man and Mouse: Animals in Medical Research*. Oxford University Press, Oxford.

PAULING, L., ITANO, H.A., SINGER, S.J. & WELLS, I.C. (1949) Sickle cell anaemia: a molecular disease. *Science*, 110, 543–548.

PERSSON, P-E., SIVONEN, K., KETO, J., *et al.* (1984) Potentially toxic blue–green algae (cyanobacteria) in Finnish natural waters. *Aqua Fennica*, 14, 147–154.

PETERS, R.A. (1957) Mechanism of the toxicity of the active constituent of *Dichapetalum cymosum* and related compounds. *Advances in Enzymology*, 18, 113–159.

—— (1963) *Biochemical Lesions and Lethal Synthesis*. Pergamon, Oxford.

PETERS, R.A. & WAKELIN, R.W. (1957) The synthesis of fluorocitric acid and its inhibition by acetate. *Biochemical Journal*, 67, 280–286.

PETERS, R.A., STOCKEN, L.A. & THOMPSON, R.H.S. (1945). British anti-lewisite (BAL). *Nature (London)*, 156, 616–619.

PETO, R., GRAY, R., BRANTOM, P. & GRASSO, P. (1991a) Dose and time relationships for tumour induction in the liver and aesophagus of 4080 inbred rats by chronic ingestion of *N*-nitrosodiethylamine and *N*-nitrosodimethylamine. *Cancer Research*, 51, 6452–6469.

—— (1991b) Effects on 4080 rats of chronic ingestion of *N*-nitrosodiethylamine and *N*-nitrosodimethylamine: a detailed dose–response study. *Cancer Research*, 51, 6415–6451.

PHILBERT, M.A., NOLAN, C.C., CREMER, J.E., TUCKER, D. & BROWN, A.W. (1987) 1,3-Dinitrobenzene-induced encephalopathy in rats. *Neuropathology and Applied Neurobiology*, 13, 371–389.

PIETERS, R.H.H., BOL, M., SEINEN, W. & PENNINKS, A.H. (1992) The organotin-induced thymus atrophy, characterised by depletion of CD4$^+$CD8$^+$ thymocytes, is preceded by a reduction of the immature CD4$^-$CD8$^+$ TcR$\alpha\beta^{-/low}$CD2^{high} thymoblast subset. *Immunology*, 76, 203–208.

PLAA, G.L. (1986) Toxic responses in the liver. In *Toxicology: The Basic Science of Poisons* (eds C.D. Klaassen, M.O. Amdur & J. Doull), pp. 286–309. Macmillan, New York.

PLESTINA, R. & STONER, H.B. (1972) Pulmonary oedema in rats given monocrotaline pyrrole. *Journal of Pathology and Bacteriology*, 106, 235–249.

PLESTINA, R., DAVIS, A. & BAILEY, D.R. (1972) Effect of metrifonate on blood cholinesterases in children during treatment of Schistosomiasis. *Bulletin of the World Health Organization*, 46, 747–759.

POHJANVIRTA, R., KULJU, T., MORSELT, A.F.W., *et al.* (1989) Target tissue morphology and serum biochemistry following 2,3,7,8-tetrachlorodibenzo-*p*-dioxin (TCDD) exposure in TCDD-susceptible and TCDD-resistant rat strains. *Fundamental and Applied Toxicology*, 12, 698–712.

POHJANVIRTA, R. & TUOMISTO, J. (1994) Short term toxicity of 2,3,7,8-tetrachlorodibenzo-*p*-dioxin (TCDD) in laboratory animals: effects, mechanisms and animal models. *Pharmacological Reviews*, 46, 483–542.

POLAND, A. & KNUTSON, J.C. (1982) 2,3,7,8-Tetrachlorodibenzo-*p*-dioxin and related halogenated aromatic hydrocarbons: examination of the mechanisms of toxicity. *Annual Review of Pharmacology and Toxicology*, 22, 517–554.

POPPER, K.R. (1974) *Conjectures and Refutations: The Growth of Scientific Knowledge*. Routledge & Kegan Paul, London.

PORTER, T.D. & COON, M.J. (1991) Cytochrome P450: multiplicity of isoforms, substrates and catalytic and regulatory mechanisms. *Journal of Biological Chemistry*, 266, 13469–13472

POSKANZER, D. & HERBST, A. (1977) Epidemiology of vaginal adenosis and adenocarcinoma associated with exposure to stilboestrol *in utero*. *Cancer*, 39, 1892–1895.

POTTS, A.M., PRAGLIN, J., FARKAS, I., ORBISON, L. & CHICKERING, D. (1955) Studies on the visual toxicity of methanol. VIII: Additional observation on methanol poisoning in the primate test object. *American Journal of Opthamology*, 40, 76–82.

PRICE, S.C., HALL, D.E. & HINTON, R.H. (1985) Lipid accumulation in the livers of chlorpromazine-treated rats does not induce peroxisome proliferation. *Toxicology Letters*, 25, 11–18.

PRINEAS, J. (1969) The pathogenesis of dying back polyneuropathies. 2: An ultrastructural study of experimental acrylamide intoxication in the cat. *Journal of Neuropathology and Experimental Neurology*, 28, 598–621.

PROUT, M.S., PROVAN, W.M. & GREEN, T. (1985) Species differences in response to trichloroethylene. I: Pharacokinetics in rats and mice. *Toxicology and Applied Pharmacology*, 79, 389–400.

PULIDO, P., KAGI, J.H.R. & VALLEE, B.L. (1966) Isolation and some properties of human metallothionein. *Biochemistry*, 5, 1768–1777.

PURCHASE, I.F.H. (1994) Current knowledge of mechanisms of carcinogenicity: genotoxins versus non-genotoxins. *Human and Experimental Toxicology*, 13, 17–28.

PURCHASE, I.F.H & THERON, J.J. (1968). The acute toxicity of ochratoxin A to rats. *Food and Cosmetic Toxicology*, 6, 479–483.

PURCHASE, I.F.H., STAFFORD, J. & PADDLE, G.M. (1987) Vinyl chloride: an assessment of the risk of occupational exposure. *Food and Chemical Toxicology*, 25, 187–202.

RAAG, R. & POULOS, T. (1991) Crystal structures of cytochrome $P450_{CAM}$ complexed with camphane, thiocamphor and adamantane: factors controlling P450 substrate hydroxylation. *Biochemistry*, 30, 2674–2684.

RAFFRAY, M., MCCARTHY, D., SNOWDEN, R.T. & COHEN, G.M. (1993) Apoptosis as a mechanism of tributyltin cytotoxicity, relationship of apoptotic markers to biochemical and cellular effects. *Toxicology and Applied Pharmacology*, 119, 122–130.

RANDERATH, K., REDDY, M.F. & GUPTA, R.C. (1981) ^{32}P-Labelling test for DNA damage. *Proceedings of the National Academy of Sciences*, 78, 6126–6129.

RANDERATH, K., RANDERATH, E., AGRAWAL, H.P., *et al.* (1985) Postlabelling methods for carcinogen–DNA adduct analysis. *Environmental Health Perspectives*, 62, 57–65.

RAO, M.S. & REDDY, J.K.B (1987) Peroxisome proliferation and hepatocarcinogenesis. *Carcinogenesis*, 8, 631–636.

RAO, M.S., THORGEIRSSON, S., REDDY, M.K., *et al.*, (1986) Induction of peroxisome proliferation in hepatocytes transplanted into the anterior chamber of the eye. *American Journal of Pathology*, 124, 519–527.

RAWLINGS, S.J., SHUKER, D.F.G., WEBB, M. & BROWN, N.A. (1985) The teratogenic potential of alkoxy acids in post-implantation rat embryo culture: structure-activity relationships. *Toxicology Letters*, 28, 49–58.

RAY, D.E., BROWN, A.W., CAVANAGH, J.B., *et al.* (1992) Functional/metabolic modulation of the brain stem lesions caused by 1,3-dinitrobenzene in the rat. *Neurotoxicology*, 13, 379–388.

REDDY, B.S., COHEN, L.A., MCCOY, G.D., *et al.* (1980) Nutrition and its relationship to cancer. *Advances in Cancer Research*, 32, 237–345.

REDDY, J.K. & KUMAR, N.S. (1977) The peroxisome proliferation associated polypeptide in rat liver. *Biochemical and Biophysical Research Communications*, 77, 824–829.

REDDY, J.K. & LALWANI, N.D. (1983) Carcinogenesis by hepatic peroxisome proliferators: evaluation of the risk of hypolipidaemic drugs and industrial plasticisers to humans. *Critical Reviews in Toxicology*, 12, 1–58.

REDDY, J.K., LALWANI, N.D., QURESHI, S.A., REDDY, M.K. & MOEHLE, C.M. (1984a) Induction of hepatic peroxisome proliferation in non-rodent species including primates. *American Journal of Pathology*, 114, 171–183.

REDDY, J.K., RAO, M.S., QURESHI, S.A., *et al.* (1984b) Induction and origin of hepatocytes in rat pancreas. *Journal of Cell Biology*, 98, 2081–2090.

REDDY, J.K., JIRTLE, R.L., WATANABE, T.K., *et al.* (1984c) Response of hepatocytes transplanted into syngeneic hosts and heteroplanted into athymic mice to peroxisomal proliferators. *Cancer Research*, 44, 2582–2589.

REED, D.J. (1990) Glutathione: toxicological implications. *Annual Reviews of Pharmacology and Toxicology*, 30, 603–631.

REEVES, P.R., CASE, D.E., JEPSON, H.T., *et al.* (1978) Practolol metabolism. II: Metabolism in human subjects. *Journal of Pharmacology and Experimental Therapeutics*, 205, 489–498.

REGAN, T. (1983) *The Case for Animal Rights*. Routledge & Kegan Paul, London.

REGGIANI, G. (1983) An overview on the health effects of halogenated dioxins and related compounds: the Yusho and Taiwan episodes. In *Accidental Exposure to Dioxins* (eds F. Coulston & F. Pocchiari), pp. 39–67. Academic Press, New York.

REID, W.D. (1972) Mechanism of allyl alcohol-induced hepatic necrosis. *Experientia*, 28, 1058–1061.

REINER, E., KRAUTHACKER, B., SIMEON, V. & SKRINJARIC-SPOLJAR, M. (1975). Mechanism of inhibition *in vitro* of mammalian acetylcholinesterase and cholinesterase in solution of *O,O*-dimethyl 2,2,2-trichloro-l-hydroxyethyl phosphate (trichlorphon). *Biochemical Pharmacology*, 24, 717–722.

RICKARD, J. & BRODIE, M.E. (1985) Correlation of blood and brain levels of the neurotoxic pyrethroid deltamethrin with the onset of symptoms in rats. *Pesticide Biochemistry and Physiology*, 23, 143–156.

RÖE, O. (1982) Species differences in methanol toxicity. *Critical Reviews in Toxicology*, 10, 275–287.

ROELS, H.A., LAUWERYS, R.R., BUCHET, J.P., *et al.* (1989) Health significance of cadmium induced renal dysfunction: a five year follow up. *British Journal of Industrial Medicine*, 46, 755–764.

ROGULJA, P.V., KOVAC, W. & SCHMID, H. (1973) Metronidazol-encephalopathie der ratte. *Acta Neuropathologica (Berlin)*, 25, 36–45.

ROITT, I.M., BROSTOFF, J. & MALE, D.K. (1989) *Immunology*. Gower Medical Publishing, London.

ROMERO, I., BROWN, A.W. CAVANAGH, J.B., *et al.* (1991) Vascular factors in the neurotoxic damage caused by 1,3-dinitrobenzene in the rat. *Neuropathology and Applied Neurobiology*, 17, 495–508.

ROSE, G.P. & DEWAR, A.J. (1983) Intoxication with four synthetic pyrethroids fails to show any correlation between neuromuscular dysfunction and neurobiochemical abnormalities in rats. *Archives of Toxicology*, 53, 297–316.

ROSE, G.P., DEWAR, A.J. & STRATFORD, I.J. (1980) A biochemical method for assessing the neurotoxic effects of misonidazole in the rat. *British Journal of Cancer*, 42, 890–899.

ROSE, M.S. & ALDRIDGE, W.N. (1968). The interaction of triethyltin with components of animal tissues. *Biochemical Journal*, 106, 821–828.

ROSE, M.S., SMITH, L.L. & WYATT, I. (1974) Evidence for energy-dependent accumulation of paraquat in rat lung. *Nature (London)*, 252, 314–315.

ROSE, M.S., LOCK, E.A., SMITH, L.L. & WYATT, I. (1976) Paraquat accumulation: tissue and species specificity. *Biochemical Pharmacology*, 25, 419–423.

ROUGHTON, F.J.W. & DARLING, R.C. (1944). The effect of carbon dioxide on the oxygen dissociation curve. *American Journal of Physiology*, 141, 17–31.

ROWLAND, I.R., MALLETT, A.K. & WISE, A. (1985) The effect of diet on the mammalian gut flora and its metabolic activity. *CRC Critical Reviews in Toxicology*, 16, 31–103.

ROYAL SOCIETY STUDY GROUP (1992) *Risk: Analysis, Perception and Management*. Royal Society, London.

RUSSELL, L.D. (1980) Sertoli-germ cell interactions: a review. *Gamete Research*, 3, 179–202.

SAFE, S. (1984) Polychlorinated biphenyls (PCB's) and polybrominated biphenyls (PBB's): biochemistry, toxicology and mechanism of action. *CRC Critical Reviews in Toxicology*, 13, 319–396.

(1990) Polychlorinated biphenyls (PCBs), dibenzo-*p*-dioxins (PCDDs), dibenzofurans (PCDFs) and related compounds: environmental and mechanistic considerations which support the development of toxic equivalency factors (TEFs). *CRC Critical Reviews in Toxicology*, 21, 51–88.

SAKAMOTO, J, KUROSAKA, Y. & HASHIMOTO, K. (1988) Histological changes of acrylamide-induced testicular lesions in mice. *Experimental and Molecular Pathology*, 48, 324–334.

SANDERMAN, H. (1992) Plant metabolism of xenobiotics. *Trends in Biochemical Sciences*, 17, 82–84.

SANDLER, M., ed. (1980) *Enzyme Inhibitors as Drugs*. Macmillan, Basingstoke.

SANDLER, M. & SMITH, H.J., eds (1989) *Design of Enzyme Inhibitors as Drugs*. Oxford University Press, Oxford.

References

SAYRE, L.M., SHEARSON, C.M., WONGRONGKOLRIT, T., MEDORI, R. & GAMBETTI, P. (1986) Structural basis of γ-diketone neurotoxicity: non-neurotoxicity of 3,3-dimethyl-2,5,-hexanedione, a γ-diketone incapable of pyrrole formation. *Toxicology and Applied Pharmacology*, 84, 36–44.

SCATCHARD, G. (1949) The attractions of proteins for small molecules. *Annals of the New York Academy of Sciences*, 51, 660–672.

SCHANNE, F.A.X., KANE, A.B., YOUNG E.E. & FARBER, J.L. (1979) Calcium, dependence of toxic cell death: a final common pathway. *Science*, 206, 700–702.

SCHAUMBURG, H.H., WISMEWSKI, H.M. & SPENCER, P.S. (1974) Ultrastructural studies of the dying back process. I: peripheral nerve terminal and axonal degeneration in synthetic acrylamide intoxication. *Journal of Neuropathology and Experimental Neurology*, 33, 260–284.

SCHELINE, R.R. (1973) Metabolism of foreign compounds by gastrointestinal micro-organisms. *Pharmacological Reviews*, 25, 451–523.

SCHMAHL, D. (1979) Problems of dose–response studies in chemical carcinogenesis with special reference to N-nitroso compounds. *CRC Critical Reviews in Toxicology*, 6, 257–281.

SCHMECHEL, D., MARANGOS, P.J., ZIS, A.R., BRIGHTMAN, M. & GOODWIN, F.K. (1978) Brain enolases as specific markers of neuronal and glial cells. *Science*, 199, 313–315.

SCHNEIDER, H. & CERVÓS-NAVARRO, J. (1974) Acute gliopathy in spinal cord and brain stem induced by 6-aminonicotinamide. *Acta Neuropathologica (Berlin)*, 27, 11–23.

SCOTT, J.K. NEUMAN, W.F. & ALLEN, R. (1950) The effect of added carrier on the distribution and excretion of soluble Be[7]. *Journal of Biological Chemistry*, 182, 291–298.

SEINEN, W., VOS, J.G., VAN SPANJE, I., *et al.* (1977a) Toxicity of organotin compounds. 2: Comparative *in vivo* and *in vitro* studies with various organotin and organolead compounds in different animal species with special emphasis on lymphocyte cytotoxicity. *Toxicology and Applied Pharmacology*, 42, 197–212.

SEINEN, W., VOS, J.G., VAN KRIEKEN, R., *et al.* (1977b) Toxicity of organotin compounds. 3: Suppression of thymus dependent immunity in rats by di-n-butyltin dichloride and di-n-octyltin dichloride. *Toxicology and Applied Pharmacology*, 42, 213–224.

SEINEN, W. & WILLEMS, M.I. (1976) Toxicity of organotin compounds. 1: Atrophy of thymus and thymus dependent lymphoid tissue in rats fed di-n-octyltin dichloride. *Toxicology and Applied Pharmacology*, 35, 63–75.

SELWYN, M.J. (1976) Triorganotin compounds as ionophores and inhibitors of ion translocating ATPases. In *Organotin Compounds: New Chemistry and Applications* (ed. J.J. Zuckerman), pp. 204–226. Advances in Chemistry Series No. 157, American Chemical Society, Washington, DC.

SENIOR, A.E. (1988) ATP synthesis by oxidative phosphorylatlon. *Physiological Reviews*, 68, 177–231.

SHARMA, R., LAKE, B.G. & GIBSON, G.G. (1988) Co-induction of microsomal cytochrome P-452 and peroxisomal fatty acid β-oxidation pathway in the rat by clofibrate and di(2-ethylhexyl)-phthalate. *Biochemical Pharmacology*, 37, 1203–1206.

SHEN, W., KAMENDULLS, L.M., RAY, S.D. & CORCORAN, G.B. (1992) Acetaminophen-induced cytotoxicity in cultured mouse hepatocytes: effects of Ca^{2+} endonuclease, DNA repair and glutathione depletion inhibitors on DNA fragmentation and cell death. *Toxicology and Applied Pharmacology*, 112, 32–40.

SHERRATT, H.S.A. & OSMUNDSEN, H. (1976) On the mechanism of some pharmacological actions of the hypoglycaemic toxins hypoglycin and pent-4-enoic acid: a way out of the present confusion. *Biochemical Pharmacology*, 25, 743–750.

SHIMADA, T., YUN, C-H., YAMAZAKI, H., *et al.* (1992) Characterisation of human lung microsomal P4501A1 and its role in the oxidation of chemical carcinogens. *Molecular Pharmacology*, 41, 856–864.

SIEBENLIST, K.R. & TAKETA, F. (1983) Inactivation of yeast hexokinase B by triethyltin bromide. *Biochemistry*, 22, 4229–4234.

SIMEON, V., REINER, E. & VERNON, C.A. (1972) Effect of temperature and pH on carbamoylation and phosphorylation of serum cholinesterases: theoretical interpretation of activation energies in complex reactions. *Biochemical Journal*, 130, 515–524.

SINGER, P. (1983) *Animal Liberation*. Thorsons, Wellingborough, UK.

SIPES, I.G. & GANDOLFI, A.J. (1986) Biotransformation of toxicants. In *Toxicology: The Basic Science of Poisons* (eds C.D. Klaassen, M.O. Amdur & J. Doull), pp. 64–98. Macmillan, New York.

SIVONEN, K., NAMIKOSHI, M., EVANS, W.R., *et al.* (1992) Isolation and characterisation of a variety of microcystins from seven strains of the cyanobacterial genus *Anabaena*. *Applied Environmental Microbiology*, 58, 2495–2500.

SKERFVING, S. & VOSTAL, J. (1972) Symptoms and signs of intoxication. In *Mercury in the Environment: An Epidemiological and Toxicological Appraisal* (eds L. Friberg & J. Vostal), pp. 93–108. CRC Press, Clevedon, Ohio.

SKILLETER, D.N. (1989) Molecular mechanisms of beryllium toxicity. *Life Science Reports*, 7, 245–283.

SKILLETER, D.N. & PRICE, R.J. (1978) The uptake and subsequent loss of beryllium by rat liver parenchymal and non-parenchymal cells after the intravenous administration of particulate and soluble forms. *Chemico-Biological Interactions*, 20, 383–396.

(1979) The role of lysosomes in the hepatic accumulation and release of beryllium. *Biochemical Pharmacology*, 28, 3595–3599.

(1981) Effects of beryllium compounds on rat liver Kupffer cells in culture. *Toxicology and Applied Pharmacology*, 59, 279–286.

SKRINJARIC-SPOLJAR, M., SIMEON, V. & REINER, E. (1973) Spontaneous reactivation and aging of dimethylphosphorylated acetylcholinesterase and cholinesterase. *Biochimica et Biophysica Acta*, 315, 363–369.

SLUTSKER, L., HOESLY, F.C., MILLER, L., *et al.* (1990) Eosinophilia–myalgia syndrome associated with exposure to tryptophan from a single manufacturer. *Journal of the American Medical Association*, 264, 213–217.

SMIALOWICZ, R.J., RIDDLE, M.M., ROGERS, R.R., *et al.*, (1991) Evaluation of the immunotoxicity of orally administered 2-methoxyacetic acid in Fischer 344 rats. *Fundamental and Applied Toxicology*, 17, 771–781.

SMIALOWICZ, R.J., RIDDLE, M.M. & WILLIAMS, W.C. (1993) Methoxyacetaldehyde, an intermediate metabolite of 2-methoxyethanol, is immunosuppressive in the rat. *Fundamental and Applied Toxicology*, 21, 1–7.

SMITH, H.V. & SPALDING, J.M.K. (1959) Outbreak of paralysis in Morocco due to ortho cresyl phosphate poisoning. *Lancet*, 2, 1019–1021.

SMITH, L.L. & NEMERY, B. (1986) The lung as a target organ for toxicity. In *Target Organ Toxicity* (ed. G.M. Cohen), Vol. 2, pp. 45–80. CRC Press, Boca Raton, Florida.

SMITH, L.L. & WYATT, I. (1981) The accummulation of putrescine into slices of rat lung and brain and its relationship to the accummulation of paraquat. *Biochemical Pharmacology*, 30, 1053–1058.

SMITH, L.L., COHEN, G.M. & ALDRIDGE, W.N. (1986) Morphological and bio-chemical correlates of chemical induced injury in the lung. *Archives of Toxicology*, 58, 214–218.

SMITH, L.W. and CULVENOR, C.C. (1981) Plant sources of hepatotoxic pyrrolizidine alkaloids. *Journal of Natural Products*, 44, 129–152.

SMITH, M.I. & ELVOVE, E. (1930) Pharmacological and chemical studies of the so-called ginger paralysis. *USA Public Health Reports*, 45, 1703–1716.

SMITH, M.I., ELVOVE, E. & FRAZIER, W.H. (1930) Pharmacological action of certain phenol esters with special references to the etiology of so-called ginger paralysis. *USA Public Health Reports*, 45, 2509–2524.

SMITH, M.I., ENGEL, E.W. & STOHLMAN, E.F. (1932) Further studies on the pharmacology of certain phenol esters with special reference to the relation of chemical constitution and physiologic action. *USA Public Health Reports*, 47, 1–53.

References

SMITH, P. & HEATH, D. (1976) Paraquat. *Critical Reviews in Toxicology*, 4, 411–445.

SMITH, R.P. (1986) Toxic responses of the blood. In *Toxicology: The Basic Science of Poisons*, (eds C.D. Klaasson, M.O. Anadur & J. Doull), pp. 223–244. Macmillan, New York.

SNOEIJ, N.J., PENNINKS, A.H. & SEINEN, W. (1988) Dibutyltin and tributyltin compounds induce thymus atrophy in rats due to a selective action on thymic lymphoblasts. *International Journal of Immunopharmacology*, 10, 891–899.

SONES, K., HEANEY, R.K. & FENWICK, G.R. (1984) The glucosinolate content of UK vegetables – cabbage (*Brassicae oleracea*), swede (*B. napus*) and turnip (*B. campestris*). *Food Additives and Contaminants*, 1, 289–296.

SPENCER, P.S. & SCHAUMBURG, H.H. (1975) Experimental neuropathy produced by 2,5-hexanedione – a major metabolite of the neurotoxic industrial solvent methyl *n*-butyl ketone. *Journal of Neurology, Neurosurgery and Psychiatry*, 38, 771–775.

SPENCER, P.S. & SCHAUMBURG, H.H. (1976) Central–peripheral distal axonopathy – the pathology of dying-back polyneuropathies. *Progress in Neuropathology*, 3, 253–295.

STANBURY, J.B., WYNGAARDEN, J.B. FREDRICKSON, D.S., GOLSTEIN, J.L. & BROWN, M.S., eds (1983) *The Metabolic Basis for Inherited Disease*. McGraw-Hill, New York.

STOLOFF, L. (1977). Aflatoxin – an overview. In *Mycotoxins in Human and Animal Health* (eds J.W. Rodrick, C.W. Heseltine & M.A. Mehlman) Pathotox Publishers, Park Forest South, Illinois.

STONER, H.B. (1961) Studies on the mechanism of shock: the activity of the reticuloendothelial system after limb ischaemia in the rat. *British Journal of Experimental Pathology*, 42, 523–538.

STUBBS, G.W., SAARI, J.C. & FUTTERMAN, S. (1979) 11-*cis*-Retinol-binding proteins from bovine retina. *Journal of Biological Chemistry*, 254, 8529–8533.

SUGIMURA, T. & WAKABAYASHI, K. (1991) Heterocyclic amines, new mutagens and carcinogens in cooked food. *Advances in Experimental Biology and Medicine*, 283, 569–578.

SUSSMAN, J.L., HAVEL, M., FROLOW, F., *et al.* (1991) Atomic structure of acetylcholinesterase from *Torpedo californica*: a prototype acetylcholine-binding protein. *Science*, 253, 872–879.

SWANN, P.F. & MCLEAN, A.E.M. (1968) The effect of diet on the toxic and carcinogenic action of dimethylnitrosamine. *Biochemical Journal*, 107, 14–15P.

SWENBERG, J.A., HOEL, D.G. & MAGEE, P.N. (1991) Mechanistic and statistical insight into large carcinogenesis bioassays on *N*-nitrosodiethylamine and *N*-nitrosodimethylamine. *Cancer Research*, 51, 6409–6414.

SWENSEN, D.H., MILLER, E.C. & MILLER, J.A. (1974). Aflatoxin B_1,-2,3-oxide: evidence for its formation in rat liver *in vivo* and by human liver microsomes *in vitro*. *Biochemical and Biophysical Research Communications*, 60, 1036–1043.

SWYGERT, L.A., MAES, E.F., SEWELL, L.E., *et al.* (1990) Eosinophilia–myalgia syndrome: results of national surveillance. *Journal of the American Medical Association*, 264, 1698–1703.

TABUENCA, J.M. (1981) Toxic allergic syndrome caused by the ingestion of rape seed oil denatured with aniline. *Lancet*, 2, 567–568.

TAKETA, F., SIEBENLIST, K., KASTEN-JOLLY, J. & PALOSARRI, N. (1980) Interaction of triethyltin with cat hemoglobin: identification of binding sites and effects on haemoglobin function. *Archives of Biochemistry and Biophysics*, 203, 466–472.

TARDIF, R., LAPARE, S., KRISHNAN, K. & BRODEUR, J. (1993) Physiologically based modelling of the toxicokinetic interaction between toluene and *m*-xylene in the rat. *Toxicology and Applied Pharmacology*, 120, 266–273.

TATES, A.D., GRIMMT, T., TORNQVIST, M., *et al.* (1991) Biological and chemical monitoring of occupational exposure to ethylene oxide. *Mutation Research*, 250, 483–497.

TATUM, E.L. (1959) A case history in biological research. *Science*, 129, 1711–1715.

TENNANT, R.W. & ASHBY, J. (1991) Classification according to chemical structure, mutagenicity to Salmonella and level of carcinogenicity of a further 39 chemicals tested for carcinogenicity by the US NTP. *Mutation Research*, 257, 209–227.

TEPHLY, T.R. (1977) Introduction, factors in responses to the environment. *Federated Proceedings*, 36, 1627–1628.

(1991) The toxicity of methanol. *Life Sciences*, 48, 1031–1041.

TEPHLY, T.R., PARKE, R.E., Jr & MANNERING, G.T. (1964) Methanol metabolism in the rat. *Journal of Pharmacology and Experimental Therapeutics*, 143, 292–300.

THOMAS, J.A. & THOMAS, M.J. (1984) Biological effects of di-(2-ethylhexyl) phthalate and other phthalic esters. *Critical Reviews in Toxicology*, 13, 283–317.

TIBS (1994) Protein phosphorylation. *Trends in Biochemical Sciences*, special issue, 19, 439–513.

TIMBRELL, J.A. (1982) *Principles of Biochemical Toxicology*. Taylor & Francis, London.

TIPPING, E., KETTERER, B., CHRISTODOULIDES, L. & ENDERBY, G. (1976) The non-covalent binding of small molecules to ligandin: interaction with steroids and their conjugates, fatty acids, bromsulphophthalein, carcinogens, glutathione and related compounds. *European Journal of Biochemistry*, 67, 583–590.

TIPPING, E., KETTERER, B., CHRISTODOULIDES, C., *et al.*, (1979) Interactions of triethyltin with rat glutathione-S-transferases A, B and C: enzyme inhibition and equilibrium dialysis studies. *Chemical Biological Interactions*, 24, 317–327.

TIPTON, K.F. (1980) Kinetics and enzyme inhibitor studies. In *Enzyme Inhibitors as Drugs* (ed. M. Sandler), pp. 1–23. Macmillan, London.

TOGGAS, S.M., KRADY, J.K. & BILLINGSLEY, M.L. (1992) Molecular neurotoxicity of trimethyltin: identification of stannin, a novel protein expressed in trimethyltin sensitive cells. *Molecular Pharmacology*, 432, 44–56.

TOLBERT, N.E. (1981) Metabolic pathways in peroxisomes and glyoxisomes. *Annual Reviews of Biochemistry*, 50, 133–157.

TORKELSON, T.R., SADEK, S.E., ROWE, D.K., *et al.* (1961) Toxicologic investigations of 1,2-dibromo-3-chloropropane. *Toxicology and Applied Pharmacology*, 3, 545–559.

TORNQVIST, M. & KANTIAINEN, A. (1993) Adducted proteins in the identification of endogenous electrophiles. *Environmental Health Perspectives*, 99, 39–44.

TORNQVIST, M., OSTERMAN-GOLKAR, S., KAUTIAINEN, A. *et al.* (1986) Tissue doses of ethylene oxide in cigarette smokers determined from adduct levels in haemoglobin. *Carcinogenesis*, 7, 1519–1521.

TORNQVIST, M., SVARTENGREN, M. & ERICSSON, C.H. (1992) Methylations of haemoglobin from twins discordant for cigarette smoking: hereditary and tobacco related factors. *Chemico-Biological Interactions*, 82, 91–98.

TRIPATHI, R.K. (1976) Relation of acetylcholinesterase sensitivity to cross resistance of a house fly strain to organophosphates and carbamates. *Pesticide Biochemistry and Physiology*, 6, 30–34.

TRIPATHI, R.K. & O'BRIEN, R.D. (1973) Insensitivity of acetylcholinesterase as a factor in resistance of houseflies to the organophosphate Rabon. *Pesticide Biochemistry and Physiology*, 3, 495–498.

TSUBAKI, T. & IRUKAYAMA, K., eds (1977) *Minamata disease*. Elsevier, Amsterdam.

VAHTER, M., MOTTETT, N.K., FRIBERG, L., *et al.* (1994) Speciation of mercury in the primate blood and brain following long-term exposure to methylmercury. *Toxicology and Applied Pharmacology*, 124, 221–229.

VAINIO, H., COLEMAN, M, & WILBOURN, J. (1991) Carcinogenicity, evaluation and ongoing studies: the IARC databases. *Environmental Health Perspective*, 96, 5–9.

VAN BLADEREN, P.J. (1988) Formation of toxic metabolites from drugs and other xenobiotics by glutathione conjugation. *Trends in Pharmacological Sciences*, 9, 295–299.

VANDEKAR, M. (1980) Minimising occupational exposure to pesticides: cholinesterase determination and organophosphorus poisoning. *Residue Reviews*, 75, 68–79.

VARTIAINEN, T. & LIIMATAINEN, A. (1986) High levels of mutagenic activity in chlorinated drinking water in Finland. *Mutation Research*, 169, 29–34.

VARTIAINEN, T., LIIMATAINEN, A., JAASKELAINEN, S. and KAURANEN, P. (1987) Comparison of solvent extractions and resin absorption for isolation of mutagenic compounds from chlorinated drinking water with high humus content. *Water Research*, 21, 773–779.

VARTIAINEN, T., LIIMATAINEN, A., KAURANEN, P. & HIISVIRTA, L. (1988) Relations between drinking water mutagenicity and water quality parameters. *Chemosphere*, 17, 189–202.

VERMEULEN, N.P.E., BESSENS, J.G.M. & VAN DER STRAAT, R. (1992) Molecular aspects of paracetamol-induced hepatotoxicity and its mechanism-based prevention. *Drug Metabolism Reviews*, 24, 367–407.

VERSCHOYLE, R.D. & ALDRIDGE, W.N. (1980) Structure–activity relationships of some pyrethroids in rats. *Archives of Toxicology*, 45, 325–329.

(1987) The interaction between phosphorothionate insecticides, pneumotoxic trialkyl phosphorothiolates and effects on lung 7-ethoxycoumarin *O*-deethylase activity. *Archives of Toxicology*, 60, 311–318.

VERSCHOYLE, R.D. & LITTLE, R.A. (1981) The acute toxicity of some organolead and organotin compounds in the rat with particular reference to the gastric lesion. *Journal of Applied Toxicology*, 1, 270–277.

VIJVERBERG, H.P.M. & VAN DEN BERCKEN, J. (1990) Neurotoxicological effects and the mode of action of pyrethroid insecticides. *CRC Critical Reviews in Toxicology*, 21, 105–126.

VINEIS, P., CAPOROSO, N., TANNENBAUM, S.R., *et al.* (1990) Acetylation phenotype, carcinogen–haemoglobin adducts, and cigarette smoking. *Cancer Research*, 50, 3002–3004.

VOLK, B., HETTMANNSPERGER, U., PAPP, T., *et al.* (1991) Mapping of phenytoin inducible cytochrome P450 immunoreactivity in the mouse central nervous system. *Neuroscience*, 42, 215–235.

WAINIO, W.W. & GREENLEES, J. (1960) Complexes of cytochrome C oxidase with cyanide and carbon monoxide. *Archives of Biochemistry and Biophysics*, 90, 18–21.

WATANABE, I., IWASAKI, Y., SATOYOSHI, E. & DAVIS, J.W. (1981) Haemorrhage in thiamine-deficient encephalopathy. *Journal of Neuropathology and Experimental Neurology*, 40, 566–580.

WATANABE, T., LALWANI, N.D. & REDDY, J.K. (1985) Specific changes in the protein composition of rat liver in response to the peroxisome proliferators ciprofibrate, Wy-14,643 and Di(2-ethylhexyl)phthalate. *Biochemical Journal*, 227, 767–775.

WEBB, M., ed. (1979) *The Chemistry, Biochemistry and Biology of Cadmium*. Elsvier/North-Holland, Amsterdam.

WEIL, C.S. (1952) Tables for convenient calculation of median-effective dose (LD_{50} or ED_{50}) and instructions in their use. *Biometrics*, 8, 249–263.

WESER, U. & RUPP, H. (1979) Physicochemical properties of metallothioneins. In *The Chemistry, Biochemistry and Biology of Cadmium* (ed. M. Webb), pp. 267–283. Elsevier/North Holland Biomedical Press, Amsterdam.

WEST, I.C. (1990) What determines the specificity of the multi-drug resistence pump? *Trends in Biochemical Sciences*, 15, 42–46.

WHO (1976) Conference on intoxication due to alkylmercury treated seed. Baghdad, Iraq, 9–13 September 1974. *Bulletin of the World Health Organization*, 53 (suppl.).

(1984) *Toxic Oil Syndrome: Mass Food Poisoning in Spain*. Report on a meeting in Madrid, 21–25 March 1983. WHO, Copenhagen.

(1988) *Pyrollizidine alkaloids*. International Programme of Chemical Safety, Geneva. Environmental Health Criteria Document No. 80.

(1991) *Toxic Oil Syndrome and Eosinophilia–Myalgia Syndrome: Pursuing Parallels in Pathogenesis*. WHO, Copenhagen.

(1992) *Toxic Oil Syndrome: Current Knowledge and Future Perspectives*. WHO, Copenhagen.

(1993) *Toxic Oil Syndrome and Eosinophilia–Myalgia Syndrome: Clinical Aspects*. WHO, Copenhagen.

WIELAND, T. & FAULSTICH, H. (1978) Amatoxins, phallotoxins, phallolysin and antamanide: the biologically active components of poisonous Amanita mushrooms. *CRC Critical Review in Toxicology*, 5, 185–260.

WILKINSON, G.N. (1961) Statistical estimations in enzyme kinetics. *Biochemical Journal*, 80, 324–332.

WILLIAMS, G.M. & WEISBURGER, J.H. (1986) Chemical carcinogens. In *Toxicology: The Basic Science of Poisons* (eds C.D. Klaassen, M.O. Amdur & J. Doull), pp. 99–173. Macmillan, New York.

WITSCHI, H.P. & ALDRIDGE, W.N. (1968) Uptake, distribution and binding of beryllium to organelles of the rat liver cell. *Biochemical Journal*, 106, 811–820.

WOLFF, M S. TONIOLO, P.G., LEE, E.W., RIVERA, M. & DUBIN, N. (1993) Blood levels of organochlorine residues and risk of breast cancer. *Journal of the National Cancer Institute*, 85, 648–652.

WOOD, C.A. & BULLER, F. (1904) Poisoning by wood alcohol: cases of death and blindness from Columbian spirits and other methylated preparations. *Journal of the American Medical Association*, 43, 972–977; 1058–1062; 1117–1123; 1213–1221; 1289–1296.

WRIGHT, P. (1975) Untoward effects associated with practolol administration: oculomucocutaneous syndrome. *British Medical Journal*, 1, 595–598.

WYLLIE, A.H. (1992) Apoptosis and the regulation of cell numbers in normal and neoplastic tissues: an overview. *Cancer and Metastasis Reviews*, 11, 95–103.

WYLLIE, A.H., KERR, J.F.R. & CURRIE, A.R. (1980) Cell death: the significance of apoptosis. *International Reviews of Cytology*, 68, 251–306.

WYLLIE, A.H., MOORS, R.G., SMITH, A.L. & DUNLOP, D. (1984) Chromatin cleavage in apoptosis: association with condensed chromatin morphology and dependence on macromolecular synthesis. *Journal of Pathology*, 142, 67–77.

WYSYNSKI, A.M., BALDWIN, L.A., LEONARD, D.A. & CALABRESE, E.J. (1993) Interactive potential of omega-3 fatty acids with clofibrate and DEHP on hepatic peroxisome proliferation in male Wistar rats. *Human and Experimental Toxicology*, 12, 337–340.

YONEMOTO, J., BROWN, N.A. & WEBB, M. (1984) Effects of dimethoxyethylphthalate, monoethoxyethylphthalate, 2-methoxyethanol and methoxyacetic acid on post-implantation rat embryos in culture. *Toxicology Letters*, 21, 97–102.

ZIEGLER, B.M. (1993) Recent studies on the structure and function of multisubstrate flavin-containing monooxygenases. *Annual Reviews of Pharmacology and Toxicology*, 33, 179–199.

ZELIKOFF, J.T., SMIALOWICZ, R., BIGAZZI, P.E., *et al.* (1994) Immunomodulation by metals. *Fundamental and Applied Toxicology*, 22, 1–7.

Index

acetylcholinesterase
  biomonitoring 174–7
  function and inhibitors of 86
  inhibition *in vivo*, signs and symptoms 86–8
  oxime reactivation of phosphylated esterases
    89–90, 119
  properties of phosphylated esterases 88
active oxygen species and glutathione 54–5
acute intoxication 29–32, 35
  cadmium 32
  carbon monoxide 31
  DDT 32
  hydrocyanic acid 29–31
  malathion, malaoxon and isomalathion
    138–40
  organophosphorus compounds 31–2
acrylamide intoxication
  exposure–response 143–6
  central neuropathy (severe poisoning) 95
  peripheral neuropathy 93–5, 126–7
  signs and symptoms 93–4
  structure-activity of related compounds 94
  threshold 148
active transport of intoxicants
  beryllium 71
  paraquat 46, 68–9
albumin 47–8
algae *see* cyanobacteria
Ames test 107, 160–2
  chlorinated mutagens in drinking water 204–6
  mutagens in cooked food 207
  significance 162
animal experimentation
  ethics 162–3
  versus *in vitro* techniques 162–3
  no animal model for human diseases 160–1
anticholinesterases, biomonitoring of dose and
    effect 174–7
apoptosis and necrosis 105–6
axonopathy 61–3
  acrylamide 126–7, 144–6, 148

1,3-dinitrobenzene 124–5
2,5-hexanedione 33, 95–6, 142–4
organophosphorus compounds 125–6
  di-isopropylphosphorofluoridate 125–6
  mono *o*-cresyl saligen phosphate 62–3
  tri *p*-ethylphenyl phosphate 63
  tri *o*-cresyl phosphate (tri 2-tolyl phosphate)
    61–3

beryllium 70–1, 102–3
  Kupffer cell uptake 71
  liver damage 70, 102–3
  lysosomal uptake (liver) 71
  phagocytic function 102
  tissue uptake 70
biliary excretion 71
bioactivation 60–5
  dimethylnitrosamine 60
  glycol ethers 101
  hexachloro-1, 3-butadiene 64–5
  methods to establish *in vivo* 72–3
  monocrotaline 61
  tetraethyllead and tetraethyltin 63–4
  tri *o*-cresyl phosphate (tri 2-tolyl phosphate)
    61
  tri *p*-ethylphenyl phosphate 63
biochemical lesion 2
biomonitoring 166–79
  dose and effect in humans
    anticholinesterase compounds 174–5
    dichlorvos 176–7
  dose in experimental animals 177
  dose in humans 169–77
    ethylene oxide haemoglobin adducts 174
    methylmercury in blood and hair 170–2
  effects in humans and animals 177–8
  general principles 150, 166–8, 169–70, 176,
    178–9
  genetically determined susceptibility 168
    pesticide resistance in insects 164
    succinyldicholine 169

brain cells
    selective vulnerability 81–3, 103–4, 124–5

cadmium 32
    binding to metallothionein 50, 191
    cadmium excretion in urine/cadmium in renal
        cortex 191, 193
    environmental exposure (Cadmibel study)
        191–3
    exposure
        accumulation *in vivo* 50
        common sources 191
    kidney lesions 32
        biomarkers for effects 191–2
    protocol for Cadmibel study 192
    threshold 148, 193–4
carbon monoxide intoxication 31, 79–81
    haemoglobin complex 31
    signs and symptoms 31
carcinogenesis, chemical 34, 106–9, 127–30,
        140–1, 147–9
    DNA modification 106–9, 127–30
    exposure–response 140–1
    humans 107–8
causality/association in epidemiological studies
        184–5, 194–5
cell necrosis and apoptosis 105–6
chemical accidents
    aetiology of chemical poisoning, methods 140
    aminorex induced pulmonary hypertension 161
    eosinophilia myalgia syndrome (USA) 132, 161
    malathion episode in Pakistan 138–9
    margarine disease (Germany and Netherlands)
        161
    methanol (USA) 156–7
    methyl isocyanate (Bhopal) 39
    methyl *n*-butylketone (USA) 142–3
    methylmercury (Iraq, Minamata and Niigata)
        170, 203
    practolol (oculmucocutaneous syndrome) 161
    toxic oil syndrome (Spain) 130–2, 161, 188–91
    triethyltin (France) 103
    tri *o*-cresyl phosphate (Ginger Jake) in USA 61
chemicals, essential and toxic 137–8
chemical carcinogenesis *see* carcinogenesis
chlorfenvinphos
    species selectivity 157–9
chlorinated mutagens in drinking water
    Ames test 204–5
    experience in Finland 204
    mutagenic activity of treated waters 205
    MX, a potent mutagen 204
    retrospective epidemiology 206
cholinergic transmitter system, perturbation of
        118–19
    therapy 89–90, 119
chronic intoxication 32–5
    acrylamide (central nervous system) 33
    carcinogenesis 34
    delayed neuropathy 32–3
    dimethylnitrosamine 34
    ethanol, liver cirrhosis 33
    2,5-hexanedione (central nervous system) 33
    hydrocyanic acid 31, 33
    organophosphorus compounds 32–3

paraquat (lung fibrosis) 33
trimethyltin 103–4
triethyllead 63–4
copper
    binding to metallothionein 50
covalent interactions with macromolecules 20–3
    analysis of data to derive rate constants 22
    chemical reactants for specific groups 26
    organophosphorus compounds and esterases
        21–4
cyanide *see* hydrocyanic acid
cyanobacteria (algae)
    anatoxin-a(S), an organophosphorus compound
        6, 88, 201–2
    strains produce different hepatotoxic peptides
        202
    hepatotoxicity of toxins 201
cysteine in proteins, reagents for 26
cytochrome P_{450}s 65–8
    mechanism 66
    steroid metabolism 67
    xenobiotic metabolism 67

DDT
    acute intoxication 32, 38, 83
    distribution *in vivo* 32, 38
    epidemiological studies 215
    experience in vector-control use 214–15
    risk of exposure
        solubility in water 38
definition of toxicology and toxicity (intoxication)
        3
delayed neuropathy
    acrylamide 143–4, 148
    2,5-hexanedione and other diketones 95–6,
        142–3
    methylmercury 126–7
    organophosphorus compounds 61–3, 90–3,
        163–4, 177
delivery of intoxicant 36–76
    decreased concentration at target (Chapter 5)
        36–57
    entry and distribution 39–51
    general principles 36–8, 39–40, 55–6
    increased concentration at target (Chapter 6)
        58–76
    membranes, movement across 41–5, 56
        endocytosis, pinocytosis and phagocytosis 45
        facilitated diffusion and active transport 44–5
        filtration and passive diffusion 43–4
        gastro-intestinal tract 45–6
        skin 36, 56
deltamethrin 82–3, 119–21
    species selectivity 154
detoxification
    by glutathione 54–6
    chemistry of 52–4
    enzymes of 52–4
        physiological role 55–6
dialkyltin compounds
    thymus atrophy 111–12
dichlorvos *see* metrifonate
    dose and effect monitoring in humans 176–7
diethylnitrosamine 9
    carcinogenesis in liver 140–1, 148–9

diethylnitrosamine (*continued*)
  exposure–response 141
γ-diketones and related compounds
  structure–response 142–5
dimethylnitrosamine 34, 60, 128–30, 141, 147–8
  carcinogenesis in liver and kidney 60,
    127–30
  exposure–response 147–8
1,3-dinitrobenzene, neuropathy 124–5
  influence of external stimuli 124–5
diquat, kidney damage 83–5
distribution of intoxicant *in vivo*, parameters of
    46–52
  adipose tissue 50–1
  binding to macromolecules 47–51
    albumin 47–8
    glutathione S-transferase 49–50
    haemoglobin 48–9
    ligandin *see* glutathione S-transferase
    metallothionein 50
  excretion of 52
DNA adducts 106–9, 127–30, 178
dose biomonitoring 169–77
dose–response
  2,5-hexanedione and clinical neuropathy
    143–4
  methylmercury and paresthesia 171

ecotoxicology *see* environmental and
    ecotoxicology
effect biomonitoring
  anticholinesterases 174–7
  biomarkers for kidney function 191–2
  humans and experimental animals 177
electrophiles, oxidants and active oxygen species
    54–5
embryonic development 101–2
energy conservation, mechanism and inhibitors
    79–81
enterohepatic circulation 71
environmental and ecotoxicology 196–208
  chlorinated mutagens in drinking water 204–6
  cyanobacterial (algal) toxins 201–2
  methylmercury 202–4
  polychlorinated biphenyls and hydroxy
    derivatives 197–201
eosinophilia myalgia syndrome 132, 191
epidemiological studies 180–95
  case-control, cohort, controlled trial cross-
    sectional, population statistics 180–4
  causality and associations 184–5, 194–5
  environmental exposure to cadmium 191–4
  epidemiology of chemical-induced toxicity
    (scheme) 181
  smoking and lung cancer 185–8, 193–4
  general principles 180–2, 193–5
  occupational exposures 184–5
  toxic oil syndrome 188–91
esterases
  aging of phosphylated 88, 92
  inhibitors of 86–9
  neuropathy target esterase (NTE) 90–3
ethanol 33, 121–2
2-ethoxyacetic acid, testicular atrophy 99–102
etofenprox 82

exposure, types of 7–8
exposure–response
  acrylamide and neuropathy 143–5
  bioassay for impurities in malathion 138–40
  cancer due to alkylnitrosamines 140–1,
    148–9
  essential and toxic compounds 137–8
  mono 2-tolyl diphenyl phosphate 148

fibrosis 33, 121–2
foetal development 101–2, 106–7

genetically determined susceptibility
  succinyldicholine 169
  insect resistance to pesticides 163–4
glutathione 54–5
  hexachloro-1,3-butadiene adduct 65
glutathione S-transferase *see* glutathione 54
  binding of intoxicants (ligandin) 49–50
glycol ethers 99–102
  bioactivation 101
  testicular atrophy 99–102

haemoglobin adducts
  ethylene oxide 174
haemoglobin, binding to
  methylmercury 170–2
  trimethyl- and triethyltin 19, 48
hazard and risk, *see* risk and hazard
hexachloro-1, 3-butadiene
  glutathione adduct and mercapturic acid
    derivative 65
  mercapturic acid derivative 65
  kidney tubular damage 64
  β-lyase 65
2,5-hexanedione axonopathy 33, 95–6
  dose–response 142–3
  threshold 148
histidine in proteins, reagents for 26
human chemical-induced disease with no animal
    model 160–1
hydrocyanic acid 29–31
  clearance *in vivo* 30
  cytochrome oxidase inhibition 30
  distribution *in vivo* 29–30
  neuronal necrosis 31, 33
  therapy 117
hypersensitivity to chemicals 111–12

immune system, function 109–11
immunotoxicity of chemicals 109–12
inflammation
  eosinophilia myalgia syndrome 132
  toxic oil syndrome 130–2
initiation of toxicity
  analogy with mutation 113–14
  general principles 77–79, 112–114
  interaction with targets 77–114
intoxication, parameters to define 30, 34–5
intramyelinic vacuoles 103–4, 147
in vitro techniques 162–4
  Ames test 160–2, 164
  development of 164
  hepatocytes (peroxisome proliferation) 159
isothiocyanates 52

kidney
  anatomy and function 51–2
  excretion of intoxicants 52
kidney intoxication
  biomarkers for effects 191–2
  cadmium 32
    environmental exposure 191–4
  dimethylnitrosamine carcinogenesis
  diquat 68
  hexachloro-1,3-butadiene 65
    uptake of *p*-aminohippurate by affected
      slices 64
kinetics and endpoints 17–28
  Michaelis constants 23–4
  physiologically based pharmacokinetic
    modelling (PB–PK) 74–5
  reversible and covalent interactions 18–23
    experimental differentiation 25–6
kinetics *in vivo* 26–7
  health (homeostasis) and intoxication 27–8
  volumes of different departments and
    distribution of 26–7
Kupffer cells, liver
  uptake of beryllium 71, 102–3

lethal synthesis 2
ligandin *see* glutathione S-transferases
liver peroxisomes 97–9, 159
liver intoxication
  beryllium 70–1
  dimethylnitrosamine 60
  monocrotaline 61
  rare earths 102
lung intoxication
  methyl isocyanate 38–9
  monocrotaline 61
  other intoxicants 85
  paraquat 83–4
  smoking and lung cancer 185–8, 193–4
  toxic oil syndrome (phase 1) 130–2, 188
  trimethyl phosphorothiates 73
lysine in macromolecules, reagents for 26

malathion
  chemical accident in Pakistan 138–9
  impurities in 138–40
  selectivity between insect and humans
    138–40
membranes, movement across
  endocytosis, pinocytosis and phagocytosis
    45
  facilitated diffusion and active transport
    44–5
  filtration and passive diffusion 43–4
  gastro-intestinal tract 45–6
  skin 36, 56
mercuric ion
  binding to metallothionein 50
metabolism of xenobiotics 74
  general principles 73–5
  hydrophilic metabolites 74
  lipophilic metabolites 74
  species differences 74, 156–9
metallothionein 50, 191
metals, absorption from GI tract 45

methanol
  ocular toxicity 156–7
  species selectivity 155–7
2-methoxyacetic acid
  testicular atrophy and foetal development
    100–101
  thymus atrophy 112
methyl isocyanate intoxication 38–9
  chemical accident in Bhopal 39
  chemical properties 38–9
  lung effects 39
  sites of action 39
methylmercury intoxication
  binding to haemoglobin 48–9
  biomonitoring in blood and hair 170–2
  chemical accidents in Iraq and Japan 170
  chemical accidents, list 203
  clearance from blood 172
  dose–response (paresthesia) 172
  from mercury in environment 203–4
  neurotoxicity of 126–7
  signs and symptoms 203
metrifonate, conversion to dichlorvos 65
  threshold 149
Michaelis constants 23–4
  analysis of data 24
mitochondria (oxidative phosphorylation) 79–81
monocrotaline 61
mono *o*-cresyl diphenyl phosphate 149
mutagens in water *see* chlorinated mutagens
mutation and carcinogenesis 106–9
  Ames test 107, 160–2

necrosis and apoptosis 105–6
neuronal necrosis
  1,3-dinitrobenzene 124–5
  specific areas of brain 103–4, 122–5
  soman 119
  tetraethyllead 63–4
  trimethyltin 122–4
neuropathy target esterase (NTE) 90–3
neurotoxicity
  cell selectivity 81–3
  central neuropathy 124–5
  intramyelinic vacuoles 103–4, 146–7
  neuronal necrosis 63–4, 103–4, 122–4, 146–7
  peripheral axonopathy 90–6, 126–7, 143–6

organophosphorus compounds 21–3
  acute intoxication 31–2, 86–90
    acetylcholinesterase inhibition 31, 86–8
    signs and symptoms 31–2, 118–19
    therapy 89–90, 119
    threshold 149
  chronic intoxication 32–3
    age dependence (rats and chickens) 93,
      163–4
    axonopathy 32–3
    delayed neuropathy 32–3, 61–3, 90–3
    dose and effect monitoring in humans 177
    neuropathy target esterase (NTE) 33, 90–3
    protectors and promoters 91–3
    threshold 148
  kinetics of reaction with esterases 21–3
oxygen species, oxidants and glutathione 51–5

paraquat intoxication 33, 84–5
  absorption from GI tract 46
  active transport by types 1 and 2 alveolar cells
    68–9
  lung and kidney damage 68, 84
  mechanism 84–5
  oxidation–reduction of paraquat ion 84
  signs and symptoms 84
peroxisomes
  composition 98
  proliferation 97–9
    species selectivity 159
physiologically based pharmacokinetic modelling
    (PB–PK) 74–5
polychlorinated biphenyls 197–201
  hydroxy derivatives 199–200
  effects on plasma retinol and thyroxine 199
  signs and symptoms of poisoning 198–9
  seals, effects on plasma retinol/thyroxine 199
  uses, properties and chemical composition
    197–8
pyrethroids intoxication 81–3
  CS- and T-syndromes 82–3
  voltage-dependent sodium channels 83, 119–21
pyridine 2-aldoxime methiodide
  absorption from GI tract 43
  therapy of organophosphorus intoxication
    89–90, 119

rare earths, fatty liver 102
research, toxicological 210–13, 217 *see* Preface
    ix–x
  current priorities 212–13
  definition 210–11
  Himsworth's globe (structure of scientific
    knowledge) 211–12
  inputs into toxicological research 211–12
reticulo-endothelial system *see* Kupffer cell
retinol, thyroxine and vitamin A
  effects of polychlorinated biphenyls 198–200
reversible interactions and analysis of data by
    Scatchard method 18–20
risk and hazard 213–17
  acceptable risk and society's attitude 214, 216
  definitions 213
  exposure to DDT 214–16
  inputs into risk assessment 213–14

selective toxicity
  metabolism of intoxicants 156–9
    chlorfenvinphos 159
    methanol 156–7
  peroxisomes in liver 159
  species dependent 74, 93, 153–65
  types and definitions 153–5, 163–5
serine in proteins, reagents for 26
smoking and lung cancer 185–8, 193–4
  aetiological agent(s) and individual
    susceptibility 188
species selectivity *see* selective toxicity
stages of toxicity (intoxication) 10–16, 167
  active transport of intoxicant (stage 2) 44–5
  binding of intoxicant (stage 2) 47–51
  biological consequences (stage 4) 115–35
  bioactivation (stage 2) 60–5, 72–3

clinical signs and symptoms (stage 5) 115–35
  decreased delivery of intoxicant to target
    (stage 2) 36–57
  delivery (stage 2) 36–76
  detoxification (stage 2) 52–6
  distribution (stage 2) 39–51
  early consequences (stage 4) 115–35
  entry (stage 1) 36–8
  excretion (stage 2) 51–2
  exposure (stage 1) 36–8
  increased delivery of intoxicant to target (stage
    2) 58–76
  interaction with targets (stage 3) 77–114
structure–activity
  acrylamide and related compounds 94
structure–response
  γ- and other diketones 142–5
  acidic phenols and phenylimino compounds
    146–7
  triorganotins 146–7
succinyldicholine, genetic susceptibility to 169

targets, general principles 77–9
  consequences of reaction with 115–16, 133–5
TCDD (dioxin)
  species and strain selectivity 154–6, 163
  thymus atrophy 112
testicular development 99–100
testicular atrophy 96, 99–102
  1,3-dinitrobenzene 102
  2,5-hexanedione 96, 102
  2-methoxy- and ethoxyacetic acids 100–1
    Sertoli cells 102
    spermatocytes (meotic, pachytene) 100–1
tetraethyllead intoxication
  signs and symptoms 63–4
therapy, prophylaxis and prevention
  general principles and examples 133–5
  cyanide 117
  organophosphorus compounds 89–90, 119
thresholds, various intoxicants 147–9
  cadmium and renal tubular damage 193–4
  definition 147
  influence of macromolecular turnover and
    detoxification 150
thymus atrophy
  dialkyltins 111–12
  2-methoxyacetic acid 112
  TCDD (dioxin) 112
thyroxine
  iodide to thyroxine action and excretion 10–11
  transport in plasma 199–200
thyroxine, retinol and vitamin A
  effects of polychlorinated biphenyls 198–200
toxicity (intoxication), parameters of 1–6
  stages of 10–16
toxic oil syndrome
  anilides in case oils 130, 189–90
  causes of death 130–32
  eosinophilia 130–32
  markers/aetiological agents in case oils
    fatty acid anilides 189
    rape seed oil constituents 189
  signs and symptoms (3 stages) 130–32, 188
  toxico-epidemiological study 188–91

vasculitis (non-necrotising) 130–2
toxicological research *see* research, toxicological
toxicology
  and molecular biology ix, 8–9, 10
  comparison with homeostasis e.g. throxine
    formation and distribution 10
  definition, historical aspects and parameters
    2–6
triethyllead intoxication
  signs and symptoms 63–4
trimethyltin compounds
  binding to haemoglobin 48
  neuronal necrosis 103–4, 122–4
triethyltin
  binding to haemoglobin 19, 48
  binding to and effects on mitochondrial
    functions 19, 80, 146–7
  intramyelinic vacuoles 103–4, 147

triorganotins 19
  intramyelinic vacuoles 103–4
  neuronal necrosis 103–4
  structure–response 147
trichlorethylene 97–8
tri *o*- and *p*-ethylphenyl phosphates 63
tri *o*-cresyl phosphate (tri 2-tolyl phosphate) 61–3,
  90–3

valine in proteins, reagents for 26
vitamin A, retinol and thyroxine
  effects of polychlorinated biphenyls 198–200
voltage-dependent sodium channels
  perturbation of 81–3, 119–21
    deltamethrin 120
    dose–response 120
    glucose, brain content and utilisation 120–21
    signs and symptoms 119–21